The Longevity Bible

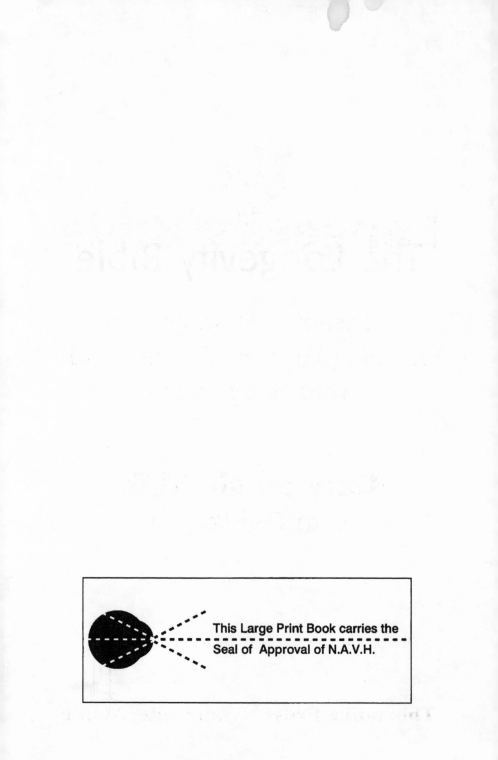

This Large Print Book carries the
Seal of Approval of N.A.V.H.

The Longevity Bible

8 Essential Strategies for Keeping Your Mind Sharp and Your Body Young

Gary Small, M.D.
with Gigi Vorgan

Thorndike Press • Waterville, Maine

Published in 2006 by arrangement with
Hyperion, an imprint of Buena Vista Books, Inc.

Thorndike Press® Large Print Health, Home and Learning.

The tree indicium is a trademark of Thorndike Press.

The text of this Large Print edition is unabridged.
Other aspects of the book may vary from the original edition.

Set in 16 pt. Plantin.

Printed in the United States on permanent paper.

Library of Congress Cataloging-in-Publication Data

Small, Gary W.
    The longevity bible : 8 essential strategies for keeping
your mind sharp and your body young / by Gary Small
with Gigi Vorgan. — Large print ed.
      p. cm.
    Includes bibliographical references.
    ISBN 0-7862-8941-4 (lg. print : hc : alk. paper)
    1. Longevity. 2. Aging. 3. Health. 4. Large type books.
I. Vorgan, Gigi, 1958– II. Title.
RA776.75.S526 2006b
  613.2—dc22   2006022784

We dedicate this book to our loving family,
especially our children,
Rachel and Harry.
Their sweet faces and enthusiasm
enrich our lives every day,
and make us grateful
for the quality of our longevity.

Contents

Note: Although some of the stories contained in this book are true accounts of individuals who have participated in UCLA research programs, others are composite accounts based on the experiences of many case studies, and do not represent any one person or group of people. In these composites, similarities to any one person or persons are coincidental and unintentional.

Readers should consider consulting with their physician before initiating any exercise or treatment program.

Acknowledgments

Many friends and colleagues provided valuable input and encouragement during the writing of this book, including Helen Berman, Susan Bowerman, Rachel Champeau, Susan Coddon, Neal Frankle, Dr. Martin Greenberger, Dr. David Heber, Dr. Robert Hucherson, Dr. Shirley Impellizzeri, Andrea Kaplan, Dr. Daniel Keatinge, Chef David Lawrence, Kimberly McClain, Dr. Michael Persky, Dr. Judith Reichman, Dr. Peter Rosen, Michele and Dr. Nathan Rubin, Dottie Sefton, Sandi Shapiro, Pauline Spaulding, and Cara and Rob Steinberg. We are also indebted to our talented photographer and friend, Sterling Franken-Steffen, and our publicists Grace McQuade and Lynn Goldberg, as well as our outstanding publishing team at Hyperion, including our wonderful editor Brenda Copeland; Zareen Jaffery; our tireless publicist Beth Dickey; and the rest of the Hyperion family. This book would not have been possible without the support of Mary

Ellen O'Neill and our longtime agent and good friend, Sandra Dijkstra, whose talent and instincts never cease to amaze us.

Gary Small, M.D.
Gigi Vorgan

Part 1

Quality Longevity – Living Longer, Younger, and Healthier

It is not enough to add years to one's life . . . one must also add life to those years.

— JOHN F. KENNEDY

You're savoring your ritual cappuccino across the street from your dentist's office when this incredibly handsome young guy sits down two tables over. Your eyes meet his and he smiles seductively — you practically choke. You could swear you know him from somewhere. . . . He gives you a little wave. Where the heck could you know him from? He's so *young*. And you've been married a *long* time. Oh my god, he's coming over! Could this amazing hunk *possibly* be hitting on you? Ridiculous. No way! Thank God in heaven you just had your teeth cleaned. He grins broadly. "Hi! Remember me?!" You're completely at a loss. "I'm Andy! Andy Carter! I was on your son's basketball team in middle

17

school." You freeze with a ridiculous smile on your face and a sudden urge to evaporate into thin air.

Age reminders happen to everyone. It could be as simple as the appearance of a single gray hair, the first time someone calls you "Ma'am," or perhaps walking into a room and forgetting the reason why. None of us can stop time, but we *can* slow down the effects of aging — and sometimes even reverse them.

A mere one hundred years ago, people were lucky to live beyond age forty. Now, life expectancy has risen to age seventy-four for men and eighty for women, and recent studies show that the average sixty-five-year-old American can expect to live another seventeen years. Modern medical science is striving to keep us alive well into our nineties and beyond, and most people say they want to live as long as possible. But who wants to live to be one hundred without their health, vitality, and faculties intact? That's where *The Longevity Bible's Eight Essentials* come in — showing us how to keep it *all* together — our brains, our bodies, and our attitudes.

The Eight Essentials

Traditionally, magazine and television advertisers have focused their marketing strategies on youthful looks and attitudes to attract consumers to their products. Recently, however, there has been a shift in tactics. Today, Madison Avenue's emphasis is not so much on youthful demographics but on "psychographics" — marketing focused toward the age group in which consumers actually *perceive* themselves as being. Try asking baby boomers how old they consider themselves, not in actual calendar years, but mentally and physically. Many will confess they still have the attitude of a twenty-five-year-old and feel nowhere near their chronological age.

Most of us protest against the idea of aging in the way our parents did and vow to fight against the process as long as possible. We are looking for a safe, convenient, medically sound way to live longer, empower ourselves, and remain healthy and fulfilled throughout that long life — what I refer to as "quality longevity."

Empowering ourselves for the future requires learning new skills, as well as honing the ones we already have. In my last book, *The Memory Prescription*, I showed how we could jump-start our brain and body fitness by focusing on four of the basic essentials: achieving *mental sharpness, physical fitness, a healthy diet,* and *stress reduction.* Now, in *The Longevity Bible,* I outline my entire program — all Eight Essentials — to allow every one of us to achieve our own maximum, quality longevity in every area of our lives. These essential strategies include keys to *keeping a positive outlook, cultivating healthy relationships, getting the most out of modern medicine,* and *adapting and flourishing in a changing environment.*

We'll look at the science behind the Eight Essentials, and at simple and practical ways for integrating them into our daily life. When practiced together, these Eight Essentials create a synergy that achieves positive results faster and far more effectively than could be achieved by doing them individually.

Fix Your Brain First: The Rest Will Follow

We begin our longevity solution by sharpening our minds (Essential 1) and maximizing our brain fitness. Fix your brain for longevity, and your body will follow in kind. By keeping our minds sharp, we are more inclined to stay physically fit, enhance our relationships, maintain a longevity diet, and follow the other healthy lifestyle strategies outlined in this book. In fact, all the Essentials contribute to keeping our brains young, fit, and cognitively strong throughout all stages of life. Simply doing mental aerobics can significantly improve memory skills and, when combined with the other Essentials, may extend life expectancy. A recent study found that mentally stimulating leisure activities such as reading, doing crossword puzzles, or playing board games lowers the risk for Alzheimer's disease by nearly a third.

Scientific evidence shows that keeping a positive outlook (Essential 2) helps us to stay healthy and live longer. In a recent study, positive and satisfied middle-aged people were twice as likely to survive over a period of twenty years, as compared to more negative individuals. Optimists have fewer physical and emotional difficulties, experience less pain, enjoy higher energy levels, and are generally happier and calmer. Positive thinking has been found to boost the body's immune system so we can better fight infection.

When we feel good, it boosts our self-confidence, which helps us to have better relationships (Essential 3). The MacArthur Study of Successful Aging found that people who are socially connected may survive up to 20 percent longer than those who live more isolated lives. Today, we have many tools to help us connect with others, shore up self-doubt, and make ourselves feel and look younger and more beautiful, both through medical and nonmedical techniques. Despite the myth that libido declines with age, several scientific studies have found that our desire and need for sex continues throughout our lives. A healthy sex life at every age helps lower blood pressure, reduce stress, ward off depression, boost the immune system, diminish pain, maintain physical fitness, and even extend life expectancy.

Stress is among the leading causes of age-related disease (Essential 4). It contributes to physical pain, as well as to the appearance of wrinkles and premature aging. Few people realize that our ability to adapt to our ever-changing environments can greatly contribute to lowering our stress levels. Whether it's traffic, smoke, clutter, noise, mold, smog, or information overload, our quality longevity depends upon our ability to adjust to these environmental influences (Essential 5). Personalizing our immediate surroundings, at home and at work, is an important environmental element that is within our control.

It is much easier to maintain a positive attitude when we enjoy good health, and the best way to ensure that is by eating a healthy diet and staying physically fit. With so many fitness options available, there is bound to be something that appeals to just about everybody. Along with the basics of tennis, jogging, cycling, swimming, and yoga, many people are getting fit with Pilates, weight training, Bosu ball, spinning, salsa dancing, ballet, trail running, and more. Essential 6 will introduce the Longevity Fitness Routine, which covers cardiovascular conditioning, balance and flexibility work, and strength training — the three vital fitness areas for maximizing health, boosting energy levels, and preventing many age-related diseases. Recent research has found that regular physical activity can add two or more years to an individual's life expectancy.

Reducing the clutter in our lives is a powerful way to lower stress levels. Just as it feels good to occasionally clean out your closet and get rid of the clutter there, it can sometimes become necessary to reduce relationship clutter — clean your emotional house — and conserve your energy for the people you love or care about. At times, relationships may become more damaging than they are enriching — old friendships that were once meaningful can become simply old habits that may have negative effects but are hard to break.

A healthy diet can have a major impact on life expectancy by lowering our risk for heart disease, cancer, and other age-related illnesses. Longitudinal studies have found that a diet that emphasizes the right food choices and helps people stay at their target body weight can increase survival rates by 50 percent or more. We'll learn about the Longevity Diet (Essential 7), a healthy diet plan that allows you to eat *all* of your favorite foods — even naughty desserts. It incorporates the best scientific data on healthful eating for longevity and weight control, combined with some of the most satisfying and delicious foods available. Just as fitness experts now tell us that for long-range health, it's best to cross-train our bodies by emphasizing aerobics one day, weight training the next, and perhaps yoga the day after that, the Longevity

Diet shows us how to cross-train our eating, allowing us to break free of the boredom and repetition of today's popular low-carbohydrate, South Florida, salmon-every-meal diets. We can enjoy a barbecued steak and a Caesar salad one day and a delicious pasta dinner with whole-grain crusty bread the next. The Longevity Diet allows our bodies to break free of today's fashionable diets and learn to process all good foods in realistic portions, while feeling sated, satisfied, and anything but deprived.

We will look at the latest in medicines and treatments designed to keep us young (Essential 8). From smart drugs to Botox to microscopic lasers, we'll learn about the options available to keep us looking and feeling youthful throughout our lives. Even simply taking drugs to lower blood pressure has been shown to increase life expectancy by at least two or more years, and scientists have found that cholesterol-lowering statin drugs can increase survival rates of heart patients by more than 50 percent.

Many baby boomers may recall the 1960s Harvard professor who traveled to India and became the guru known as Ram Dass. His "Be here now" message became the mantra for staying in the moment, neither worrying about the past nor stressing over the future. His message echoes that of many other teachers, ranging from Martin Buber to Lao-Tzu.

We don't have to become spiritual gurus to live a long, healthy life, but attempting to stay in the moment helps us to achieve quality longevity. Mindfulness or *mindful awareness* — the subtle process of moment-to-moment awareness of one's thoughts, feelings, and physical states — is key to sharpening memory and staying mentally fit. Initial research suggests that this ability not only reduces stress and anxiety, but also boosts the immune system and promotes health and healing for a variety of medical illnesses and conditions, including heart disease, diabetes, arthritis, and chronic pain.

This underlying principle of mindful awareness can be applied to nearly all of the Eight Essential Strategies. Having an awareness of our bodies and what is going on around us helps us maintain balance and avoid danger. Awareness of our internal sensations reminds us to stop eating when we are sated — a key to maintaining our target body weight. By integrating mindful awareness into our daily lives, we not only enjoy ourselves more and live longer, we take better care of ourselves, have a more positive outlook, and feel more empathy toward others.

Mindfulness often fosters a sense of spirituality, and several studies have found that people who pursue some form of spirituality live longer. Recently, investigators found that visiting a house of worship just once a week can extend life expectancy by nearly a decade. Studies of patients with chronic physical illnesses have found that those who believed in God had a 30 percent lower mortality rate as compared with those who felt abandoned by God. The increased longevity benefits of spirituality result from many of its forms, including religion, meditation, a personal belief in a higher power, and more.

Many of the benefits of *The Longevity Bible*'s Eight Essentials can be achieved in a remarkably short period — as little as fourteen days. My research team at UCLA conducted controlled studies to test how well volunteer subjects could improve their brain and body fitness by focusing on just four of the essential strategies: *mental aerobics, physical fitness, stress management,* and *a healthy diet.*

We found that after just two weeks, the

Shirley I., a thirty-four-year-old social worker raising a young daughter on her own, had always been fastidious and fiercely independent. She lived with a certain level of stress in her life, but it was constant, and she had developed habitual ways to cope. Sometimes she let off steam by shopping. But why not? Imelda Marcos had more than three hundred pairs of shoes and it didn't kill her.

As she had planned, Shirley went back to graduate school and became a licensed psychologist. It was at the outset of her career that she met and began dating a hugely successful investment banker. The attraction was strong and Shirley was falling in love, but she felt he was pressuring her to give up her independence, move in, and get engaged. In time, his sense of humor, intelligence, and "old-fashioned" courting style — flowers, candlelight dinners, Mediterranean cruises — won her over. Eventually she agreed, and they set up a household together with her daughter.

With the added stress of a new

career, the pressing needs of a pre-teen daughter, and the heavy social demands of her fiancé weighing on her, Shirley found herself becoming forgetful for the first time in her life. Little details began falling through the cracks and she actually mixed up a patient's appointment and missed one of her kid's sports events. When her daughter started making jokes about "Mommy losing her memory," Shirley decided to do something about improving her memory and reducing her stress. She came to UCLA and volunteered for our Fourteen-Day Healthy Longevity Study.

After just two weeks on the program, her memory scores improved significantly, she lost three pounds without trying, and felt more relaxed and better able to deal with both her job and her responsibilities at home. Shirley was able to comfort herself with her old, familiar coping styles, and she was happy. So were the shoe departments at Saks and Neiman Marcus.

volunteers who followed the healthy longevity lifestyle program (as opposed to the
control group who merely continued their
usual behavior) experienced improved
memory performance and brain efficiency.
They also reported greater levels of relaxation and lower levels of stress.

We observed significant physical health
benefits as well. Many volunteers on the
program lost weight and experienced a significant decline in blood pressure and cholesterol levels.

Shirley's experience was similar to that
of many other subjects in the study for
whom these essential longevity strategies
improved memory and reduced stress, as
well as lowered blood pressure and cholesterol levels. Scientific evidence indicates
that adopting these lifestyle strategies not
only lowers the risk for Alzheimer's disease, but actually increases life expectancy — *making us live longer* — while
adding to the quality of those years.

Quality Longevity for the Long Haul

Large-scale, longitudinal aging studies,
including the MacArthur Study of Successful Aging, the Baltimore Longitudinal

Study of Aging, the Leisure World Cohort Study, and many others, have yielded scientific findings that add to the foundation of *The Longevity Bible*'s strategies. The MacArthur Study found that staying connected through social relationships as we get older is linked to longer and better living. A healthy emotional life — founded on intimacy and strong relationships — is associated with a more positive mental state as well as improved physical health and function. Another key finding is that it's almost *never* too late (or too early) to make healthy lifestyle choices and instigate changes to achieve quality longevity.

Whether we are approaching our forties, fifties, sixties, or more, we all face the challenges and rewards of aging. Studies on successful aging have shown that only one third of what predicts how well we age is controlled by genetics. Approximately two thirds is based on our personal lifestyle choices and, therefore, under our own control.

As we learn about the Eight Essentials, we will see how our psychologist, Shirley, and several others tackle the bumps and hurdles that so many of us face as we get older. We will learn how to apply the Eight Essentials, quickly and easily, and begin living a quality longevity lifestyle. If it's true that we're only as young as we feel, then it's time to start feeling, looking, and acting younger today.

Part 2

The Eight Essentials

Essential 1

Sharpen Your Mind

Memory is the mother of all wisdom.
— AESCHYLUS

The newspaper's daily crossword puzzle had long been the high point of Michele R.'s morning routine. Monday's easy puzzle she could do quickly, and in pen. But as the clues got harder throughout the rest of the week, she felt challenged enough to get that "puzzler's high" whenever she could solve them all and complete the puzzle. That all changed when Michele started working the newspaper's new brainteaser — Sudoku. There was nothing easy about it. How could arranging a bunch of numbers in a grid possibly hold her attention for more than a few minutes? Words were so much more interesting than numbers, and she had always been lousy at math.

It only took a week for Michele to get hooked on the new puzzle, as she began to pick up its patterns and logical challenges. She grabbed for the entertainment section of the newspaper before anyone could get near it — Sudoku had become Michele's new obsession. But instead of being fun and challenging like the crossword, it was often frustrating and sometimes enraging. She absolutely couldn't start her day off right if she failed to solve that morning's Sudoku. Her kids joked that if Michele kept up this fixation with the puzzle, she might have to join a Sudoku Anonymous group to kick the habit.

Soon Michele's husband began doing Sudokus as well. They would copy the one in the morning paper and race each other to see who could finish it first. As Michele got better at Sudoku, she began to get that puzzler's high back, and the added excitement of beating her husband every morning made it all the more fun.

Most people enjoy mentally challenging puzzles, especially when they are able to solve them. As Michele did, it's good to find mental challenges and leisure activities that are fun and engaging, but not ones that are so tough that we *strain,* rather than *train* the brain. Staying mentally active sharpens the mind, improves memory, and protects the brain from future decline. This first Essential is the key to following all the Essentials, which empowers us to take control of how we age.

A study published in the *New England Journal of Medicine* found that participating in leisure activities, such as playing board games, reading books, or doing crossword puzzles, cuts the risk for developing Alzheimer's disease by nearly a third. When scientists study animals raised in mentally stimulating cages — those with lots of toys, mazes, and other distractions — the animals not only have an easier time remembering how to navigate their mazes, but their brains' memory centers are much larger than those of animals brought up in standard-issue cages.

Several large-scale studies have found that people who engage in mentally stimulating leisure activities, along with other quality longevity strategies, not only feel happier and function better, but also tend to live longer. The most well-known longitudinal investigation of healthy aging, the MacArthur Study, found that people who remained mentally active — doing puzzles, reading books, playing cards or other games — had better quality of life and longer life expectancy than those who had less mental stimulation.

When scientists compare college-educated volunteers with those who have not attended college, they consistently find a lower risk for Alzheimer's disease among the more educated study volunteers. A recent brain imaging study found that with more years of education, we are better able to use the front part of the brain to augment mental prowess. This is a good argument for continuing education throughout our lifetimes.

The Sharper Mind

According to the scientific evidence, whenever we push ourselves to solve problems in a new way, we may be strengthening the connections between our brain cells. Each brain cell has dendrites. These minute extensions — similar to branches of a tree — pass information along from brain cell to brain cell. Without use, our dendrites can atrophy or shrink; but when we exercise them in new and creative ways, their connections remain active, passing new information along. Basically, any conscious effort to exercise your brain can potentially create new brain cell connections. And, remarkably, new dendrites can still be created even if old ones have already died.

Over the years, we learn more complex mental skills that eventually become automatic, so that our minds can perform certain mental tasks with less effort. As we gain experience, our minds become able to automatically take in the big picture without having to focus on every little detail. Take a look at the following paragraph:

Dont alwyas blveiee what yor'ue rdanieg becusae the hmuan mnid has phaoenmneal pweor. Aoccdrnig to uinervtisy rsceearchers, it deosn't mttaer inwaht odrer the ltteers in a wrod are plcead. Waht is improtnat is taht the frist and lsat letetrs rae in the corerct pclae.

You probably understood the message, yet the delivery was a mess. Our minds have learned to automatically perceive the meaning of something, even if details are missing or wrong. Systematic studies have found that older, healthy people with more experience are better and quicker at assessing an overall scene or picking out a face in a crowd than younger people, who tend to focus on details.

We can fine-tune these skills at any age with mental exercise. To make the most of our brain power and optimize mental sharpness, it is helpful to keep in mind what I call the *P's and Q's for Sharpening the Mind: Presence, Persevere, Quality,* and *Question.*

- *Presence.* Staying focused on the present makes us more efficient in any given mental task. What is key to remaining present and on task is not just the ability to take in what's going on around us, but also being able to shut out what's not important.
- *Persevere.* Sticking with a specific mental task builds learning and memory skills. You may start piano lessons today, but unless you continue to practice over the following weeks and

months, you won't gain the mental benefits or the enjoyment of mastering the instrument. With perseverance, your memory skills will improve and you'll enjoy heightened confidence in your cognitive abilities.

- *Quality.* When our minds focus on the qualities, details, and meanings of new information, we retain it longer and have a greater sense of control. This control allows us to organize the information and improves our learning abilities. If our hobbies and leisure activities have qualities that we value, they become more fun and fulfilling. Many people like to get involved in competitions, keeping a prize they value in mind during their activity. This may explain why competitive sports are so exciting for both the participants and the fans.

- *Question.* Curiosity allows us to expand our mental horizons. Reading stimulating books and magazines, exploring unfamiliar places and hobbies, and continually probing and asking questions will keep our mental skills intact.

Applying the *P's* and *Q's* not only helps

keep our mental lives active, but it allows us to develop *resilience,* the ability to recover from negative experiences. When we take chances and reasonable risks, explore new opportunities, and learn new skills, we also become better at bouncing back if we should fail in an endeavor. Being able to set and achieve new goals leads to greater self-confidence, personal strength, and a positive outlook (see Essential 2).

Risk-taking and thrill-seeking taken to the extreme are behaviors typical of adolescence, and with maturity most people learn to avoid dangerous activities, thus lengthening their life expectancy. The key is to find a balance — a way to pursue novel experiences that expand the mind without going overboard. The following are a few activities to consider for keeping mentally sharp over the years.

- *Travel.* If your inclination is to head for the beach and plug yourself into a lounge chair during your holidays, consider trying a different kind of vacation, maybe a sightseeing adventure to a destination you've never visited, or perhaps a stay at a self-realization spa or a dude ranch. Many vacation packages and cruises take visitors to new and exotic locations and enrich their experience with informative lectures on the region. Elderhostel (*www.elder hostel.org*) is one of the world's largest educational and travel organizations for people age fifty-five and older.

- *Get creative.* Learning a musical instrument or taking up oil painting are great ways to stimulate the artistic side of the brain, especially if you tend to be an analytical, left-brain type of person. Exploring your talents in right-brain creative pursuits will help keep your brain cells active and possibly protect them from future decline.

- *Challenge yourself.* Take your mental pursuits to the next level. If you do only the easy newspaper crossword puzzles on Mondays and Tuesdays, push yourself and try the more challenging Thursday and Friday puzzles. If you're a whiz at putting together five-hundred-piece jigsaw puzzles, buy a thousand-piece puzzle and get to work.

- *Take on a new hobby.* Whether it's collecting stamps, knitting, climbing rocks, or French cooking, getting involved in a new hobby is a great way to expand the mind. Hobbies distract us from everyday worries and allow us to gain a sense of mastery in whatever area we choose to pursue. People who engage in hobbies are less likely to experience mental decline as they age than those who spend most of their spare time in front of the television.

- *Join a study group or book club.* Some people like to study on their own, while others enjoy the interaction of a group experience. Book clubs and study groups are a popular way to expand your mental horizons and enjoy the company of like-minded learners.
- *Go back to school.* Most colleges and universities have extension classes for part-time students of all ages. Our UCLA Center on Aging has a Senior Scholars Program that makes it easy for older adults to audit undergraduate classes. The intergenerational component of the program enriches the experience for both generations: The undergraduates benefit from the wisdom of their older classmates, who in turn enjoy the youthful energy of returning to a college campus and interacting with a new twenty-something generation.
- *Flex your brain.* Try some Web sites, books, or magazines with puzzles de-

signed to flex your brain muscles. Check out the upcoming mental aerobic exercises, as well as those in the Appendix, which will give you a taste of the range of mental teasers and encourage you to pursue more puzzles. Enjoy some mentally challenging games such as Scrabble or Trivial Pursuit, activities that also can be a fun social event.

Building Brain Mass

A recent study published in the journal *Nature* found that three months of mental training can alter brain structure and, in essence, build brain muscle. After the study volunteers were given MRI brain scans, they were taught to juggle — a mentally challenging task. After three months of juggling, the brain scans were repeated. This time the scans showed significant increases in the volume of gray matter — the outer rim of the brain that is responsible for thinking and complex reasoning. Either their brain cells had grown larger and developed more extensive connections, or the number of brain cells had increased enough to build brain bulk. However, when the volunteers gave up their new hobby, their brains shrank back to their previous sizes. You can build brain muscle but you have to continue your mental activity to sustain the benefits.

In the first study of its kind, our UCLA research team found that when mental aerobics and memory training are combined with other *Longevity Bible* Essential Strategies, not only do volunteers improve their memory abilities but their brains become more efficient. We studied a group of volunteers who had only very mild age-related memory complaints — the kinds of occasional slips typical of people in their forties and fifties: walking into a room and forgetting the reason why, or having trouble recalling a word without a delay. Half of the group spent about twenty minutes each day on a mental aerobics program — learning memory techniques and solving puzzles — and kept physically active and ate a healthy diet. The other half of the study volunteers served as a control group and did not make any lifestyle changes during the two-week period. All volunteers received PET scans to measure their brain activity before and after the study.

Those who followed the healthy longevity lifestyle program had a highly significant change in brain efficiency in a region in the front part of the brain that controls everyday memory tasks, or "working memory." Working memory allows people to keep a limited amount of information in their minds for a brief period — such as when you get a phone number from Directory Assistance and remember it just long enough to dial it.

Just as athletes build physical stamina and muscular efficiency when they work out with a trainer at the gym, the healthy-lifestyle volunteers appeared to be building more efficient "brain muscle." Our study results suggested that focused mental activity and memory training can lead to greater brain efficiency — those on the program needed to use *less* brain energy to perform *better* on mental tasks.

For some study volunteers, this effect was dramatic. Michele R., a forty-six-year-old retired pharmacist and mother of three school children, admitted to having too many responsibilities on her plate. She was constantly carpooling, volunteering, and attempting to keep up with her endless list of chores and errands. Before entering the healthy longevity research study, she had begun to notice her memory slips, particularly when she was under pressure or multitasking. Her memory test scores showed that her verbal memory was typical for a woman of her age — not quite as good as it was when she was in college or pharmacy school, but about average for her age group. When we performed a brain stress test — a functional MRI scan that monitored activity during a memory task — the scanner showed a large area of the brain working hard while she performed the memory tasks.

After practicing *The Longevity Bible*'s memory techniques and spending time exercising her brain with mental aerobics each day, the brain stress tests showed that she needed to use very little of her brain's memory centers to successfully recall new information, and her verbal memory scores had increased by 200 percent — a dramatic improvement that made her memory more typical of a twenty-five-year-old than of a forty-six-year-old. With just two weeks of practice, Michele had subtracted more than twenty years from her brain age.

Memory Training 101

Memory defines who we are, now and at every moment. It also defines our future,

On Nancy G.'s fortieth birthday, she came home from work to find her husband's gift: a beautifully typed divorce petition. Unable to discuss the divorce rationally with her own mother, who was in the early stages of Alzheimer's disease, Nancy was forced to spend the ensuing years nursing her mother as well as her two teenage daughters through the trauma of Daddy going to live with his new, pretty "friend." Because she had to bump her part-time marketing job up to full-time, Nancy gave up her yoga classes and morning hikes with friends.

Nancy was already too busy or exhausted to read her novels or do the crossword puzzle at night, and it now seemed like the girls needed hours of help with their studies. Nancy's mother's health was declining daily, and Nancy's boss was insisting that she begin traveling for work. And though she finally met someone she was interested in dating, even that was causing tension because he was constantly asking for more time alone with her.

Nancy began getting stress head-aches like those she'd had in college. But what really worried her was how forgetful she was becoming — a client's name here, an appointment there, mixing up one of the girls' teacher conferences with another school function, and so on. Nancy had always prided herself on being responsible and prompt, and now she was panicked — was she getting Alzheimer's disease like her mother?

When Nancy came to UCLA seeking help, she learned about *The Longevity Bible* Essential Strategies. She almost immediately improved her memory abilities using simple techniques like *Look, Snap, Connect*, along with some other, more advanced memory techniques. Nancy came to understand that genetics accounts for only one third of what predicts whether or not someone will get Alzheimer's disease. She learned that she could stave off and possibly prevent symptoms even if it turned out she was genetically at risk. She began to feel more empowered, which sharply lowered her stress levels. The reduction of Nancy's anxiety levels not only helped improve her memory, it relieved her headaches and gave her more energy for all aspects of her life.

because without memory ability, we cannot make plans and think ahead. And, of course, without memory, it's as if we have no past. Staying mentally sharp requires optimum memory performance, the foundation for any quality longevity program.

The memory techniques that I taught Nancy are simple and easy to learn. Whether you need to remember a shopping list, the name and face of a new acquaintance, or the heights of the ten tallest buildings in the world, you can accomplish any of those tasks with my three basic memory techniques: *Look, Snap, Connect.*

Look reminds us to focus our attention. The most common explanation for memory loss is that the information never gets into our minds in the first place, usually because we are distracted or multitasking. Reminding ourselves to focus our attention will dramatically boost our memory power.

Snap stands for creating a mental snapshot or visual image — in our mind's eye — of the information to be remembered. For most people, visual images are much easier to remember than other forms of information.

Connect means we need to link up the visual images in a meaningful way. These associations are the key to drumming up memories when we want to recall them later.

Getting interested in what you are trying to learn and infusing the information with personal meaning will make these techniques more effective. Experiments with expert chess players have shown that they can readily memorize the chess pieces on the board if the pieces are placed as they would be during a match, but the players' ability to recall a pattern of pieces placed at random is almost impossible. One arrangement of chess pieces has meaning, while the other does not.

If I were to briefly introduce you to my friend Sylvia at a crowded party, it is quite possible you would forget her name. However, if you were to mention that she reminds you of your college roommate who also happened to be named Sylvia — giving my friend's name personal meaning for you — you would probably always remember my friend Sylvia's name.

When linking up your mental snapshots, create a story that has action and detail. If a picture is worth a thousand words, then a Technicolor motion picture is probably worth a million. Try memorizing the following eight words using Look, Snap, Connect. Create eight visual images and link them together in a story.

> Whistle
> Grandmother
> Sweater
> Juggler
> Cherries
> Ping-Pong
> Poodles
> Bow tie

Spend a moment coming up with a story before reading on.

Almost everyone's story will come out differently. If you like ridiculous stories, as I do, then you might be imagining a grandmother blowing a whistle as she knits a sweater. She gives the sweater to her grandson, who is juggling three cherries. One of the cherries gets away from him and interrupts his poodles' Ping-Pong game. Look closely, because the poodles have on bright red bow ties.

Notice my story's detail, action, and attempt at humor. All these elements make it easier for me to learn the words and recall them later. If you prefer more logical stories, then you might have the juggler wear the bow tie and let the grandmother eat the cherries. This technique works well for remembering everyday memory tasks and errands such as grocery lists or picking up a package at the post office after work.

Name That Face

Nancy G.'s memory complaints included difficulty with names and faces, and she is not alone: That is the most common form of forgetfulness as we age. Nancy was able to improve her ability to recall a person's name after recognizing his or her face by applying a variation of Look, Snap, Connect.

Whenever she met someone whose name she wanted to remember, she imagined a *Name Snap* (visual image reminding her of the person's name) and a *Face Snap* (a distinguishing facial or other body feature), and then used Connect to link the two Snaps together. When she met new coworker Lucille, she noticed her bright red hair (Face Snap), which reminded her of Lucille Ball (Name Snap). To connect these two Snaps, Nancy imagined Lucille Ball working in the next cubicle over, where the new Lucille would now be working.

Some names automatically trigger a visual image — meet Mrs. Taylor and you can picture her sewing a dress. Mr. Baker could be checking on his cake. Ms. Hill might be standing on top of a knoll. Other names evoke the image of a famous individual with the same name. You may visualize Mr. Fields on his tractor or eating his wife's chocolate chip cookies.

Not all names readily lend themselves to mental snapshots, so you may need to substitute visually evocative words that sound like or rhyme with the name. For Ms. Balisok, perhaps you see a ball of socks. When you meet Mr. Haft, you might see him floating on half a raft.

Try to come up with a visual image for each of the following names so you can create a Name Snap:

Herzog
Gambhir
Potvin

There is no right answer, but you could imagine seeing Mrs. Herzog driving a hearse with a hog as a passenger. Perhaps Mr. Gambhir is playing a Monopoly game while drinking a beer, and Ms. Potvin may have landscaped her yard with pots full of growing vines.

Memory Masters Reveal Their Tricks

For some motivated individuals, their memory feats become a competitive sport. These memory mavens challenge each other at international contests and manage to memorize remarkably large numbers and amounts of trivia.

Scientists at University College London found that these master memorizers are not that different from the rest of us. Their IQs are not extraordinary and their brain structures are unremarkable. What they do share are the strategies for accomplishing these memory feats, as well as the way their brains function when performing these mental tasks. The memory strategies activate a network of brain regions known to be involved in spatial navigation and memory.

One of the most commonly used memory techniques is called the Roman Room Method, wherein you visualize yourself walking through a familiar route, such as a sequence of rooms in your home, and mentally place images of the items to be remembered at specific points on the route. When you want to recall the items, you simply retrace your steps. This strategy has been around since ancient Roman orators used it to help them recall the specifics of their speeches.

We all can become memory masters by learning this technique. Start with your apartment or house and take a mental walk through the rooms. In each room, mentally deposit an object you want to remember, such as your blue suit hanging on the back of the front door, ready to go to the tailor's, or your phone book on the bathroom counter, open to the number of your dentist, whom you need to call for an appointment. Before long, your routes can include your office, your sister's beach house, and so on, until you have committed to memory more information than you ever wanted to know. I may have to name my next book *How to Forget What You Don't Want to Remember* in order to help some people reset their overstuffed memory storage units.

It's Never Too Late to Boost Memory Power

Nancy's mother was already suffering from the early stages of Alzheimer's disease. She had shown some improvement after treatment with Aricept and Namenda (see Essential 8), but even with the medicine, Nancy's mom was not the same woman she had been just a few years earlier. Nancy had heard that some of the mental exercises that she herself had been practicing could be simplified so that her mother would find them stimulating and not too challenging.

Recent studies suggest that people who have early stage Alzheimer's disease may be capable of learning more than previously thought. Dr. David Loewenstein and associates at Mount Sinai Medical Center in Miami Beach, Florida, taught Alzheimer's patients memory skills to improve name and face recognition over a three-month period. They found that the intervention improved recall of faces and names by 170 percent, and the improvement was sustained over the following three-month period. In another study of Alzheimer's patients, an eight-week mental stimulation program, in combination with the anti-dementia medicine Aricept, significantly improved patient interactions and overall functioning levels.

Mental Aerobics

Whether you are a puzzle fanatic or just a beginner, I've included some mental aerobic exercises to get you started and help you to advance to the next level of challenge. Keeping the mind active and alert is an essential component of any comprehensive quality longevity program, so start out at the level you think matches your needs, whether it's beginning, intermediate, or advanced.

Brain teasers and puzzles often involve *lateral thinking,* which means that we are trying to solve a problem from many angles instead of tackling it head on. When you get stumped with a puzzle, try thinking "outside the box" — see if you can come up with a new and creative solu-

tion. When you do, you'll not only be forti-
fying your brain cells, you'll probably
experience a sense of intellectual gratification.

It's also a good idea to cross-train your
brain. For right-handed people, the right
side, or hemisphere, of the brain controls
spatial relationships and the left side specializes in verbal skills and logical analysis.
I've labeled most of the puzzles according
to the hemisphere that tends to work the
hardest when you're searching for the solution. Cross-train by exercising both sides
of the brain.

You'll find the answers to the exercises at
the end of each section. If you come up
with an alternative answer, be sure to let
me know at *www.DrGarySmall.com*.

Beginning Exercises

1. Warm-up Exercise. Brush your hair
using your nondominant hand (i.e., if
you're right-handed, use your left hand).
You'll notice that it is awkward at first, but
practice this exercise over the next few
days and you'll see how much easier it
gets.

2. Beginner's Number-Placement Puz-

zle. Fill in the grid so that every row, every column, and every two-by-two box contains the digits 1 through 4.

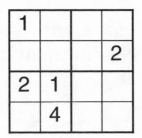

3. Whole-Brain Exercise. Say "silk" six times. What do cows drink?

4. Left-Brain Exercise. See how many words you can spell from the letters below. No letter may be used twice, and each word must contain the letter *L*.

L I G O B A E

5. Left-Brain Exercise. How many months have twenty-eight days?

6. Left-Brain Exercise. All of the vowels have been removed from the following proverb, and the remaining consonants are in the correct sequence, broken up into groups of two to five letters. Replace the vowels and figure out the proverb.

STRK WHLTH RNS HT

7. *Right-Brain Exercise.* Figure out which object does not match the others.

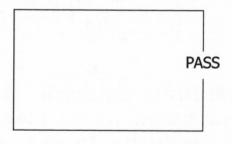

A   B   C   D   E   F   G   H   I

8. *Whole-Brain Exercise.* Figure out the word suggested by the message below.

PASS

Answers to Beginning Exercises

1. *Warm-up Exercise.* No right answer.
2. *Beginner's Number-Placement Puzzle.*

1	2	3	4
4	3	1	2
2	1	4	3
3	4	2	1

OR

1	2	4	3
4	3	1	2
2	1	3	4
3	4	2	1

3. Whole-Brain Exercise. Cows generally drink water, unless they are like me and sometimes prefer sparkling water. If you said "milk," then you might need to slow down a bit and focus your attention.

4. Left-Brain Exercise. I came up with the following words:

Agile, Ail, Ale, Bagel, Bail, Bale, Blog, Boil, El, Gail, Gale, Gel, Glib, Glob, Globe, Goal, Goalie, Lab, Lag, Lea, Leg, Lego, Lib, Lie, Lob, Lobe, Log, Loge, Oblige

5. Whole-Brain Exercise. All of them.

6. Left-Brain Exercise. Strike while the iron is hot.

7. Right-Brain Exercise. E (the angle is wider than that in all the other figures).

8. Whole-Brain Exercise. Pass Through.

Once you feel you have mastered the above exercises, continue to aerobicize your brain by moving on to the more challenging exercises on the next page.

Intermediate Exercises

1. Warm-up Exercise. Sit down at the computer and try using the mouse with your nondominant hand. Browse the Internet and see how well you do. This is an excellent exercise for anyone suffering from tendonitis due to mouse overuse. Practice over the next few days to see if you can improve your skills.

2. Letter-Placement Puzzle. Now we're going to substitute letters for the numbers, to make it slightly tougher. Fill in the grid so that every row, every column, and every two-by-two box contains the letters A, B, C, and D.

	C	
A		D
	D	B

3. Left-Brain Exercise.

See how many words you can spell from the letters below. No letter may be used twice, and each word must contain the letter "M."

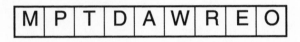

M	P	T	D	A	W	R	E	O

4. Right-Brain Exercise.

The following arrangement of sticks forms six squares. Try to remove four sticks so that the remaining unmoved sticks form two rectangles.

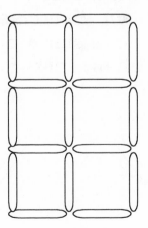

5. *Left-Brain Exercise.* Starting with the word WARM, change one letter at a time until you have the word FILE. Each change must result in a proper word.

WARM

. . . .

. . . .

. . . .

FILE

6. *Whole-Brain Exercise.* Count up the number of *F*'s in the following sentence.
Fresh fish is an excellent source of Omega-3 and a better source of antioxidants than many realize.
7. *Right-Brain Exercise.* By making just one move in a single direction, see if you can make all the sticks form a triangle.

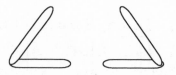

8. Whole-Brain Exercise. Figure out the word suggested by the message below.

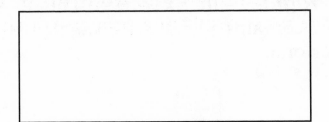

COVER

Answers to Intermediate Exercises

1. Warm-up Exercise. No right answer.

2. Letter-Placement Puzzle.

3. Left-Brain Exercise. Here are some of the words I found:

D	C	A	B
A	B	C	D
B	A	D	C
C	D	B	A

Admire, Am, Dam, Dorm, Dram, Dream, Dreamt, Em, Ma, Mad, Made, Map, Mar, Mare, Mart, Mat, Mate, Mated, Meat, Met, Mew, Mop, Moped, More, Mow, Mower, Pram, Ramp, Ram, Roam, Rome, Romp,

Tame, Tamed, Tamp, Team, Tempt, Term, Tram, Wam, Warm, Warmed, Worm

4. Right-Brain Exercise. The solution below contains a smaller rectangle within a larger one.

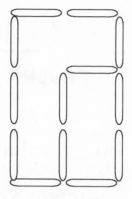

5. Left-Brain Exercise. Warm, Farm, Firm, Film, File, or Warm, Farm, Firm, Fire, File.

6. Whole-Brain Exercise. Many people count two, but the correct answer is four. Our brains often just don't process the word "of."

7. Right-Brain Exercise. If you slowly bring the page closer to your face, you will see an image of a triangle.

8. Whole-Brain Exercise. Undercover

Now take a two-minute stress-release break and breathe deeply and slowly, so you will be prepared for the brain-busters below.

Advanced Exercises

1. Warm-up Exercise. See if you can draw the three-dimensional figure below, using your nondominant hand:

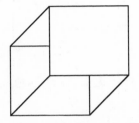

2. Advanced Number-Placement Puzzle. Now we're going to make it tougher by jumping from four to six numbers. Fill in the grid so that every row, every column, and every three-by-two box contains the digits 1 through 6. Unless you are an off-the-charts genius or an idiot savant, you will need a pencil with an eraser.

1		2	6		
	5			1	
2	6	4			
				4	6
			1		
5	2			6	3

3. *Whole-Brain Exercise.* Add two lines to complete the sequence below.

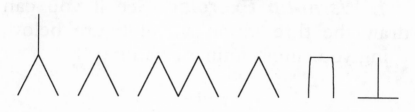

4. *Left-Brain Exercise.* Which is the odd one out?

Grouper Catfish Puffer Angelfish

5. *Whole-Brain Exercise.* Figure out the message suggested below.

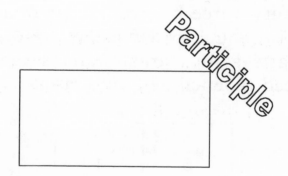

6. *Left-Brain Exercise.* How many tri-angles of any size are in the figure?

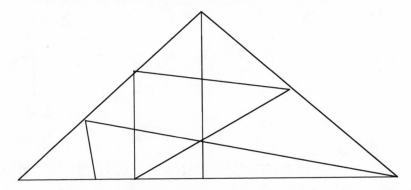

7. *Whole-Brain Exercise.* A truck that is one hundred feet long is moving one hundred feet per minute. It must cross a bridge that is one hundred feet in length. How long does it take the truck to cross the bridge?

8. *Mental Aerobics Word Finder.* Find and circle the words in the grid on the next page, which appear forward, backward, up, down, and diagonally.

P	O	H	S	I	F	E	S	A	C	N
F	O	D	D	O	O	F	O	R	I	O
O	S	N	O	F	R	O	M	A	N	W
C	O	O	Y	Z	G	E	E	S	O	H
I	A	X	T	E	E	B	G	A	M	E
B	R	A	I	N	T	E	A	S	E	R
O	E	R	E	D	I	B	T	O	N	E
R	L	L	A	C	E	R	H	O	M	E
E	A	U	X	T	E	A	R	E	E	D
A	X	O	T	S	A	C	E	N	T	I
B	A	S	S	N	E	V	E	R	I	R

Axon	Game	Reed
Bass	Mnemonic	Relax
Brainteaser	Never	Roman
Doze	Nowhere	Stress
Fish	Omega three	
Foci	Oxide	
Forget	Recall	

Answers to Advanced Exercises

1. Warm-up Exercise. No right answer.

2. Advanced Number-Placement Puzzle.

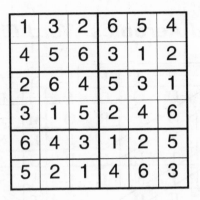

1	3	2	6	5	4
4	5	6	3	1	2
2	6	4	5	3	1
3	1	5	2	4	6
6	4	3	1	2	5
5	2	1	4	6	3

3. Whole-Brain Exercise. Create an "X" with the two lines to complete the inverted letter sequence.

4. Left-Brain Exercise. Catfish is the only freshwater fish. All the others are salt-water fish.

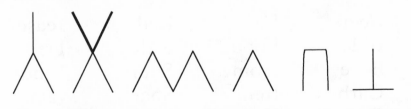

5. Whole-Brain Exercise. Dangling participle.

6. Left-Brain Exercise. Twenty-four.

7. Whole-Brain Exercise. Two minutes.

During the first minute, the front of the truck will cross the bridge, and during the second minute, the rest of the truck will cross it.

8. Mental Aerobics Word Finder.

P	O	H	S	I	F	E	S	A	C	N
F	O	D	D	O	O	F	O	R	I	O
O	S	N	O	F	R	O	M	A	N	W
C	O	O	Y	Z	G	E	E	S	O	H
I	A	X	T	E	E	B	G	A	M	E
B	R	A	I	N	T	E	A	S	E	R
O	E	R	E	D	I	B	T	O	N	E
R	L	L	A	C	E	R	H	O	M	E
E	A	U	X	T	E	A	R	E	E	D
A	X	O	T	S	A	C	E	N	T	I
B	A	S	S	N	E	V	E	R	I	R

For extra credit, see if you can find these other words.

Beet	Foe	Red	Tease
Bide	Food	Ride	Tie
Bore	Home	Shop	Tone
Carb	Item	Soar	Vat
Cast	Lace	Sore	Yet
Cent	Omen	Soul	Zen
Even	Pony	Tear	

Keeping Your Mind Sharp

- To get the most out of your mental workouts, apply the *P*'s and *Q*'s for Sharpening the Mind: 1) maintain *presence* and focus; 2) *persevere* in your endeavors to further sharpen your mind; 3) look for the *quality* and meaning in things; and 4) always *question* to learn more.
- Try a different approach to expanding your mental horizons, whether it's traveling to new destinations, learning a musical instrument, taking up ballroom dancing, or going back to school.
- Learn and use the three basic memory techniques:
  - Look: Focus attention on what you want to remember.
  - Snap: Imagine a mental snapshot of the information.
  - Connect: Link the snapshots together in your mind's eye.
- Practice other memory strategies for remembering names and faces.
- Stay mentally active through puzzles, games, reading, and other stimu-

lating hobbies, but be sure to train and not strain your brain — find the level of challenge that keeps you interested without frustrating or exhausting you.

Essential 2

Keep a Positive Outlook

A positive attitude may not solve all your problems, but it will annoy enough people to make it worth the effort.
— HERM ALBRIGHT

You're throwing a dinner party for the new boss and his wife, and everyone from the office is coming. You nabbed the best caterer in town, your house is spotless, and your wife looks fantastic. The bartender is the only staff that's arrived so far, and he's handing out cocktails to the earliest guests. But where the hell is the caterer? Your wife tells you not to worry — he'll get there any minute.

An hour later, the party is hopping and the boss is laughing, but you are freaking out because you just learned that the caterer's truck broke down and the food may not arrive for another two hours. Your wife hands you a drink and tells you to relax, she's got it completely under control.

Your wife walks calmly into the kitchen, wondering "What the X#@!?$* am I going to do now?!" The boss's wife follows her in and says she overheard the whole thing and wants a peek at the pantry. They pull out several boxes of linguini, grab some fresh garlic, butter, and frozen shrimp. Two other women join them and start chopping tomatoes for bruschetta, which they start blowing out of there on crackers as hors d'oeuvres. The bartender brings them a bottle of wine and a few glasses, and suddenly it's a cooking party in the kitchen.

Later, you're eating this pasta your wife threw together, the boss is making toasts to his hosts, everybody *seems* to be having a great time, but *you* know they're all just faking it in a futile attempt not to hurt your feelings over this giant bomb of a dinner party. That caterer is toast.

On Monday, you slink into the office, avoiding all eye contact, especially with the boss — you may have to say good-bye to your corner office after that party fiasco. But the boss follows you down the hall and throws his arm around you. "What an evening! And your wife is incredible! The food was amazing." You look at him dumbfounded. He goes on effusively. "I really admire you — you're a guy who can make the most of a tough situation — like when a caterer blows you off when the new boss is coming over! I love it! I know you're going to move up in this company."

Here's a cheerful thought: Science shows that keeping a positive attitude helps us stay healthy and live longer. A recent Mayo Clinic study found that individuals scoring high in optimism on the MMPI (Minnesota Multiphasic Personality Inventory) were 50 percent more likely to survive the next thirty years than pessimists were. These optimists also had fewer physical and emotional difficulties, were less limited by pain, enjoyed higher energy levels, and were generally happier and calmer.

Everyday stressors from work, family, health issues, social commitments, and countless other challenges can make it tough to stay upbeat, and many factors contribute to whether one has a tendency toward optimism or pessimism. Genes play a role, but so do our early childhood experiences, family background, self-esteem, and degree of spirituality — all of these influences affect our ability to think in a positive way. However, in the pursuit of quality longevity, it is possible to train ourselves to see the cup half *full* instead of half empty. Maintaining a positive attitude, like any other skill, can be learned.

Optimists Win the Longevity Game

Positive thinkers tend to avoid depression, which is known to shorten one's lifespan, especially when not adequately treated. Optimists are also more likely to get timely medical help because they anticipate that they can improve or prevent their health problems. Researchers at Aarhus University Hospital in Denmark considered another possible mechanism for the connection between positive thinking and health — the immune system, the body's means for fighting off infection. In looking at more than three hundred volunteers between the ages of seventy and eighty-five, they found that those who continually ruminated on negative thoughts had higher counts of white blood cells, as if their bodies were trying to fight off a disease. This suggests that negativity may have an adverse effect on health by actually stimulating a physiological response.

People with a prevailing positive outlook are also more inclined to feel content with their lives, and self-satisfaction has been associated with longer life expectancy. Scientists in Finland studied the impact of a sense of well-being and happiness on longevity and found that satisfied people were twice as likely to survive after twenty years compared with individuals who claimed to be dissatisfied.

Those of us who have a generally positive attitude toward aging live longer than those who do not. Dr. Becca Levy and her associates at Yale University explored the influence of attitude on life expectancy in a study that followed over seven hundred individuals for more than two decades. They found that older people who viewed aging in a positive light lived seven and a half years longer than those who saw aging as a more negative experience. If you anticipate a vital, healthy, and fulfilling future, that perception may indeed come true.

In Pursuit of Happiness

Some scientists believe that our brains may be hardwired in ways that determine how happy we tend to be. Dr. Richard Davidson and his colleagues at the University of Wisconsin have pinpointed an area in the front part of the brain that controls positive feelings, optimism, and happiness. His group studied one of the most powerful positive sets of emotions — a mother's feelings toward her newborn baby. Using functional MRI brain scans, they found that when mothers viewed photos of their babies, their brain activity increased dramatically in this front brain region, as compared with the brain activity of mothers viewing photos of unfamiliar infants.

Research also shows that joyful individuals share certain personality traits and habits. For generally upbeat people, happiness is associated with a personality type that emphasizes independence, self-esteem, competence, and close relationships.

Fortunately, even if there is some hardwiring that predisposes us to joy, much of what determines our happiness is under our own control. Although some people pursue it through fancy vacations, expensive cars, jewelry, or other material things, the thrill of these quick-fix gratifications is generally short-lived. Sustained contentment is more likely to result from healthy relationships and meaningful accomplishments.

Ironically, a tragedy or loss can sometimes set individuals on a path to sustained happiness. Many people who survived the 9/11 disaster but were close enough to experience the destruction firsthand were initially devastated, but they eventually got a clearer perspective on what is truly important in their lives — family, friends, and sustaining a purpose in life. Through adversity, people often become more aware of their own survival skills, resilience, emotional strength, and power to help others as well as to be helped. Nobody's life is free of misfortune, but through adversity we can become more aware of little things we often forget to appreciate, and sometimes gain new positive perspectives and insights for the future.

Dr. Ronnie Janoff-Bulman and colleagues at the University of Massachusetts have studied the way profound life events — both positive and negative — may influence an individual's ability to enjoy *sustained* happiness and fulfillment. They compared the well-being of two groups: lottery winners and people who had suddenly become paralyzed. Though the lottery winners experienced initial euphoria following their new wealth, in the long run many were no happier than the accident victims, in part because normal, everyday pleasures now paled next to the thrill of winning the "big one." In contrast, many of the people who became paralyzed learned to adjust to their new disabilities, and were eventually better able to appreciate small pleasures and accomplishments, as compared with the nouveau riche in the study.

Longevity Through Spirituality

Throughout history, various forms of spirituality and religion have been a way for people to embrace a more positive outlook and find deeper meaning in life. Although organized religion is a major influence in many people's lives throughout the world, spirituality is a broad concept and isn't necessarily connected to a specific belief system or form of worship. Some people satisfy their spiritual needs though meditation, music, or art, while others seek harmony with nature or the universe. Whatever form your spiritual expression takes, it can not only help you to feel more secure and manage your stress, but can also extend your life expectancy.

Several scientific studies have found that regular church attendance is associated with longer life. One recent study showed that visiting a house of worship just once each week extends average life expectancy by seven years. The scientists found that this churchgoing/longevity connection held up even when they factored out the influences of the social support and healthy lifestyles associated with organized religion.

Some people believe that their faith in a higher power keeps them healthy and heals their illnesses. Dr. Kenneth Pargament and his associates at Bowling Green State University in Ohio studied nearly six hundred medical patients and found that those who believed in God had a 30 percent lower mortality rate as compared with those who felt abandoned by God. However, not all studies demonstrate a connection between faith and health. For example, faith has not been found to improve recovery from serious injuries or acute illnesses, or slow the growth of cancer cells. But faith seems to help people face their injury or illness in a way that nurtures acceptance of their human frailty.

Although scientific studies have not definitively confirmed that faith heals, when faced with crises or illnesses beyond their control, many people find that prayer helps them cope, and research points to other health benefits as well. Dr. Harold Koenig and colleagues at Duke University interviewed over eight hundred medical inpatients and found that those embracing religious beliefs or some type of spirituality had better social support, less depression, and higher cognitive function.

The chanting and prayer that is typical of organized religions share many of the mental and physiological qualities of meditation, and scientists have pointed to studies on meditation to explain how faith and religion may help heal our bodies. Research has demonstrated that meditation can positively modify brain activity, immune function, and the body's stress response, as well as lower heart rate and blood pressure. It can also help people achieve a state of mindful awareness, allowing them to stay more present and attuned to what is going on around them. This often leads to a more positive outlook, particularly for people who are easily distracted or habitually multitasking.

Mainstream medicine is recognizing the importance of the interaction between spirituality and health. Neuroscientists have been able to pinpoint specific areas of the brain that are activated when people pray. The meditative state typical of intense prayer has been found to lower blood pressure and heart rate, which reduces the body's stress response (see Essential 4). Nearly two out of every three U.S. medical schools now offer courses on spirituality. Some medical students actually follow the hospital chaplains on their rounds to learn firsthand how the clergy help people who are suffering from physical illnesses.

Confidence — the Longevity Benefits

Having a positive attitude often leads to increased self-confidence, because with a positive attitude we are more likely to believe that we can solve problems and exert control over our environment and ourselves. In the MacArthur Study, investigators found that study volunteers who rated high in self-confidence were more likely to believe that they could improve and maintain their memory skills. Self-confidence was also associated with better physical performance and a greater sense of empowerment. Older people who were able to meet challenges and solve problems had a much better sense of their abilities to live independently, regardless of their actual abilities. These positive self-perceptions greatly improved their quality of life.

Self-confidence and self-esteem are character traits that form early in our development. Our sense of self is often influenced by our childhood experiences. At a young age, we begin to compare ourselves to others. One might have been stronger, taller, cuter, or smarter than one's playmates in the sandbox, but those playmates might have had more doting grandparents or better handball skills or longer curls. This kind of competitive comparison of our own attributes to those of others can either bolster or deflate our self-esteem. An abusive parent or even a negative comment at the wrong time or place can erode our confidence, whereas our early successes or encouragement from parents can positively shape our future self-perceptions.

Self-esteem affects almost every aspect of life. When we feel good about ourselves, we have more fulfilling relationships, we're more resilient, we feel more upbeat and are better able to cope with adversity. Unfortunately, too often people focus much of their self-esteem on physical appearance and the attainment of wealth rather than on values, personality traits, integrity, and behavior. Certainly, living a quality longevity lifestyle — eating healthfully, limiting stress, and staying fit — helps people not only to feel younger, but to look younger as well.

But it is sometimes hard to live up to the perfect, youth-obsessed images constantly bombarding us in magazines, television, and films. This becomes an increasing challenge as we age. Although no one can stop time, with the latest preventive measures and modern medical treatments, we *can* take years off our appearance (see Essential 8). Older people sometimes complain of feeling invisible or overlooked, as if they are "fading into the background." The sooner a person can shake off the desire to conform to an idealized, unrealistic, and usually unattainable "supermodel/ super-wealthy image," the healthier they will be physically and emotionally, and the greater their self-esteem.

Building Self-Esteem

Anyone who has ever experienced a period of low self-esteem knows it can certainly fuel a negative outlook. Some simple exercises can help provide a positive spin and clearer perspective on negative perceptions one might have about oneself.

Doing the Right Thing

Matching your actions to your beliefs is a great self-esteem builder. As much as possible, make choices and act in ways that fit with your beliefs about moral behavior. Perform a small act of kindness to a stranger or to someone you care about, make a charitable donation, or perhaps pledge your time for a good cause. Helping others and supporting causes one believes in usually makes people feel good about themselves.

Inner Critic and Rebuttal Exercise

The following chart has two columns, Inner Critic and Rebuttals. Under Inner Critic, write down three examples of ways in which you might criticize yourself. Next to each criticism, list several rebuttals. For example, you might write that you're not very good at your job because you didn't get a promotion and you haven't been giving it your all lately. In the rebuttal column, you can dispute this negative perception by listing your professional achievements; things you enjoy about your job; and recognition you may have received from your boss or coworkers in the past. You may find that your critical belief is a distortion when you recall your work achievements, the aspects of your job that you really like, and how much your coworkers respect you.

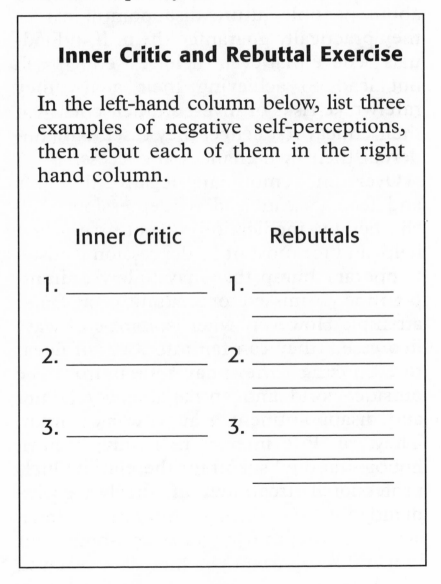

Inner Critic and Rebuttal Exercise

In the left-hand column below, list three examples of negative self-perceptions, then rebut each of them in the right hand column.

Inner Critic	Rebuttals
1. _____	1. _____
	_____
	_____
2. _____	2. _____
	_____
	_____
3. _____	3. _____
	_____
	_____

Drinking from the Half-Full Cup

Some people get more wrapped up in sadness, worry, and negative thoughts than others. By always anticipating the worst, some of these individuals don't just worry about possible future disappointments — they practically guarantee them. If individuals believe that even their best efforts will not lead to achieving their goals, they rarely take risks or invest all their energy in their endeavors; hence, they essentially undercut their own chances at success.

Over time, embracing negative thoughts and feelings can lead to depression. Psychotherapy, medication, or both can often help, and for most of us depression is just a temporary bump that may follow a disappointment, missed opportunity, or failed attempt. However, when some people get depressed, they can fall into a rut of negative thinking. They may retreat from the outside world and anticipate only failure and disappointment around every corner. They can lose interest in family, friends, hobbies, and jobs, and for these individuals professional treatment is firmly recommended.

Jim S., fifty-seven, a successful trial attorney, was respected by his colleagues and well known for his high-profile celebrity cases. Although he truly enjoyed helping his clients when they needed him the most, his "day job" was getting a little bit dull. Jim had always liked new challenges, and he was searching for a way to be more creative. After being asked to write a couple of articles for a trade journal, Jim found he really got a creative charge out of it. And it was much more fun than the tedious legalese of his case material. When he met a literary agent at a dinner party, she encouraged Jim to consider writing a proposal for a book featuring some of his most noteworthy trials.

Jim was pumped up about the book proposal and started working on it every night. He had fantasies of taking time off from the firm and launching a literary career — maybe he would try a mystery novel after his first book hit the best-seller list. After all, John Grisham started out as a lawyer — and his books even became movies! The more Jim got into the book proposal, the less he enjoyed going to work at his law firm.

Jim finally turned in his proposal and anxiously waited for the agent's response. When she called, she was enthusiastic about it and sent the proposal out to over a dozen New York editors. Jim could already see himself doing a national book tour, appearing on the morning talk shows, and having gala book-signings. Maybe he would give up trial law altogether — he certainly wouldn't miss the pressure and the long hours.

Although a couple of editors expressed some initial interest in his proposal, no solid offers came in; just rejection letters saying there were already too many books out on the same topic. One editor suggested that if the cases in Jim's book focused on political figures, there might be some interest, since a major election was coming up next year. Jim's agent encouraged him to rewrite the proposal with this political spin.

Jim initially agreed, but every time he sat down to do the rewrite, he felt overwhelmed and frustrated. He was a harsh critic — as soon as he put something down on paper, he'd re-read it and cross it out. The "charge" he'd gotten from writing the proposal was gone, and it had become a daunting endeavor. He couldn't keep his mind on it and kept procrastinating. He finally admitted to himself that he was never going to write the thing.

Jim felt humiliated for getting carried away with his fantasies of literary fame. He'd become distracted from his job as a trial lawyer, and even though he tried to throw himself back into it, that work now seemed even duller than before.

Worst of all, Jim had lost his confidence — not just in writing, but in his law practice as well. If his chance of becoming a famous author could vanish so quickly, maybe he would lose the next case, too. Soon his pessimism was tainting everything he did

— if his wife planned a picnic on the weekend, he would ruminate about rain. If he had a meeting across town, Jim fretted that the traffic would make him late. He felt anxious and easily agitated, and he wasn't sleeping well. Jim's wife grew concerned that he was becoming depressed and pressed him to seek professional help.

After a couple of months of psychotherapy, Jim was able to gain some insight into his negativity and pessimism. He realized that his current reaction to the book letdown was similar to the way he'd reacted to disappointments and insecurities he'd experienced as a child. To avoid the discomfort of any more disappointments, he was seeing everything in the future as negative — that way there would be no surprises.

To help Jim regain his optimism, his therapist suggested he refocus his attention on his "day job." He helped Jim learn ways to rediscover what had excited him about practicing trial law when he started out. Jim also decided to do something fun he had put off for years — he enrolled in a creative art class. He found that painting allowed him to express his creative side without the stress of trying to get a book published. His wife and friends said his paintings were really good. Jim was beginning to think so, too. Hey, maybe one of the local galleries would be interested in showing his early oils . . . In fact, Jim seemed to recall Matisse was a lawyer before he became a famous artist.

A recent study from Wake Forest University found that when we make a conscious effort to experience joy and happiness, it pays off. Dr. Will Fleeson and colleagues found that study volunteers actually felt happier when they *acted* more extroverted — singing aloud, walking over and talking to someone, or being more assertive and energetic — and other people perceived them as happier, too.

Psychotherapists use several approaches to help patients minimize negative thinking. In *cognitive therapy,* negativity is seen as resulting from conscious, negative assumptions and thoughts. Patients are taught to recognize their habitual negative thoughts and learn ways to break the habit.

By learning new cognitive skills, pessimists can, in fact, become more optimistic. Drs. Martin Seligman, Albert Ellis, and others have described systematic cognitive approaches for learning optimism. Generally, a person first focuses on how a particular event triggers a negative feeling in them. They learn to recognize the assumptions they make about those feelings, and the consequences and outcomes of their responses to those feelings. For example, your boss chooses another executive to handle a new account. You immediately feel hurt and rejected, and assume you are about to be fired. With that unsubstantiated and negative assumption tainting your mood and attitude, your performance at work slides. Your boss eventually calls you into her office tomorrow for "the talk." You spend a sleepless night worrying that you'll be fired at tomorrow's meeting with the boss, when actually she plans to hand another new account to you — possibly one you will value even more.

It's not just events that evoke feelings inside us, but the assumptions we assign to those events: I feel so bad for picking my date up late again — *and* I know she'll never go out with me again because of it. To break negative patterns and outcomes, we need to challenge those assumptions and especially to avoid the tendency to generalize negative thoughts. One error at work doesn't mean your job is in jeopardy; a single traffic citation doesn't lead to losing your driving license; and a minor argument with your spouse doesn't spell divorce. If you tend to think in this generally negative manner, remind yourself of your years of work accomplishments, outstanding driving record, or bonds of love and trust; this may help put such negative thinking into perspective.

It is possible to put concerns, worries, and fears into perspective *before* they get us into a rut of negativity. The following exercise can be helpful.

When doing this exercise, focus on only one feeling or situation at a time, then repeat the exercise for other concerns you may have. Afterward, talking with a friend, spouse, or other empathic listener about the process will often provide even more insight.

Exercise for Staying Positive

1. Think of a situation that brings up anxiety or fear for you. Start out with a simple daily concern — having a disagreement with a friend, fear of misplacing something, or perhaps being late for work. In your mind, play out the likely outcome of this situation, such as hurt feelings, anger, guilt, sadness, etc.

2. While thinking about this situation and its potential outcome, concentrate on your breathing. Breathe deeply and slowly. As you focus on your rhythmic breathing, feel yourself relaxing — physically and mentally.

3. Continue breathing as you consider the feared situation and try to see the bigger picture: With all the good times you and your friend spent together, it is unlikely that one spat will unravel that. You will probably find or be able to replace the item you lost. Stepping back, learning to relax, and putting worries into perspective allows you to recover a positive attitude more quickly.

Forgive and Forget

The ability to let go of angry feelings and turn the other cheek lowers stress levels and fosters a positive attitude. Dr. Neal Krause of the University of Michigan found that people who are readily able to forgive others experience enhanced psychological well-being and less depression than grudge-holders. The next time someone wrongs you and triggers feelings of anger, try writing them a candid letter; but after you finish it, put the letter away until the next morning. Often the simple process of writing about feelings helps dissipate them. Reading the letter after a night's sleep frequently provides another dose of perspective that helps distance us from the negative feelings — possibly enough to make sending the letter unnecessary.

Many times we hold on to angry feelings over a confrontation we had with someone long after we forget the details of what the dispute was about. This is common between spouses, long-term friends, partners, and family members. The next time you have trouble forgiving someone, even though you'd like to, keep in mind that over time you probably won't recall the actual quarrel anyway. That realization often helps people to get over their anger. Also, trying to understand what the other person is feeling — guilt, embarrassment, frustration, etc. — may help you empathize with the person's point of view and forgive him or her more readily (see Essential 3).

Sometimes we also need to forgive ourselves. Dwelling on feelings of remorse or guilt for past errors rarely solves problems, and it certainly doesn't make us feel any better. Learning to forgive ourselves and let go of our mistakes allows us to gain wisdom from them and move forward.

Keeping a Positive Spin for Quality Longevity

- Make a conscious effort to be extroverted and energetic — happiness is contagious.
- Forgive yourself and others who wrong you — letting go of grudges lowers stress levels and fosters a positive outlook.
- Build self-esteem by making moral choices. Keep in mind your accom-

plishments and successes to help rebut your inner self-critic.

- If you don't already have an active spiritual or religious life, consider getting one, whether it's through meditation, organized religion, seeking harmony with nature, or any other form.
- Learn to be optimistic through simple, systematic approaches. Recognize what your negativity triggers are, and challenge any negative assumptions you are quick to make.
- Avoid pessimistic thinking by focusing on your strengths and setting achievable and realistic goals.
- Don't be a loner — ask others for support and get professional help if you need it.

Essential 3

Cultivate Healthy and Intimate Relationships

Friendship is born at that moment when one person says to another, "What! You too? I thought I was the only one."
— C. S. LEWIS

Shirley I. was finally taking her long-awaited getaway from her patients, daughter, boyfriend, parents, and friends. She had an experienced psychologist covering for her, and her daughter knew how to reach her in case of an emergency. This was *her* week to chill out at her favorite spa — catch up on her reading and not answer to anyone about anything. She warned them all that morning: "If it's not life or death, don't call me — I don't want to talk to *anybody* for

---

seven days!" Once she got to the spa, Shirley stashed her cell phone, turned off her BlackBerry, and hid behind her giant sunglasses as she settled in at the pool with a novel.

"Hi, mind if we take this lounger?" Shirley glanced up at two smiling young women. "Sure, go ahead," Shirley said, and then went back to reading as the ladies spread their towels on the lounge chairs next to hers and chatted as they ordered drinks from a passing waiter, put suntan lotion on each other's backs, and got out their own books to read. Shirley noticed the blond woman's book and said, "I read that one. I loved it." The blonde smiled. "Really? Thank goodness. I hate going on a trip without a really good book." Shirley sat up. "Me, too. I mean, I've been so excited about getting away for a week of solitude, I actually brought six books just in case I didn't like any of them." All three women laughed. "That's why I love this place! I can really relax here and be alone. I am so exhausted from dealing with

> everyone in my life that my jaws actually hurt from talking. I'm Shirley, by the way." They introduced themselves all around and continued to chitchat. When the drinks came, Shirley put them on her tab and ordered everybody lunch as they continued to gab.

Humans are naturally social. We not only enjoy being with others, we thrive on it. Our need for intimacy, emotional connectedness, and social support begins in infancy and lasts for the rest of our lives. Dr. Rene Spitz and others found that a high proportion of adequately nourished infants who were not held or caressed by their mothers frequently experienced developmental delays.

Adults have a similar need for contact. Research has shown that people exposed to periods of sensory deprivation, such as prisoners in solitary confinement, may hallucinate and lose their ability to differentiate between fantasy and reality. It is critical to our well-being that we remain intimately connected — through talking, touching, and relating honestly to people we care about. Anyone experiencing quality longevity will credit healthy and intimate relationships as among the most meaningful and important elements of their life.

Social Butterflies Live Longer

Dr. Thomas Glass and his associates at Harvard University showed that spending enjoyable time with others actually extends life expectancy. They looked at approximately three thousand older Americans to see how much time they spent in a variety of social activities, such as playing games, attending sports events, and going out to restaurants. Their decade of research showed that the chance of longer survival was 20 percent *greater* for people who spent more time socializing than for those who socialized very little or not at all.

Several recent studies have demonstrated the direct *physical* benefits of social support. Dr. Elizabeth Brondolo and her colleagues at St. John's University in New York City studied a group of the city's traffic officers as they faced the daily stress of confronting violators and issuing tickets. They looked at how the repeated threats and insults from disgruntled drivers affected the officers' blood pressure and other physical measures, and whether or not receiving support and encouragement from their colleagues would reduce these stress effects.

By monitoring the officers' physical responses throughout the day, the researchers found that job stress spiked blood pressure. However, when colleagues offered friendly support, especially during high-tension moments, blood pressure remained stable.

Staying connected reduces anxiety and lowers the amount of stress hormones released into the body. This is important because stress hormones are known to contribute to heart disease, diabetes, Alzheimer's, and many other age-related diseases. The MacArthur Study of Successful Aging found that long-standing emotional support was associated with significantly lower blood levels of cortisol and other stress hormones. Socially connected volunteers in that study also required less pain medication following surgery, recovered more quickly, and followed their doctor's post-op advice more closely.

When we are close to a group of people, it makes us feel part of something and gives us a sense of belonging. It lifts our spirits and builds self-esteem. There are practical benefits as well — friends, family members, coworkers, and neighbors are there for each other, available to help each other out if needed. Whether it's borrowing a cup of detergent or getting a ride to the auto mechanic, it's nice to have others to lean on.

Good Habits Are Catchy

We usually meet and get to know people through a common denominator — we are parents at the same school, neighbors on the same block, or coworkers at the same company — so we're predisposed to having at least one or more things in common. Just how much influence any individual or group has upon us depends on our prior experiences with them, as well as our history of relationships with others. Social scientists describe an "inner circle" — the people whom we consider closest to us, usually spouses, children, siblings, or other close family and friends. For most of us, the size of this influential inner circle, whether it includes a spouse or several friends and relatives, tends to remain stable over the years, even if the people in that circle change.

When we spend a significant amount of time with certain people, we tend to adopt and share the same attitudes and lifestyle habits. Often we don't realize the impact these lifestyle influences are making on the quality of our longevity. If we surround ourselves with a health-conscious crowd, we are perhaps more likely to meet for a game of golf on a Sunday morning rather than a Saturday afternoon of cocktails and munchies at the club lounge.

Kimberly L., a forty-two-year-old personal stylist, met Richard T., an architect, at her tennis club. He was charming and funny, and she hadn't met anyone else she wanted to date in almost a year. At first he joined her in tennis and hiking, her favorite pastimes, but that soon gave way to late-night dinners and parties with Richard's large circle of friends.

Kimberly enjoyed being with Richard, but the more time she spent with him, the less time she spent at the tennis court, hiking trail, or gym. She began losing sleep and gaining

---

a few pounds, and she'd even been late for work a couple of times. Her best friend, Alice, mentioned that she was looking a bit worse for wear.

One evening as they finished a late supper at a French restaurant, Richard suggested that they go to his favorite bar for a nightcap. Kimberly said she'd had enough to drink for a weeknight and perhaps they should go home and try to make it to the gym in the morning. Richard got defensive and said he didn't need a "mommy" to tell him what to do. Not wanting to start an argument, Kimberly gave in and joined Richard for a drink with his friends.

The next morning Kimberly woke up a little hungover and was late for work. After a long talk with Alice, Kimberly decided to give Richard an ultimatum: Either they lighten up on the partying, or they stop seeing each other. Richard got angry and said, "Fine. Let's take a break." Kimberly was hurt, but she stuck to her guns. The first few days were rough, but she knew she was doing the best thing for herself, and Alice was there to lend support.

A week late, Richard called and apologized. He said he missed her and was ready to clean up his act. He asked if they could meet sometime for a round of tennis. Kimberly said sure, and she'd buy the drinks afterward — at the smoothie bar.

As in Kimberly's case, we can often influence others just as they can influence us. Some of us have advised our children to choose their friends wisely, and perhaps we could benefit from that same wisdom.

Clearing Out Relationship Clutter

Sometimes we hold on to relationships long after they become not just nonessential, but detrimental or even toxic. Unhealthy relationships can complicate our lives and lead us to repeat negative patterns that can bring on frustration and guilt. When we have too many of these toxic friendships or even one that has become prominent in our lives, we suffer from *relationship clutter.* It may be time to clean house — emotionally.

Clearing out relationship clutter often requires spending less time with some individuals and more with others, or perhaps severing an unhealthy relationship completely. If an acquaintance places unreasonable and heavy demands on our time and resources, it can consume our energy and leave us emotionally drained.

Sometimes people remain in unhealthy relationships simply out of habit. The negativity or uncomfortable feelings from the toxic friendship may have been going on for so long that they don't even realize they *can* unburden themselves from the feelings by getting distance from the other person. Once we change or sever such a relationship, the reduction in stress alone can go a long way toward improving the quality of our longevity.

On the other hand, it is possible to reenergize a relationship with someone when it has gotten off track. The surest way to reconnect with someone is by carving out some dedicated time to be together — alone — during which both people can share their thoughts and feelings. When deciding whether or not to try to repair a friendship, you might consider

113

how long you've known the person, if you and this person have been successful at resolving differences in the past, and whether or not this person has been or will be a positive influence in your life.

Any real and satisfying relationship takes time to nurture, and for most of us, time is limited. We need to make wise choices about the people we spend our precious free time with — and, ideally, choose people with whom we can have mutually nurturing relationships.

Barbara and Greg W., midfifties, were coming up on their thirtieth anniversary. While they were out to dinner with old friends Jane and Alan, Jane insisted on helping them plan a big party to celebrate their anniversary — especially since Barbara and Greg had done "absolutely nothing" to mark their twenty-fifth. Clearly, Jane didn't consider Barbara and Greg's romantic twenty-fifth-anniversary trip to Rome as very significant. Jane said the party *had* to be at the new luxurious hotel she had just decorated — the caterer was to die for! And they

---

had to start working on the guest list ASAP!

That night Barbara was all fired up about Jane's party idea: She'd have to get a new outfit, and Greg would definitely need a new suit. Oh, and did she mention that Jane knew the most fabulous stationer to make the invitations? Greg put up his hands. "Whoa, there. Weren't we going to spend our anniversary visiting the kids? I thought you wanted to play with your new granddaughter?" "I *do!*" Barbara said defensively. "We'll just fly all the kids out here for a week. That's what Jane and Alan did. It'll be great!" Greg glanced around the sleek and modern condo they had downsized to after their youngest was out of the house and married, and wasn't so sure. And, except for their daughters' weddings, he and Barbara had never been so keen on throwing big parties.

Over the next two weeks, Jane put Barbara through an abridged version of "Party Planning 101" — menus, flowers, music, invitations, and the most important thing of all: compiling the guest list. Barbara either couldn't make up her mind or didn't really care about many of the details, so she left several decisions in the willing hands of Jane. The bills, however, were placed wholly and firmly onto Barbara's credit cards, and Greg was *not happy* with the situation.

One night, as Barbara was getting ready for bed, Greg lay propped up, reviewing the bills. "You booked a photographer for fifteen hundred dollars? Why can't your sister take the pictures? She's good with a camera." Barbara replied from the bathroom, "This guy shot Jane's son's wedding! He's incredible! We're lucky to get him!" Greg mumbled something about his "great luck" as Barbara got into bed and said, "I just hope we can fit everyone into the Terrace Ballroom at the hotel." Greg took a deep breath. "Just how many people are we talking about?" Barbara took out the guest list Jane had printed out for her. "Hopefully no more than 150." Greg reached for the list. "May I see that?" He looked it over. "You're inviting the Franks? We haven't even spoken to them in maybe three years." Barbara got defensive. "Judy Frank goes to the same hairdresser as Jane, so she's going to know about the party. And I have to invite Jane's sister and brother-in-law, and her parents, too. They can sit with Dr. Robertson." Greg was dumbfounded. "Our old pediatrician?!" Pouting, Barbara responded, "He was Jane's pediatrician, too! And they're still really close!"

Greg continued to peruse the list, annoyed. "I thought you didn't like Christine Fowler. Didn't you say she was a meanspirited gossip queen?" Barbara snorted. "She is. But I'd rather have her out broadcasting what a great party I had instead of what a witch I was for not inviting her." Greg sighed. "That sounds like Jane talking." Barbara turned away, angry, turned off her bedside lamp, and started to cry. Greg put down the list and took her in his arms. "I'm sorry, honey. I know you've been working really hard on this thing, and I didn't mean to upset you." She sniffed. "I know. It's okay. I guess I'm just stressed out. Putting this thing together, spending all this money, having all the kids and the grandkids coming here — I just feel over-whelmed." Greg kissed her lightly. "It's *our* thirtieth anniversary, honey. We can always blow off this shindig and run away to some tropical para-dise . . ." Barbara turned to face him. "Are you kidding? Jane would never speak to me again!"

The following week was another whirlwind of activity surrounding the party — airline flights had to be booked for the kids, clothes had to be tailored, shopping had to be done, and home repairs had to be com-pleted. On Friday afternoon, Jane called Barbara and announced that she needed to add four more people to the guest list — the Kleins and the Ruperts from the tennis club — they all just adored Barbara and Greg, and Jane just *had* to invite them to the party. Barbara balked. "Jane, the maximum for the Terrace Room is 160, and we're already at that." Jane took a moment, then calmly said, "Barbara, darling, your sister and her family haven't committed yet. That's six people! And they live three thousand miles away, for Pete's sake. You don't *have* to encourage them to come . . ." Barbara was shocked. "But she's my *sister*. She was maid of honor at my wedding. I *want* her there." Jane, unfazed, replied, "Just offering a suggestion, doll. Take it or leave it."

That night, Barbara decided to leave it. The next day she and Greg called the stationers, the florist, the hotel, and the photographer, and were able to retrieve most of their deposit money. Barbara's stress melted away as she came to realize that the party had become more about Jane's need to be a social butterfly, and less about Barbara and Greg celebrating their thirty years of love and commitment. They didn't need the Kleins or the Ruperts, or a demanding pushy friend to remind them of what was important and worth honoring in their lives.

Two days before their anniversary, Barbara and Greg boarded a plane for the East Coast to visit their kids and grandchildren. Barbara's sister's family — all six of them — drove down for a night of celebration. Then the whole clan saw Barbara and Greg off on their romantic tropical voyage to the Bahamas. Barbara remembered to bring her "A" list of people to send island postcards to, and neither the Kleins nor the Ruperts made the cut.

Empathy: The Basic Social Skill

To imaginatively see things from another person's perspective and be able to understand his or her feelings is commonly known as "empathy." The ability to convey this understanding back to the other person is the emotional glue that keeps us socially connected. With empathy, we feel less alone in the world and are able to build closeness, friendship, and love.

By participating in groups that empathize together, and share a common cause, goal, or purpose, we become part of a social network. College fraternities, book clubs, alumni associations, school PTAs, charity boards, neighborhood watch committees, and political action groups are just a few examples of the ways in which people group together around similar empathic interests.

Social networks can increase our sense of belonging, purpose, and self-worth, all of which promote a positive outlook. They can help us get through difficult and stressful times, such as a divorce, a job loss, or the death of a loved one, as well as the happy types of stressful times, such as a wedding or the birth of a baby. And we don't necessarily have to lean on family and friends for support to reap the benefits. Simply knowing they're available can give us a sense of confidence when we face stressful events or other problems.

Scientists recently found that helping other people actually improves the helper's mental and physical health. Study volunteers who mentored young children experienced greater physical strength and stamina, better social interaction, and more mental stimulation than a control group that was not mentoring.

Some people are natural-born empathizers. They instantly put their own needs aside in order to be emotionally available for a friend or family member. However, not everyone is heavily weighted with this gift. Many of us have to make more of an effort, especially when distracted by the seemingly never-ending complications of our own lives. Although we'd like to think we would drop everything for a friend in need, it might require some effort to give up floor seats to a basketball playoff game the moment your friend calls and wants to spend a few hours talking about being stood up for a date.

Most of us know one or more people who seem to have no empathy skills at all, and were it not for work, family, or social obligations, we might choose to avoid these people altogether. This kind of person typically does not listen nor remember what we've told them, or even what they've told us. They appear unmoved by other people's suffering and unable or unwilling to share in their joy. It is hard to feel connected to those who lack in empathy, and they are often labeled as bores or narcissists. Luckily, most people — even the empathy-challenged — can improve their skills with a little work and some simple techniques.

We first begin learning empathy as infants by observing it in our parents. They nurture and care for us, which helps us develop our sense of self and ability to identify with and relate to others. From our parents' caring caresses, understanding words, smiles, nods, and other nonverbal communications, we learn to regulate our own emotional responses. These early experiences help shape our ability to get close to others on an emotional level.

As we mature and become more independent, we turn away from our parents and look to get our "empathy fix" from like-minded peers who share our interests, desires, and values. Eventually, we develop more intimate relationships outside of the family and aspire to deeper levels of sustained empathy in marriage and other long-term relationships.

The powerful form of loving empathy that jolts many of us when we have our own children leads us to an intense closeness and bonding with our kids. Most parents would sacrifice their own lives instantly to protect their children.

Many people agree that one of the most effective ways we become empathic toward others is by experiencing our own pain, loss, or elation. Anyone who has lived through the death of a sibling, spouse, or parent knows all too well how difficult it is for someone else going through that same experience. On the other hand, knowing the joy of holding your first child or grandchild, or perhaps watching your eldest daughter get married, is a feeling that is wonderful to share with a friend who may be experiencing it for the first time.

Our capacity for empathy is often challenged when our parents age and we are thrust into the unfamiliar role of caring for them. Although it can be emotionally confusing to care for the people who have always cared for us, many adult children lovingly care for their parents if the need arises.

Empathy has likely given the human species an edge in natural selection. Our ancient ancestors' empathy gave them connective social glue that provided a survival advantage against the adversities of their environment. By banding together, they were better able to fend off predators and nurture their offspring, whereas alone they would have been less likely to survive. Current science indicates that our social connectedness has more than a survival advantage — it has a biological basis as well.

Hardwired to Connect

With recent neuroimaging studies, doctors are discovering what appears to be the hardwiring of empathy in our brains. Dr. Tania Singer and her team studied couples in love at the Institute of Neurology at University College in London. They measured brain activity in volunteer couples when one partner experienced a pain stimulus, such as a brief electric shock. That person later observed their partner appear to be experiencing the same brief pain. Whether a volunteer actually felt the painful stimulus or whether they believed their lover felt it didn't matter. The same emotional brain centers were triggered, suggesting that these emotional brain centers may be the root of empathic experiences.

We don't have to be in love to experience empathy. Just seeing someone's facial expression — whether it's painful or pleasurable — sets off a sophisticated network of neuronal wires that fires the message through a preset pathway and triggers a response in us. This brain hardwiring for emotion is not set in stone, and we can exert some control over what we feel. Neuroscientists at the UCLA Ahmanson

Lovelace Brain Mapping Center found that when volunteers observed emotional facial expressions, certain brain areas lit up on their MRI scans. Afterward, by simply imitating those emotional facial expressions, the volunteers were able to light up the identical brain areas on their MRIs.

These findings are in line with the earliest concepts of empathy. When the German psychologist Theodore Lipps originally coined the term in the late nineteenth century, he postulated that we actually imitate another person's actions when we empathize. This "chameleon effect" has been observed in empathic individuals when they unconsciously mimic mannerisms and facial expressions of others, as opposed to people who show little empathy — sometimes referred to as "stone-faced."

Higher Education in Empathy

In school, we are taught a variety of subjects, from reading and writing to physical education and even music appreciation. But as yet, there is no standard curriculum on empathy to help us communicate effectively with important people in our lives.

Empathy, however, is becoming widely accepted as an ability that can be learned in order to enhance our social connectedness. It strengthens our sense of closeness and fulfillment in our relationships. We begin learning empathy, like language, during early childhood. And just like language, we can continue to hone those skills throughout our lifetime. The empathy process involves several components that can be fine-tuned with practice.

Recognizing Other People's Feelings

By age twelve, most of us are aware of our own various emotions and can recognize those same emotions in others. We can learn to empathize with others by drawing upon our own experiences that were similar to what the other person appears to be going through.

Some people have more trouble differentiating among subtle emotional states. The ability to recognize the subtleties of facial expression as well as body and verbal language can be learned, practiced, and improved upon. Some psychologists have their patients view and study photographs or drawings that convey a range of facial expressions of various emotions such as anger, guilt, fear, or sadness, to help them learn to recognize those emotions. Once we are able to recognize another person's emotional state, we can more readily empathize with that person's feelings.

Attentive Listening

When we are engaged in a conversation, it's natural to want to jump in when a thought or reaction gets triggered in us. However, interrupting somebody in midsentence or midthought may distract or frustrate that person, and we could end up not hearing how they really feel. Great conversationalists are often people who say little, but listen a great deal. Empathic individuals tend to give the other person enough time to relate their experience as fully as possible. This type of attentive listening requires self-control — not just over interrupting the speaker or allowing your mind to wander, but also over unnecessary movement or fidgeting that can distract the speaker.

The following exercise not only helps build listening skills, it can be used as a regular tool to "check in" with your partner or close friend after a long day or other period of time apart. Sometimes just five minutes of uninterrupted attentive listening is all it takes to connect with someone you have been merely passing rushing in the hallway for days — even if you live under the same roof.

Attentive Listening Exercise

This exercise can help us learn to avoid being distracted by our own thoughts and reactions, including the desire to jump in and participate while the other person is speaking. You can do this exercise with a friend, spouse, family member, or even someone you don't know very well. Set aside fifteen minutes so you both can take a turn.

- *One Person Talks.* For three to five minutes, one partner talks about something that is going on in his or her life right now. It could be a crisis, chronic issue, or perhaps a past or upcoming event. Beginners may choose to start by discussing feelings or situations that do not involve the listener directly. If the topic does involve the listener, the speaker should be careful to discuss only his or her *feelings* about the situation, individual, or relationship, and avoid criticizing the listener. This exercise is *not* about attacking and defending, it is about talking, listening, and being understood.

- *Other Person Listens.* The listener should not interrupt or coax. Rather than jump in and say, "I know just what you mean! I've felt exactly like that!" the listener should maintain eye contact and stay focused on what the other person is saying. Even if the listener's mind wanders momentarily to thoughts like, "What am I going to say when it's my turn?" the listener should push those thoughts away and bring his or her attention back to what the speaker is saying.

- *Switch Roles.* After three to five minutes, the *listener* now talks about something he or she is going through, and the other person becomes the attentive listener. The topic may be completely unrelated to the first speaker's discussion. If it is related to the first person's discussion, the second speaker should be careful not to retaliate or attack, and instead focus on his or her own feelings.

- *Discuss the Experience.* After both partners have had a chance to speak and listen, they should spend the next few minutes discussing what the experience felt like. Many people find that by simply listening attentively, they develop an almost immediate sense of empathy and understanding for the other person. By being listened to thoughtfully, most people feel understood and cared about. It may take practice to break the habit of interrupting the speaker with encouraging thoughts, feelings, and one's own experiences, but it gets easier with practice.

Communicating Your Empathic Response

Understanding what another person is going through is a large part of empathy. *Conveying* that understanding back to the other person is just as important, and is what truly draws people together and keeps them close. Communicating with another person about his or her concerns, without criticizing, makes that person feel understood. This kind of exchange involves basic communication skills — both verbal and nonverbal — including eye contact, facial expression, and body language. Even people who are born great communicators can enhance these skills.

One way to communicate your understanding after attentively listening is to clarify what you heard the other person tell you. You could try saying things like, "I want to make sure I understand this . . ." or "Let's see if I have this right." You can then restate the other person's feelings or situation and try to paraphrase their words. Asking for more detail is also helpful. Follow-up questions show the other person that you have heard them, you're interested, and you would like to know more.

If your partner is trying to cope with a difficult situation, you might start by acknowledging his or her efforts. If there is nothing you can do to help, let your partner know that you understand and are willing to listen. Sometimes just lending a nonjudgmental ear can be far more supportive than trying to fix the situation.

Communicating our understanding and compassion to our mates not only brings us closer, but can also enhance our sexual fulfillment. A satisfying sex life contributes to overall quality longevity — physically and emotionally — and really brings people together.

Good Sex for Longer Life

Researchers the world over have reported a positive link between sexual activity and life expectancy. A recent study determined the level of sexual activity of nearly one thousand men from a town in South Wales, and then followed their health outcomes over the next ten years. The life expectancy for the sexually active men — those reporting orgasms twice or more each week — was 50 percent greater than for the men who experienced orgasms less than once a month.

One of the longevity-increasing benefits

of remaining sexually active may be its association with lower rates of heart attacks, which researchers speculate is related to the release of the hormone DHEA during orgasm. Testosterone, the hormone that stimulates sex drive in both women and men, has been found to help reduce the risk of heart attack, as well. Sexual activity also helps maintain physical fitness by burning calories and fat.

Engaging in sexual activity may also bolster immune function, the body's ability to fight off infection. A study of college students found 30 percent higher immunoglobulin A levels in those having sexual intercourse once or twice a week, as compared with abstinent students. (Of course, this doesn't apply to my own teenage daughter, who will have no time for such activities due to constant studying and then conducting the New York Philharmonic Orchestra, until she marries the perfect young man who meets my complete approval.)

Research shows that besides improving physical health and potentially adding years to one's life, healthy sexual activity adds quality to those years, as well. Sexual satisfaction reduces tension and helps us sleep better, perhaps through the release of endorphins and other hormones. Studies have also found it to relieve chronic back pain, anxiety, and headaches. Positive sexual experiences often increase self-esteem, and many religions and cultures view sexual expression as a tool for spiritual enlightenment.

Love the One You're With

A healthy sex life fosters intimacy, feelings of affection, and closeness between partners. Expressing our sexual desire is a basic ingredient in bonding as a couple, and sexually satisfied couples have a greater probability of long-term stability.

Although sexual intimacy is good for our health, emotional state, and longevity forecast, many people find it challenging to keep passion alive over the course of several years. Family needs, work pressures, illnesses, and a multitude of distractions may leave some people physically exhausted and emotionally depleted at the end of the day, and sex may be the last thing on their minds. The following simple strategies can help couples communicate better, strengthen intimacy, and ultimately lead to a more satisfying sex life.

First, Love the One You Are

It's very easy to blame a partner for his or her lack of sexual interest. Because he or she no longer dresses or acts sexy, initiates intimate contact, or perhaps even mentions sex, our own desire has shut down.

Before pointing at a partner, however, one should try focusing on oneself. Letting go of negative feelings like anger, guilt, and fear gives us a more positive outlook and helps bolster our sexual self-esteem. As we age, our bodies change, but it is a myth that sexual quality and desire necessarily decline. In fact, as we gain more experience and wisdom, lovemaking can become more pleasurable than ever before. By practicing mindful awareness — staying in the moment and remaining aware of all the sensations going on in our bodies — we are likely to be more playful and emotionally available to our partner, which in turn can help our partner to overcome his or her own distractions and fears.

Talking Sex

Talking with a partner about sexual desires and fantasies can be difficult, especially when one is unaccustomed to doing so. But the benefits can be so great that a little discomfort is usually well worth the effort. Partners might start by discussing sexual experiences they have had together that were particularly satisfying. Try the following simple exercise:

1. Tell your partner something he or she has done in the past that really turned you on. Your partner may not be aware that it was so enjoyable for you.
2. Your partner now tells you something you have done that really turned him or her on.

This kind of discussion can begin a sexual dialogue that leads to sharing of fantasies and more fulfilling sexual intimacy.

Show That You Listened

Responding positively and nonjudgmentally to your partner's sexual wishes promotes greater intimacy. If you have told your partner about something that excites you in bed and he or she responds by trying it, you know that your partner has listened, cares, and wants to please you. That's as good a description of love as any. Whether it's lighting a few candles, buying new sexy pajamas, or massaging your partner's back, taking the initiative is another way to show your partner that you are interested and want to please him or her.

More Tips on Staying Intimately Connected

Even the closest of couples may find that the challenges of work and family can leave them mentally and physically exhausted by day's end — thus derailing their goal of being sexually intimate with each other. There are several positive steps people can take to overcome these and other common barriers that sometimes arise in relationships. Consider some of these suggestions:

Schedule an intimate date. Plan ahead for time alone with your partner — perhaps dinner at your favorite restaurant followed by a romantic night at a hotel, or even a cozy evening at home alone. The anticipation alone can be exciting.

Set the mood. Before going to bed, spruce up the bedroom with some candles, play soft music, and if you enjoy incense, light some.

Time your medicines. Many of us experience aches and pains that may restrict our movement and distract us from "the mood." Discover the time it takes for your medicine to take effect — whether it's an anti-inflammatory, a sexual-function enhancer, or even a Tylenol — and be sure to take it accordingly.

Try a "quickie." Not all lovemaking has to be a major event preceded by candlelit dinners and roses. Sometimes a brief sexual encounter — complete with excitement and urgency — can be a spicy variation. Whether it is a spontaneous encounter in the bathroom while the kids are watching TV, or a brief midday rendezvous at lunch, these get-togethers often have a fun and sneaky quality that can be exhilarating.

Indulge your fantasies. Try telling your partner some private thoughts that turn you on. Almost everyone has sexual fantasies and exploring them with your partner can bring you to a new level of intimacy.

The Value of Vows

According to information from the Centers for Disease Control and Prevention, marriage may increase life expectancy by as much as five years. Numerous studies have found that married people live longer, happily married people live the longest, and married couples who continue to be sexually active (with each other, of course) are *most* satisfied with their lives, overall.

New research from the University of Warwick in England found that a spouse's happiness spills over to the partner's state of mind. The study looked at over 9,700 married couples and compared them to 3,300 couples who lived together out of wedlock. A happier husband made for a happier wife and vice versa, but this did not hold true for the unmarried couples. The study showed that the cohabitating couples who remained unmarried had a greater sense of personal autonomy at the cost of their emotional connection.

The national divorce rate has nearly doubled during the last forty years, and a growing industry of "marriage educators" has attempted to remedy today's fractured families. Typically, there are three types of couples-counseling techniques that assist partners in improving their communication skills and satisfaction with their relationships. In the traditional and most common technique, behavioral marital therapy, the therapist helps the couple learn communication skills and ways to resolve their differences in a kinder, more empathic manner. A second form, insight-oriented marital therapy, uses both behavioral techniques and strategies for understanding the other person's reasons for becoming angry and defensive in the relationship, in order to defuse chronic power struggles.

A third, newer approach — emotionally focused therapy — helps people recognize that their partner has needs and coping styles that may differ greatly from their own. Partners learn to appreciate and accommodate these differences, rather than attempting to change them. Dr. Susan Johnson of the University of Ottawa has studied this form of relatively brief therapy — usually eight to twelve sessions — and has found significant gains that last at least three years for most couples, even those at high risk for divorce. This is a much higher success rate than that reported for the more traditional forms of couples therapy.

Many couples don't need formal therapy to help resolve their conflicts and keep their relationships on track. However, even contented, successful couples can benefit from some simple strategies to help them stay connected and happy for the long haul.

Set aside time. Many people are so busy multitasking throughout their waking hours that they may have little time left to talk about their day-to-day concerns and personal issues with their partner. Make it a daily ritual to spend some time together — without kids, friends, television, or other distractions. This time can be used to talk about what's on your mind and how you're really feeling. Sometimes just holding your partner and *not* talking may be what is needed.

Keep a sense of humor. All couples argue. What defines a successful marriage is *how* the couple argues. Try to punctuate a disagreement with an occasional smile or some humor to convey your understanding of the other person's idiosyncrasies.

Stay in touch. An effective way to maintain emotional closeness during a period apart can be a quick phone call or voice mail to let your partner know you are thinking about them. An e-mail works well, too.

Don't criticize. Focusing solely on your partner's weaknesses may make him or her defensive and sabotage your attempts to feel connected. Try talking about the feelings that your partner's actions trigger in you, rather than simply criticizing his or her actions. Instead of saying, "Why do you have to be so thoughtless and slam the door while I am working?" try "When you slam the door while I'm working, I lose my train of thought and I feel frustrated and powerless."

Socialize as a couple. Find things you and your partner like going out and doing together, and try to do them with other people you enjoy spending time with — particularly other like-minded couples. Sharing views and new ideas with other people carries over into your own relationship and keeps things lively — even if it's only a few private laughs after everyone else has gone home.

Take care of yourself. Most people in long-term relationships understand that their partner cannot meet all of their personal needs. Besides taking responsibility for your own medical health, you need to care for yourself emotionally and socially. Regular tennis games, poker nights, book clubs, support groups, community theater, sporting leagues, and involvement with religious or charity groups are just a few of the ways we can refuel ourselves independently of our partners. When we come back together, we are often emotionally energized and ready to enjoy each other's company.

Table for One

Most people spend a good portion of their adult lives as single people, whether they're unmarried, divorced, or widowed. And despite progress in defining the individual with greater independence in today's society, there is still an emphasis on couples, as well as security in groups. If you've ever eaten at a table for one at a fine restaurant, you may know how it feels — people smile sympathetically or act like you're contagious, while the waiters constantly inquire, "Will someone else be joining you?"

Coupling is not the social solution to quality longevity for everyone. There are advantages to being single and able to make decisions based on one's own needs and desires, without having to compromise to suit another person's whims. But the need for social connectedness remains, and single people who maintain strong relationships with family, friends, and community groups live longer than those who do not. In fact, single women, who tend to have stronger and longer-lasting relationships with friends and family, outlive their male counterparts by several years. It benefits single people to remain out there and connected, whether it's through sports, work, dating, volunteering, or other social activities.

Man's Best Friend

Many people love pets, but most don't realize that pets may contribute to their owners' longer life expectancy. Studies of patients with heart disease have found that pet owners live longer — often more than a year — than those without a pet. A UCLA study showed that dog owners required less medical care for stress-induced aches and pains than the study subjects with no dogs, and these therapeutic effects are not limited to canines. Having cats, parakeets, turtles — even just watching a tank full of tropical fish — have all been shown to lower stress levels, thus contributing to quality longevity.

Some studies have found that pet owners have reduced blood pressure and cholesterol levels, as well as increased life satisfaction levels. Exactly how pets help us reduce stress is not known; however, we definitely bond with our pets, and they can be good and true companions. There are also practical benefits to pet ownership, such as having a walking companion, an alarm that sounds when visitors approach the door, and, as in the case of my dog, a little friend who happily keeps the kitchen floor clear of any food scraps that might happen to fall.

When considering a pet, think about what is practical for you and your family, your living space and surroundings, and your personal preferences. Even people with strong allergies can usually find a hypoallergenic pet they can tolerate and love.

Parent Care

Thanks to advances in medical technology, adult children and their older parents are both enjoying longer life and better health. Still, the risk for chronic disease increases with age, and some adult children, often still dealing with the needs of their own kids, can find themselves simultaneously thrust into the unfamiliar role of caring for their parents.

Because most people continue to look to their parents for emotional support throughout adulthood, it can be psychologically difficult to have that role reversed. For the parents, the idea of turning to their children for help can sometimes be tinged with humiliation.

On a practical level, many older parents and adult children are not prepared to cope with the medical, financial, legal, and geographical challenges that can emerge when parents need the help of their children. It is important to prepare in advance for this possible transition. Most of us who have had a good relationship with our parents and our children want those caring relationships to continue, even if the roles should reverse. Here are some issues and strategies to consider during the transition period associated with parent care.

Be empathic. Parent care may stir up a variety of feelings, such as anxiety, fear, and guilt. Try to anticipate some of the concerns of the other generation. Among the many issues at hand, the adult child needs to consider their parent's possible discomfort about receiving care from them. The parent may want to take into account the sense of loss his or her adult child is experiencing now that the roles are reversing. Remaining empathic will make it easier to talk about mutual feelings and maintain closeness.

Ask for help. Both parents and adult children are often reluctant to ask for help. Parents don't want to burden their children, and many "sandwich-generation" adult children — busy caring for parents and children simultaneously — don't turn to other family members or caregivers for assistance. Traditionally, an adult daughter takes on the greatest responsibility of care, but if she is overburdened and unwilling to let others help, the entire family suffers.

Money matters. Between parents and children, money can be a symbol of love, power, caring, revenge, or a variety of other motives and feelings. Concentrate on clarifying practical questions such as: What are the actual assets and the real needs of the family members? Getting good legal advice on wills, trusts, and other financial issues well in advance of the inter-family discussions of these matters can help families avoid conflicts in the future.

Housing. If a parent can no longer live alone, questions emerge about how to provide the best living arrangement. Some adult children welcome their parents into their homes, which often works out well, especially if the parent has enough privacy and sense of purpose within the family. For others, an assisted-living arrangement or skilled nursing home may be a more feasible alternative. Many resources are available to help families sort through the many alternatives (see Appendix 3).

Health care. Many adult children get involved with their parent's health care if the parent is unable to make all necessary decisions on his or her own. The key is to respect the parent's privacy, yet understand when it's important to step in and help. Having advance directives in place is a good way to make sure the parent's wishes are being followed.

Keeping Relationships
Healthy and Intimate

- Stay connected and involved socially, whether you are single or in a couple. Try to spend time with a healthy crowd, because good habits are contagious.
- Clear out relationship clutter by cutting loose unsatisfying or "toxic" friends and acquaintances.
- Develop and maintain your empathy skills. Listen to others, try to identify with their feelings, and let them know that you understand.
- If you are in an intimate relationship, make efforts to nurture it: Schedule time together, share feelings without criticizing, and stay in touch with friends and other couples. A healthy sex life adds to quality longevity.
- Having a pet may contribute to longer life expectancy. Pets can also be enjoyable, stress-reducing companions.
- Planning ahead for the emotional and practical challenges of parent care can make a possible role-reversal much less stressful for both older parents and their adult children.

Essential 4

Promote Stress-Free Living

Reality is the leading cause of stress among those in touch with it.
— LILY TOMLIN

Alan F., fifty-three, gently awakens Monday morning to his favorite classical music station on the clock radio. He feels rested and calm as he recalls the fantastic weekend he spent with his family at the beach. The weather was outstanding, everyone got along great, and he didn't think about his work as a hotel-chain executive at all. During breakfast, Alan promises himself he will *not* let job pressures get to him this week. He's halfway through his shower when the water turns icy cold. Okay, so sharing the hot water is not a concept his kids have yet grasped. He towels off and tells himself it's no big deal, it's still a beautiful morning. Just then he cuts himself shaving — again. Apparently, his wife still hasn't stopped using his razor to shave her legs. Okay, maybe his wife is right and he has a problem sharing, too. His wife, the *expert* sharer, leans in and reminds Alan that he has to stop by the bank today to sign those papers, okay? As he quickly gets dressed, he has no idea how he'll fit the bank into his hectic afternoon. He's already late as he frantically searches for his keys, which are next to his cell phone — which has a dead battery. The housekeeper must have unplugged the charger again when she vacuumed yesterday. Fine, he tells himself, no problem, he'll just charge it at work. Finally, he's relaxing in traffic to the classical music station, dodging between lanes on the freeway, when he notices the flashing red police lights behind him. Alan mutters a profanity and feels his back muscles tensing up as he pulls over on the shoulder. He hears the radio DJ cheerfully report that the weather at the beach is going to be even better than it was on the weekend. As the policeman walks up to his car, Alan wishes his damn cell phone were charged so he could call in sick and head back to the beach.

Stress — a major contributor to age-related diseases — cannot be avoided entirely. Most people, including Alan F., experience stress from work pressures, annoyances at home, and any number of other daily aggravations. However, by learning to minimize stress, as well as our responses to it, we can begin to limit its impact on our lives and increase our quality longevity.

Stress isn't only due to crises or problems. Sometimes positive events — having a new child in the family, being promoted, or planning a big celebration — can stress us out. Other times it can be a loss — the death of a friend or family member, a physical illness, or perhaps a divorce. Even a trivial incident can set us off, whether it's a passing criticism, a misplaced car key, or a broken fingernail. Whatever the cause, science has shown that stress weakens our bodies and accelerates aging.

Under intense stress, our bodies mobilize energy and release stress hormones such as cortisol. As a result, our heartbeat, blood pressure, and breathing rate increase causing more oxygen to be delivered to our muscles. During this acute reaction, nonessential functions such as digestion are suppressed. This "fight or flight" response is an ideal physiological survival tool and useful in many dangerous situations. However, when stress becomes chronic, constant worry or aggravation can keep this stress response turned on, and the continual release of stress hormones can damage the body.

A recent study found that chronic stress may accelerate the very aging of our cells. Scientists from the University of California in San Francisco found that volunteers with higher stress levels had cellular markers of aging equivalent to at least one decade of additional aging, as compared to low-stress volunteers.

Over time, elevated levels of cortisol and other stress hormones can literally shrink the memory centers in our brains and increase our risk for Alzheimer's disease. Ongoing stress has also been associated with an increased risk for high blood pressure, irregular heartbeats, and some forms of cancer.

A twenty-year study of approximately thirteen thousand people found that chronic stress increased the risk of dying from stroke or heart disease. Stress has been shown to undermine our immune system, which diminishes our ability to fight off colds and infections. For some people, stress affects the digestive system and leads to conditions ranging from ulcers to irritable bowel syndrome. Stress can also raise blood sugar levels — a known risk for developing diabetes. Body weight and obesity rates are increased by chronic stress, because stress can stimulate both the appetite hormone leptin and the mood-altering chemical serotonin.

Although what triggers our stress is often beyond our control, how we perceive a stress-provoking event and the way in which we react to it directly determine its impact on our health. We *can* learn simple stress-reduction techniques to greatly improve our responses to stress and reduce its effects on us. Many of the other essential strategies, such as getting regular exercise and eating well, enjoying healthy relationships, and maintaining a positive outlook, also help reduce stress.

How Stressed Out Are You?

Understanding yourself — what stresses you out the most and how you instinctively react — is a first step to figuring out how to possibly avoid or detoxify your most stressful situations, as well as how to manage your reactions. The symptoms of stress are not always obvious, since they can be both physical and mental. If you can link up the specific stress symptom to the cause of the stress, you have taken a big step toward low-stress living. Answer the following questions to get a better idea of how stressed out you are and what triggers your stress response.

Stress Level Questionnaire

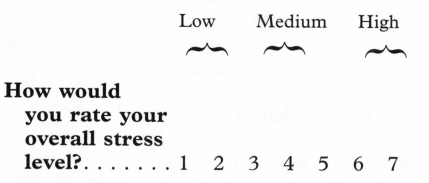

	Low	Medium	High
How would you rate your overall stress level?	1 2	3 4 5	6 7

To what degree do the following situations make you tense or irritable?

	Little		Somewhat		Very		
Argument with friend or relative	1	2	3	4	5	6	7
Waiting for a table in a restaurant	1	2	3	4	5	6	7
Arriving late for an appointment	1	2	3	4	5	6	7
Anticipating work deadlines	1	2	3	4	5	6	7

How easy is it for you to relax when you . . .

	Easy		Medium		Difficult		
Watch a television show or movie	1	2	3	4	5	6	7
Read a book or magazine	1	2	3	4	5	6	7
Take a walk, jog, or do other physical exercise	1	2	3	4	5	6	7

How often do you experience each of the following?

	Never		Sometimes			Always	
Insomnia	1	2	3	4	5	6	7
Shortness of breath	1	2	3	4	5	6	7
Rapid heart rate	1	2	3	4	5	6	7
Cold hands or feet	1	2	3	4	5	6	7
Impatience or irritability	1	2	3	4	5	6	7
Headaches	1	2	3	4	5	6	7
Apologizing for snapping at people	1	2	3	4	5	6	7
Tension or worry	1	2	3	4	5	6	7

Add up your total score, which can range from 16 to 112, and record it below:

Stress Level Total Score: _____

If your score is less than 40, then your stress levels are manageable, but you will still benefit from doing some stress-relief exercises. If you scored between 41 and 80, then you are experiencing mid-range stress levels. Learning and practicing stress-relieving techniques will be an essential strategy for improving your quality longevity. If you scored between 81 and 112, then you are in the high-stress group and will definitely benefit from the stress-reduction strategies outlined in this section.

Because people respond differently to the same environmental stimuli, some individuals seem to cope with stress better than others. However, anyone willing to challenge the control stress has on his or her life can lessen its harmful effects. Try the following strategies to lower your stress levels and increase your quality longevity.

Mindful Awareness

Mindful awareness, or mindfulness — the subtle process of moment-to-moment awareness of one's thoughts, feelings, and physical states — is a tool we use to achieve many of the *Longevity Bible* Essentials. By practicing mindful awareness, we are more likely to notice when we have had enough to eat, which helps control body weight. We are able to listen and communicate better, which often improves our relationships. And mindfulness leads to a more positive outlook, which increases our enjoyment of life.

Meditation as a means to achieving mindfulness gained popularity with Westerners when the Beatles and other celebrities began following Maharishi Mahesh Yogi, who founded the Transcendental Meditation movement in the late 1960s. With its roots in ancient Buddhist traditions, mindful awareness is not only the basis of meditation but of many other stress-management techniques as well, including self-hypnosis, biofeedback, and yoga. It also has been used to treat a variety of conditions, including hypertension, chronic pain, and anxiety.

Scientific evidence shows that the act of practiced mindfulness promotes health and mental calm. Systematic EEG brainwave studies of meditation techniques have found significant effects during and after meditation, as well as improved immune system response to vaccines. And the greater the brain wave changes from meditation, the more effective the immune response. A recent study found that regular meditation increases the size of a brain region that regulates memory and attention. Calming the mind through meditation also appears to improve physical healing. One study found that patients with psoriasis who listened to a meditation tape during ultraviolet light treatments healed four times faster than patients who did not meditate during their treatment.

Meditating on a regular basis may also extend life expectancy. Scientists spent approximately eight years following over two hundred middle-aged and older volunteers with mild forms of high blood pressure — a common illness often worsened by everyday stress. They found that those who meditated regularly had a 23 percent lower mortality rate. Deaths from cardiovascular disease were 30 percent lower and mortality rates from cancer were 49 percent lower in those who meditated, as compared with nonmeditators

Meditation and other forms of mindfulness bring about what Dr. Herbert Benson of Harvard University has termed the relaxation response — a state of deep mental and physical relaxation. Not only does it create a feeling of calm, it alters our physiology: Heart and breathing rates decrease, blood pressure lowers, and muscles relax. Many of these techniques focus on a mantra or a repeated sound that works like a hypnotic rhythm. People are also taught to observe and let go of their habitual mental chatter, and not to focus on distracting body sensations.

The goal is to keep the mind focused on one peaceful thought from moment to moment (see box). It can be frustrating at first, since our minds naturally swing from past ruminations to future worries. Initially, many people get impatient, feeling that they can't stay focused — their minds drift off to mundane thoughts, such as cleaning the garage or what they need from the market. But you needn't reach nirvana each time to benefit from simple mindful awareness exercises. The objective is simply to train yourself to take a rest from your usual ruminations so you can break some of your old, possibly negative or nonproductive thought patterns. When practiced on a daily basis, it will likely improve your state of mind, general health, and life expectancy.

Meditation Break

To jump-start your path into this ancient practice, pick a mantra — a sound, word, or phrase that is comforting to you, whether it is "world

---

peace," "love," "hmm," "om," or what-ever soothes you. Sit in a chair or cross-legged on the floor and rest your hands on your upper thighs, palms up. Close your eyes, relax your muscles, and breathe slowly and naturally. With each exhale, repeat your mantra si-lently to yourself. Try to keep focused on your mantra and your breathing, and ignore the impulse to let your mind wander. If outside thoughts do drift into your mind — "Did I mail that letter?" "Did I return that phone call?" — don't fret over it; allow those thoughts to drift through and away as you return to your mantra. The more you practice, the easier it will become to allow outside thoughts to pass through quickly. After about five min-utes, open your eyes and sit quietly for another minute or so, as you ease yourself back into your day. Do this ex-ercise daily and build up to ten-minute sessions.

Multitasking — Minds Under Stress

The term "multitasking" originally referred to a computer's ability to carry out several tasks simultaneously. For many people, multitasking has become a way of life and even a key to success. In fact, some excellent mental aerobic exercises involve engaging the brain in two or more challenging activities at a time. Although checking one's portable e-mail device while talking on a cell phone and reading the newspaper may be second nature for some people (not advisable while driving), many times multitasking can make us less productive, rather than more. And studies show that too much multitasking can lead to increased stress, anxiety, attention deficits, and memory loss.

In order to multitask, the brain uses an area known as the prefrontal cortex. This "executive" brain center controls our ability to assess and prioritize various tasks. Ironically, chronic stress causes its greatest damage to this prefrontal cortex. Brain scans of volunteers performing multiple tasks together show that as they shift from task to task, this front part of the brain actually takes a moment of rest between tasks. You may have experienced a prefrontal cortex "moment of rest" yourself if you've ever dialed a phone number and suddenly forgotten who you called when the line is answered. What probably occurred is that between the dialing and the answering, your mind shifted to another thought or task, and then took that "moment" to come back. Research has also shown that for many volunteers, job efficiency declines while multitasking, as compared to when they perform only one task at a time.

Multitasking is easiest when at least one of the tasks is routine, habitual, or requires little thought. Most people don't find it difficult to eat and read the newspaper at the same time. However, when two or more attention-requiring tasks are attempted simultaneously, people sometimes get sloppy or make mistakes.

We often don't remember things as well when we're trying to manage several details simultaneously. Without mental focus, we may not pay enough attention to new information coming in, so it never makes it into our memory stores (see Essential 1). That is one of the main reasons we forget people's names — even sometimes right after they have introduced themselves. Multitasking can also affect our relationships. If someone checks their e-mail while on the phone with a friend, they may come off as distracted or disinterested. It can also cause that person to miss or overlook key information being relayed to them.

For chronic multitaskers, I suggest that you schedule a regular time or times each day when you shut out phone calls and other distractions and complete a few priority chores, be it organizing your office or closet, sifting through your in-box, catching up on correspondence, or other tasks. The sense of having made some headway on finishing one or more tasks can make a person feel less pressured to catch up later by multitasking.

Multitasking often sneaks up on us, and even though we think we are getting a lot done, we may be operating less efficiently and can become disorganized. To combat this problem, try to put aside all but the most important task and complete it before moving on. You can also try making a list of your tasks and either complete them one-by-one in order of importance, or simply assign yourself particular tasks at certain times throughout the day. With practice, most people can become more aware of when they begin and finish a task, making them less likely to take on multiple duties simultaneously.

The Power of "No"

"No" — it's often a child's favorite word, yet many adults have a hard time saying it. When we use the word effectively, it can go a long way toward lowering stress levels.

When people don't say "no" enough, they can find themselves taking on too many responsibilities. They may then feel anxious, resentful, and perhaps a little bit "trapped" by all the tasks they have committed to but cannot possibly complete. Even requests that seem minor at first, or are set way in the future, eventually roll around and have to be piled on to one's list of responsibilities and tasks. Because time is a limited commodity for many of us, agreeing to do too many favors, chair another luncheon, be on another committee, volunteer for yet another cause, or even give someone a ride to an appointment can sometimes become overwhelming and a major source of stress.

At seventy-three, Anna, Shirley's mother, was the adored matriarch of the family. Throughout her life, she had always taken care of everyone, and hadn't stopped yet. Although she had been a straight-A student in high school and could have gone on to any college she chose, Anna instead took a job as a secretary to support her new husband through business school. She single-handedly reared their four children without the nannies and the maids that her own kids seemed to require for *their* children. If one of her grandkids ever wanted a special something, whether it was a snack, a CD, or the hottest new toy, she raced to at least three stores until she found the right item or at least brought back an assortment for them to choose from.

Anna cultivated an image of herself as the ultimate earth mother — she prided herself on helping others and had a terrible time turning down any request from her family and friends. But lately, Anna seemed irritable, and it seemed to her family that she resented doing some of the things she did. Perhaps driving her husband, Frank, everywhere since he had developed phlebitis and caring for her sister who had Alzheimer's was becoming too much for her, with all her other self-imposed duties.

Anna wasn't big on asking for help, either, much to the exasperation of her daughters. When her youngest, Shirley, asked what she could bring to Thanksgiving dinner, Anna responded, "Oh, you don't need to do that, dear."

"But, Mom, I really want to bring something to help out," Shirley insisted. "How about some dessert? I'll stop by the bakery on my way up, okay?"

"Oh, honey, I don't want you to spend any money, but if you insist, just bring anything you want . . . Maybe your chopped cucumber salad . . . or your homemade bread, but please no raisins or nuts in it. You know how Daddy is."

The family knew that something was seriously wrong when Shirley got to her mother's home on Thanksgiving.

She walked into the kitchen with the cucumber salad and a store-bought loaf of crusty French bread, and said hello to her mom, sister, and her two sisters-in-law. Suddenly, in front of them all, Anna grabbed the salad plate from Shirley and threw it on the floor, yelling, "You couldn't even *make* the bread?! I've been slaving all week, *and* taking care of your aunt and your father, and not one of you girls even *offered* to have Thanksgiving at your house!" Anna stormed out of the room sobbing, leaving the others stunned.

For people like Anna, saying "no" contradicts their perception of who they are, just as asking for help might never enter their minds. Anna was unable to gauge when the expectations she had put on herself had become unrealistic. This led her to feel a sense of desperation, and her difficulty in asking for help only made it worse. After her family convinced her to see a psychotherapist, Anna became more aware of her own needs, which helped her to say no when the requests of others were just not reasonable for her to fulfill. She also got into a support group for caregivers of Alzheimer's patients and enlisted her children's help with driving her husband around.

Often, learning to take better care of ourselves increases our enjoyment in assisting others. To help you feel more comfortable saying "no" when it makes sense, try some of the following strategies.

The upside of "no." Keep in mind that when you say no to a request, you are saying yes to something else. Not taking on the extra assignment at work will give you more time to enjoy the weekend with your family.

Make the rules and keep them. If a friend or colleague asks for a loan or favor that makes you uncomfortable, you might try telling them that "as a rule" you don't loan money to friends, help people move, and so on. This minimizes potentially hurtful feelings and may save your friendship or work relationship. This "as a rule" technique also works well with teenagers who tend to repeat the same requests often. You can eventually resort to merely saying, "You know the rule . . ."

Ignore pressure. If you're not sure about how to respond to a request, stall. Politely tell the requester that you'll get back to them after checking your schedule. That way, you can take more time to weigh the pros and cons of the request. If you are being pressured for a decision at that very moment, then you could simply deny the request due to the decision-making time constraint.

Be straightforward. Everyone gets busy from time to time, be it scrambling to meet a work deadline, planning an event, or caring for a sick friend or family member. Sometimes it can become stressful to keep commitments we've already made, and being straightforward about the situation is often the best approach. Most people can empathize with being overcommitted and can usually find an alternate solution.

A Mad, Mad World

Anger is a common and sometimes healthy response to stressful situations. People frequently report experiencing a sense of relief after getting their angry feelings "off their chest," and sometimes a reasonable expression of anger can lead to the resolution of a stressful situation. Neuroscientists recently pinpointed a specific brain region that is stimulated when people get insulted and prepare to exact revenge. This is the same area of the brain that gets stimulated when people prepare to satisfy hunger and other cravings — mostly pleasurable. This research backs up the idea that "revenge is sweet." However, just as a very hungry person may overeat at a buffet, a person who feels wronged may occasionally overindulge in their payback. Sometimes forgiveness and empathy can help an angry person rise above his or her desire for revenge, and this is almost always the best path to a peaceful resolution (also see Essential 3).

When we get angry, we can also get upset, and uncontrolled anger can lead to rage, hostility, and unhappiness. People who get angry quickly with little or no provocation may actually have a shorter life expectancy. Expressing anger arouses the nervous system and can increase heart rate, blood pressure, and risk for strokes. There is also evidence that people with an angry temperament have a greater risk for heart disease.

Holding our anger inside is not the answer, either. People who hold in their emotions and suffer silently tend to have higher stress hormone levels than those with healthy anger outlets. Systematic studies point to an optimal, intermediate level of anger expression, somewhere between unbridled outbursts and complete containment. In that way, we are able to modulate the stress hormone release that accompanies controlled anger expressions without blowing our tops, and perhaps saying things we can't take back.

There are various approaches to managing anger. Most techniques are aimed at helping people become aware of their underlying triggers, learn to control their angry feelings, and use relaxation techniques to minimize their physical responses to those feelings. Uncontrollable anger can sometimes be a symptom of another problem, such as depression, excessive drinking, or drug abuse. Regardless of the cause of chronic temper tantrums, a person must first admit to having a problem before any approach can succeed. Almost everyone can learn how to be assertive and appropriately express anger without becoming aggressive or destructive.

Laugh in the Face of Stress

Everyone likes a good laugh. Humor allows us to release tension and let go of fearful or angry feelings, even if just for a little while. Norman Cousins was a champion of using humor to battle his painful and crippling arthritic disease, and systematic research has supported such health-promoting effects of humor.

Japanese scientists recently studied a group of volunteers who watched a popular comedy show while dining, and compared them to another group eating the same meal but watching a boring lecture (not mine, I swear). After dinner, the group that laughed more had more stable blood sugar levels, and stability of blood sugar is known to lower the risk for diabetes.

Laughter may protect us against heart disease, as well. In a recent study of three hundred volunteers, scientists found that the people *without* heart disease were 60 percent more likely to see humor in everyday life. Other studies have linked watching a daily half-hour sitcom with lower blood pressure and improved heartbeat regularity, both of which lower risk for heart attacks.

Apparently, just anticipating a humorous situation has health benefits. Volunteers who were told that they would see a favorite comic in three days had a drop in their stress hormone levels and a boost in levels of chemicals that strengthen the immune system. Other research has found that laughter improves our ability to tolerate pain. Whether you prefer old W. C. Fields movies, hanging out at comedy clubs, or simply reading the Sunday funnies, a regular dose of laughter may not only lift your spirits but bolster your longevity.

Muscle Relaxation Exercise: Wind Up and Unwind

Do this lying down or in a comfortable chair. While the rest of your body remains comfortable and relaxed, slowly clench your right fist as tightly as you can. Focus on the tension in your right fist, hand, and forearm. After five seconds, relax your hand, let your fingers and wrist go limp, and relax for fifteen to thirty seconds. Notice the sensations of tension and relaxation in those muscles. Now repeat with your left fist, then relax. Next, bend your right elbow, tense your biceps muscle, and hold that tension for five seconds. Then let your arm straighten and drop gently to your side and relax for fifteen to thirty seconds. Repeat the exercise for your left side. Continue this sequence of tensing and releasing different muscle groups sequentially up your arms, through your shoulders, chest, face, back, abdomen, buttocks, legs, and feet. After you have completed moving through to your toes, tense your entire body for five seconds and then fully relax. Take several deep breaths and savor the feeling of muscle relaxation.

Sleep On It

An estimated 100 million Americans suffer from the stress of insomnia, which can cause memory impairment, fatigue, irritability, and a variety of other problems. The National Highway Traffic Safety Administration estimates that drivers falling asleep at the wheel cause more than

100,000 auto accidents each year. Cheating on your sleep may also grow your waistline. Researchers recently found that not getting enough sleep elevates blood levels of appetite-stimulating hormones and is associated with a greater risk for being overweight.

The average person needs about seven to eight hours of sleep each night, but our sleep needs decline as we age. People who are sleep deprived tend to lack energy and motivation; they often feel "fuzzy headed" or confused the next day. Although getting enough hours of sleep is a stress-reduction goal, not all sleep is equal. For sleep to be restorative, we need to *remain* asleep throughout the night. Even subtle noises that don't actually awaken us can be disruptive enough to affect the quality of our sleep. That is why falling asleep with the TV on may leave us feeling tired the next day.

The following are a few tips that can help people get the sleep they need:

- *Stay on schedule.* Our bodies naturally adjust to regular daily cycles. Sometimes sleep problems result from our schedule being temporarily out of sync with our normal lifestyle require-

178

ments. Try to get into bed the same time each evening, and set your alarm for the same time each morning. To keep your body on its routine, don't sleep too late on the weekends and avoid napping during the day.

- *Quiet down before bedtime.* Once in bed, try avoiding TV or eating. If you read, try to skip overly exciting stories that might hype you up. Those who listen to music before bed should stick with the more serene sounds and save the heavy metal for the daytime activities. Caffeine, and liquids in general, should be avoided. Also, remain mindful of when you first notice fatigue — that's the moment you want to turn out the light, get yourself in a comfortable position, and let yourself relax.
- *Take to the tub.* Many people find that a warm shower or bath before bedtime relaxes their muscles and helps them get to sleep.
- *Create a comfort zone.* Arrange the bedroom furniture, light, and sound level so they maximize calm and comfort (see Essential 5).
- *Get active during the day.* One of the best ways to sleep through the night is

to make sure you get plenty of physical activity during the day. Plan your workout sessions well before bedtime so they don't leave you overenergized, which can make it difficult to relax.

- *Talk with your doctor.* Chronic insomnia may be a symptom of depression or other medical conditions, so consult your physician if your efforts at promoting sleep are ineffective.

Acupuncture: Meet the Needles

This ancient Chinese therapy has been used as a treatment for several forms of pain and a variety of stress-related conditions. During acupuncture, thin needles are inserted into the skin at specific points on the body. Some forms of acupuncture use heat, pressure, or mild electrical current to stimulate the energy at these points, instead of needles.

The Chinese theorize that *chi* energy flows through the body along pathways, or *meridians,* and blockage of this energy causes illness. Traditional practitioners believe acupuncture unblocks these pathways and balances the flow of chi, restoring health. Some Western medical practitioners suggest other explanations for how acupuncture might work. Dr. Hélène Langevin of the University of Vermont reported that acupuncture points correlate with areas of thick connective tissue, which also contain high concentrations of nerve endings. Stimulating these regions might affect nerve areas that transmit pain signals. The treatment boosts levels of endorphins, which can have analgesic effects. Acupuncture also elevates levels of the brain chemical serotonin, the body's natural antidepressant.

In a recent study of over fifteen thousand headache sufferers, those receiving a three-month course of weekly acupuncture treatments experienced significantly less pain than headache sufferers who received only conventional treatments. Other studies have found that acupuncture relieves pain and improves function in patients with arthritis, as compared with the control, nonpiercing treatments. Although not all studies have been positive, there is enough evidence to suggest that this age-old intervention has the potential to help many people suffering from various types of pain.

Growing Your Nest Egg

Since we are living longer, it's important to plan for it financially. By preparing ahead and getting the most value from our money, we may be able to alleviate much of our stress over financial concerns for the future. Research indicates that most people are not saving enough money to comfortably enjoy their retirement years. In fact, according to a recent survey done by the AARP, one in three retirees are forced back to work after they retire either because they failed to save enough to fully retire or because they suffered catastrophic losses with their investments. Only one out of every three Americans contributes to a tax-deferred savings account such as an IRA or one based at their job, like a 401(k) plan, to help with their retirement, and those who have a plan usually contribute less money than they could or should.

Neuroscientists may have a biological explanation for this phenomenon. Neuro-imaging studies suggest that our brains are hardwired to prefer immediate gratification — enjoying the present versus saving for the future. Using functional MRI scanning, researchers at Princeton University studied the brain activity of volunteers making choices about different monetary reward options. They found that financial decisions involved two areas of the brain: the prefrontal cortex, a highly evolved decision-making brain region, and a primitive brain region known as the limbic system, which responds to decisions involving instant rewards. Study subjects who tended to be immediate gratifiers showed greater activity in this limbic region; therefore, their brain's predisposition for immediate gratification may cloud their long-term decision-making. Other studies have found that when given a choice, most people will put off what is difficult or painful, even if logically they know it is good for them in the long run.

Investment companies have been working to create new approaches to saving for the future to help people overcome the tendency to play now and save later. The sooner we get our financial planning in order, the less stress we will feel about the future. Here are a few strategies that may work for you.

- *Calculate your actual needs.* Getting a realistic idea of how much money you will have for retirement, based on your current saving habits, can either be a comforting stress-reliever or a wake-up call to make changes. An accountant, financial planner, or investment consultant can help you accurately calculate these figures.

- *Get tough about current spending.* Take a serious look at how you are spending your money today. While reviewing your patterns, look for an item that you pay for on a regular basis that you could possibly cut back on. It can actually be a fun challenge to try to save money by skipping an unnecessary foray to the shoe department or the makeup counter and instead, taking a nice, *free* walk in the fresh air.

- *Opt for the plan.* Employees are often presented with company savings-plan options in a way that lets inertia get the better of them — the default position is *no* plan, and people need to make an extra effort to opt *for* a plan. When companies switch from optional to automatic enrollment and people must opt *out* instead of opt *in* to a plan, there are dramatic increases in the proportion of people who put some of their money away for retirement.

- *Push yourself.* If you are currently contributing one percent of your earnings to a 401(k), try to notch it up to two or three percent — you may not even feel the pinch too badly. The next time you get a raise or your expenses go down, seize the opportunity to sock away more for retirement.

- *Make your contributions automatic.* That way you don't have to think about contributing at regular intervals. With future savings, out of sight means out of your hands to spend now. Whether or not your work has a retirement plan available, there are several other mechanisms you can use, such as IRAs or savings bonds purchase plans. A professional financial planner can help you choose one that meets your needs.

- *Keep an eye on your investments.* Saving and investing is an excellent start, but you also have to avoid taking undue risk with your investments. Suffering capital losses can create financial and emotional stress. Most financial advisors recommend avoiding risky investments as people approach retirement age.

Workplace Stress

People rarely do their best work under pressure, yet almost everyone has experienced stress at work at some point. Stress on the job can have a major impact on our health and well-being. Workplace stress can come from a variety of sources, including relationships, unrealistic job expectations, and even the actual physical workplace environment (see Essential 5).

Stress arising directly from an issue with the boss has been found to negatively affect the employee's health. Scientists recently found that when health care personnel worked for a boss they thought was unfair, their systolic blood pressure (when the heart contracts) increased by thirteen points and diastolic (between contractions) increased by six points on average. That's enough to increase risk for a stroke by nearly 40 percent. When the employees worked for a boss whom they respected and trusted, one who supported them with praise and feedback, the workers' blood pressure actually decreased slightly.

Other studies have found that the risk of dying from a heart attack doubles among employees during times of major company downsizing. One analysis of more than twenty-four thousand Swedish workers found that during periods of large-scale mergers, workers were more likely to take sick leave or to go to the hospital because of illness.

Much of an employee's stress on the job appears to arise from the combination of high job demands and a limited sense of control. When people feel they do have some control in their workplace — a sense of power to direct their own actions — they feel more satisfied, experience less stress, and have better health outcomes. Because we are often unable to eliminate the source of our workplace stress, finding other ways to relax can help us avoid some of the negative physical and emotional consequences.

- *Organize and avoid procrastination.* At the start of each day, spend a few minutes setting priorities and organizing the day ahead. Be realistic about what you can accomplish and avoid putting off difficult tasks. Making this a regular morning habit can help anchor you and keep you focused. It also helps minimize multitasking.
- *Fine-tune your communication skills.*

One of the greatest sources of workplace stress can be communication problems and misunderstandings. Try to be specific in formulating questions or complaints and avoid getting into conflicts that do not directly involve you. When conflicts do arise, listen carefully before explaining your own position. If possible, don't involve your superiors in a conflict with a colleague unless your own attempts to work it out have failed. Keep in mind that everything you put in writing — particularly e-mail — can become a permanent, public record, so choose your written words wisely.

- *Cool it on the caffeine.* Though modest amounts of caffeine can increase alertness, too much leads to irritability and anxiety, which only adds to stress. Avoid running to the coffeepot when the pressure is on.

- *Take regular stretching and relaxation breaks.* Get up and stretch or do a breathing exercise at regular intervals. If possible, try going outdoors or opening a window to get some fresh air during work breaks. Set your watch alarm to remind you to stretch and move around. Relaxing your muscles

188

throughout the day is a preemptive strike against stress.

- *Delegate*. People who have a hard time delegating often feel unnecessarily stressed-out. Asking people to help you by doing tasks that they can handle allows you more time to complete the work that perhaps only you can do.
- *Adapt your personal environment*. Photos and other personal items add character and a homey feeling to your workspace, which can contribute to a sense of calm. To increase comfort and avoid injury, read up on workplace ergonomic principles (see Essential 5). Sometimes simply adjusting the angle of your chair and the position of your keyboard, or perhaps propping your feet up on a box, can ease muscle tension and reduce stress.
- *Power nap*. For people who are behind on their sleep, a few winks in the afternoon can often make them more alert and energetic throughout the rest of the day. A recent study of volunteers who were allowed to nap for thirty minutes demonstrated that they had greater job productivity afterward, as compared with those who did not nap (see box).

189

Tips for Effective Power Napping

1. Limit your nap to no more than thirty minutes. Longer naps generally leave us feeling tired and groggy. Aim for the twenty-minute power nap.

2. Many people avoid daytime napping because they fear they will oversleep. Use a timer or alarm so that won't happen.

3. People with private offices only need to close the door and turn off the phone to get some quiet time. Those with more public workspaces may need to be creative in finding a quiet, private spot. Some people like to nap in their car or a shady spot in a park during their lunch break.

4. Don't worry if you cannot fall asleep. Just relaxing with your eyes closed can help you to feel more rested after nap time.

More Proven Stress Busters

There are a variety of other approaches that not only reduce stress, but also improve fitness, balance, and mental clarity. The following list includes a few examples.

- *Yoga.* This ancient Indian practice promotes health and relaxation through a sequence of physical poses and breathing exercises that build strength, balance, and flexibility. It is effective in reducing stress and increasing mental clarity. Yoga has also been found to lower cholesterol levels and blood pressure, and a recent scientific study found that yoga combined with meditation in a six-week stress-reduction program led to significant improvements in cardiac health.
- *Tai chi.* Pronounced *"tie-chee,"* this Chinese form of exercise can reduce stress, increase strength, improve balance, and help prevent falls in seniors. Many of the movements, originally derived from martial arts, are performed slowly and gracefully, and emphasize deep breathing and relaxation. Scientists recently found that tai chi can improve heart and lung function.

Researchers at the Semel Institute for Neuroscience and Human Behavior at UCLA reported that fifteen weeks of tai chi helped protect older adults against the shingles virus (the same virus that causes chickenpox), suggesting that the practice may boost immune function. Chi gong (pronounced *"chee-gong"*) is a related ancient Chinese practice that shares many similar exercises that improve mental focus, movement, and breathing.

- *Self-hypnosis.* This method generally combines relaxation techniques with visualization and imagery to induce a hypnotic state, which is essentially a very deep form of relaxation. Self-hypnosis has been found to lower stress levels, reduce pain, and alleviate some allergy symptoms. It can also improve concentration and memory ability.
- *Massage.* Besides reducing stress, massage therapy has been used to relieve symptoms of various conditions, including migraine headache, back and neck pain, and fibromyalgia. Some experts speculate that massage may do more than just provide temporary pain relief and may actually activate the body's immune system. The National

Institutes of Health has a Center for Complementary and Alternative Medicine that is pursuing systematic studies on the health benefits of massage, and initial results are encouraging.

- *Get active and social.* Physical activity not only improves health and strength, but helps us relax — partly due to the hormone endorphin — the natural antidepressant our bodies secrete during aerobic exercise. Enjoying a game of tennis or a brisk walk with a friend may reduce stress through the emotional benefits of social interaction.

- *Control clutter.* Many people are unaware that a disorganized, overly cluttered home, work space, kitchen, closet, or any other place in which we spend time can lead to stress and heightened levels of the stress hormone cortisol. Reducing the clutter around us is a lifelong challenge that is best handled on a daily basis — by putting things where they belong and tossing anything we don't need — before clutter gets out of hand (see Essential 5).

- *Open up.* One of the most effective ways to reduce stress is to talk about feelings with someone you trust. Whether it's your spouse, a best friend, or a professional, getting things off your chest can often help put problems into perspective and detoxify a stressful situation.

- *Plan ahead.* Sometimes we know about or can anticipate a stressful situation before it occurs. It may be an upcoming holiday dinner at the home of a relative who always insults you, or having to show up at work Monday morning and report to an underling who got *your* promotion. Try looking at these situations as *advance notices* — opportunities to arm ourselves emotionally to cope with the stress, and possibly avoid repeating mistakes we've made in similar situations when we didn't have time to prepare. Of course, whenever feasible, simply steering clear of a stressful situation altogether is a good longevity choice, but in many cases it just isn't possible.

Because everyone will respond differently to the various stress-reduction techniques available, it's a good idea to try several approaches until you find one or more that works best. Documented evidence shows that many of these techniques not only help you relax, but will benefit your health and longevity as well.

Living Stress Free

- Practice mindful awareness — staying in the moment and being aware of what is going on inside your body — through meditation, relaxation techniques, yoga, or other exercises you enjoy. Take stress release breaks throughout the day.
- Avoid multitasking by scheduling a regular time each day for completing priority chores; try finishing one task before beginning another.
- Learn to say "no" when you need to.
- Modulate stress with healthy expressions of anger.
- Use humor to gain perspective on stressful situations.
- Get a good night's sleep every night. Take simple steps to beat insomnia without medication.
- Discover ways to limit stress on the job.
- Place emphasis on saving for the future.
- Reduce stress by decluttering your personal environment.
- Plan your strategy for dealing with stressful events you know about in advance.

Essential 5

Master Your Environment

It isn't pollution that's harming the environment. It's the impurities in our air and water that are doing it.

— DAN QUAYLE

Barbara W. brought cookies and tea up to her husband Greg's study as he worked late on a case he was trying in the morning. He had to shift two large piles of papers and a stack of legal files, but still knocked the phone and a tray of correspondence off his massive desk just to make room for the teacup. Barbara anxiously helped him pick up the papers. She always hated coming into this room — the crazy, cluttered disarray of binders, folders, documents, and scribbled notes made her skin crawl. "How can you work in this mess?" she asked him

---

for the millionth time. He shrugged. "I know, I know, as soon as I close these two cases, I'm going to clean up in here and organize things." He relaxed back in his chair, propped his feet on another pile of files, and returned to work.

The next night, Barbara cleared the dinner dishes as Greg excused himself to his study. Twenty seconds later he shrieked, "Barbara!" She came running in to find him standing in the center of his now clean, organized, glistening study — files all tucked in the drawers and the desk polished and clear — with phone, computer, and fax machine neatly arranged on its surface. "What the hell happened?!" he demanded. "You like it?" she asked excitedly. "Maria and I cleaned up in here today." Panicked, he rifled through the desk. "Where's the Mitchelson file?! I can't find the Mitchelson file!" Barbara went to the file cabinets. "I'll help you find it." "No!" he yelled. "You've already wrecked my entire organizational system! The Mitchelson file was on

top of the third pile from the left, behind the phone, next to the fax machine! It had two yellow paper clips!"

Our environment, everything around us,
directly influences not just how we feel,
but also how well we function and how
long we live. The places where we reside,
work, and play affect us both physically
and emotionally — and each of us responds differently to various environmental factors. Whether it's features of the
environment at large, such as traffic, noise,
and smog, or more personal environmental
issues, such as clutter, smoke, or aesthetics, our quality longevity requires that
we adapt to these influences, or *adapt
them,* to meet our individual needs.

Aesthetic Living

When creating a comfortable home or
work environment, we need to focus on
function *and* the emotional impact of the
space. Everyone has his or her own tastes
in style and aesthetics; successful interior
designers often get to know their clients

personally in order to be able to evoke certain feelings in the rooms they design for them.

A sparsely decorated, modern living room may instantly relax one person, whereas a shabby chic/country decor may be just the ticket to make another person feel cozy and at home. Choices of art and color can generate an atmosphere that enhances or detracts from our emotional state. A warm color like red might alert one person to danger, while for another it evokes passion. Blues, greens, and neutral browns often produce a calming ambience.

A popular approach to home decorating, feng shui (pronounced *"fung schway"*), is the ancient Chinese art of arranging home or work environments to promote health, happiness, and prosperity. Feng shui consultants advise their clients on many details of their surroundings — from color choices to furniture placement.

Although feng shui is unfamiliar to some Westerners, many of its recommendations utilize common sense to enhance environments. One principle takes note of the importance of one's first impression upon entering a home. Creating a warm and welcoming feeling may be as simple as placing a large vase of flowers in the corner of the entry room. Also, moving beds, desks, and couches from under any overhead beams can help to avoid the feeling that something is "hanging over you." For cramped spaces, a feng shui expert may recommend hanging mirrors and eliminating any unnecessary furniture to create the impression of roominess.

The sounds and noises around us, as well as the music we listen to, have an important impact on our mood and quality of life. Listening to music has been found to increase surgeons' speed and accuracy during their procedures. A specific type of sound, in a process known as vibroacoustic therapy, has been used to reduce stress and pain symptoms. Listening to classical music has been found to lower stress-related elevations in blood pressure, and individual music choices, whether it's country music, rock, or rap, may improve mood and quality of life. Fountains or other water treatments are soothing to the ear, visually calming, and effective at masking annoying traffic sounds.

Surrounding ourselves with artwork, appealing textures, and comfortable furniture not only adds to the warmth of our environment, it also helps to lower stress and give us a sense of sanctuary. Displaying photos and gifts from people we love will help to remind us of their presence. Natural light and plants, as well as areas for quiet time and reflection, indoors and outdoors, all contribute to the aesthetics and function of our surroundings.

The Bedroom: The Final Frontier

We spend nearly one third of our lives sleeping. The way in which we arrange our bedroom environment can foster or hinder the sense of security and comfort that helps us get to sleep. The amount of sleep we get each night has a much greater impact on our health and quality longevity than many of us realize.

Although not getting enough sleep has health risks, getting too much sleep may be harmful as well. In a survey of more than 100,000 people, Japanese scientists recently found that people who slept eight or more hours each night had higher mortality rates compared with those sleeping only seven hours. However, sleeping less than four and a half hours was found to increase mortality risks as well.

Sleep also affects appetite. When we don't get enough sleep, our bodies produce inadequate amounts of a hormone that helps us to feel sated after we eat, so lack of sleep can actually lead to increased appetite and weight gain. For most people, somewhere between six and seven hours of sleep each night is associated with good health and quality longevity.

To help ensure a restful and peaceful sleep setting, pay attention to some of the following details:

Mattresses. You may swear by a certain mattress, while your partner swears *at* it. Perhaps the most important consideration in choosing a mattress is to test several different ones and determine what feels right, keeping in mind both comfort and firmness. Encasing the mattress with an allergen-blocking cover will protect you against small particles and dust mites.

Bedding. High-count cotton linens tend to be softer, making it easier for many people to fall and stay asleep. Thread-counts can range anywhere from two hundred to eight hundred, but the extremely fine sheets (those with higher thread-counts) are more expensive and tend to fall apart or need replacement after repeated washings. Your pillow choice is important, as well. Wool or goose down pillows may provide more contoured neck and shoulder support, but people with allergies might do better with a molded foam pillow. Keep in mind that even synthetic pillows can harbor dust mites. The best protection is an allergen-blocking cover. Also, for people with low-back pain, an additional pillow under the knees (for people who sleep face up) or between the knees (for side sleepers) helps to reduce muscle strain and improve comfort levels.

Lighting. If you enjoy reading in bed, be sure you have enough illumination to avoid eyestrain or headache, although not *too* much lighting, because glaring high-wattage may not be conducive to helping you drift off to a restful night's sleep. If your bedroom gets direct sun exposure in the mornings, consider window treatments that block the light if you don't want to awaken too early. When you do get up, be sure to let sunlight into the room. This is a great way to start the day and can protect against seasonal mood swings or winter depression.

Noise and temperature. Take into account noise that might awaken you, whether it's the roadside traffic, a barking dog, or a snoring spouse. Excessive snoring might be a symptom of sleep apnea, an often treatable condition. For other unavoidable noises, try ear plugs or a "white noise" machine that plays waves or other calming sounds. Make sure that your wake-up alarm is gentle, rather than shrill or high-pitched. You might try soothing music to help start your day off right.

Most people prefer a comfortably cool room for sleeping, approximately sixty-five to sixty-seven degrees Fahrenheit, allowing one or more blankets to give warmth and coziness to the bed. Try opening a window, using a fan on a low setting, or, if the weather demands it, air-conditioning or heating.

Reading and TV. Experts suggest winding down with an enjoyable, relaxing activity during the hour before bedtime. It is best to avoid watching exciting television shows or reading thriller-type books during that period because they may stimulate you instead of the opposite. If TV helps you to nod off, attempt to use an automatic shut-off button so you won't be awakened in the middle of the night by a blaring infomercial. Insomniacs often do best by eliminating TV from the bedroom altogether.

Clutter Control

Often it's subtle: You walk into a room and begin to feel uneasy, confused, or edgy — yet you haven't a clue why. The next time this happens, scan your surroundings. You may be suffering from clutter overload — the psychological effects of a disorganized, overly packed room, home, closet, or work space.

Scientists have found that laboratory animals in crowded, cluttered cages become ornery, agitated, and antisocial. Chronic crowding, clutter, and disorganization can lead to high levels of the stress hormone cortisol, which can impair memory and concentration and aggravate a wide range of age-related diseases.

Reducing clutter and maintaining an organized home and work space is a lifelong daily challenge. Typically we come home after a busy day, grab the mail, maybe drag in some packages, and never get around to putting everything away — a stack of magazines and junk mail stays on the counter, a jacket gets draped on a chair instead of hung in the closet, and so on. There's also a tendency to surround ourselves with papers, computer accessories, files, photographs, CDs, clothes, books, laundry, dishes, magazines, and more. Over time, clutter may build up until we can no longer find what we need. Some people would rather drive to the hardware store and buy a new screwdriver than dig through the garage to find the one they know they have buried somewhere.

In its extreme, clutter can escalate to pathological levels. We've all heard of those "pack rats" that cannot help but collect old newspapers, magazines, or clothes to the point that their personal clutter overtakes their surroundings. This form of obsessive-compulsive disorder can be treated professionally, but many clutter junkies adamantly resist letting go of their precious collections.

Most of us, thankfully, can easily manage our surroundings by using some of the following clutter-control tips.

- *Think small.* Reorganize and declutter one room or area of that room at a time. Trying to take on the entire house or office is overwhelming and reduces the likelihood that you'll stay with the task.
- *Box it.* Separate items and place them into one of three boxes: Designate one as a *donation* box, a second for *things*

to keep, and a third as the *uncertain* collection. Use these same boxes for each area of your home or office that you tackle.

- *Let things go.* Get your "donation" box items out of the house ASAP. Next, go through your "uncertain" box — if you haven't used something in the last twelve months, move the item to the donation box now — no whining.

- *Sort now.* When you receive mail or bring in groceries, sort them right away. For junk mail, try returning the postage-paid envelope with a note asking to be removed from the mailing list.

- *Arrange by similarities.* Take your "keep" piles and search for similarities among items, whether by function, color, or texture. Organize and put away these similar items together, so they will be easy to find later. It will be much easier to find the key to the gate padlock if it's in the designated key box, rather than "somewhere in one of the kitchen drawers." Labeling the key would be helpful, as well.

- *Put away rarely used items.* Your ski clothes don't need a prominent position in your closet during the summer months. Rarely used or seasonal items should be stored in less frequented places, such as a spare bedroom closet or attic.

- *Isolate necessary clutter.* None of us can entirely remove all the clutter from our lives, but we can reserve smaller spaces for clutter control. Whether it's a classic "junk drawer" in the kitchen, a closet in that extra bedroom, or a box in the attic, make sure it's an area that is out of sight. Also, sift through the isolated clutter at regular intervals and dispose of things, especially if the clutter is filling up that area or becoming unmanageable.

- *Schedule declutter time.* Train yourself to spend five to ten minutes each day to sort through any gathering clutter. Carry a paper bag around the house and scan your major living spaces. Are books, magazines, or mail beginning to pile up? Is your closet, desk, or pantry becoming disorganized? Sorting and tossing a bit each day helps you avoid the need for organization marathons.

Information Overload:
Managing Technology

Over the last few decades, technological developments in computers, telecommunications, and more have transformed our environments. Futurists predict that soon we will be able to exchange video calls as commonly as e-mail. Everything from tracking medical records to operating home appliances to making dinner reservations will be carried out by our rapidly emerging global networks.

What we're seeing is an explosion of information technology, and our computers are becoming not just more enjoyable but also more useful. Even psychotherapy is available online. At a recent conference sponsored by the U.S. Department of Health and Human Services, scientists reported that "talk therapy" delivered via the Internet on hand-held organizers was effective in treating patients with anxiety and social phobia. However, recent studies suggest that automation advances are often coupled with inefficiencies. With increasingly complex programs, we are seeing more software glitches and computer crashes that waste time and reduce productivity.

The resulting information overload is

creating a new form of clutter mania. Computer desktops and file systems collect clutter as much as our jam-packed closets and drawers. It's not just electronic data, but hard copies, as well. The average American consumes more than two tons of paper each year.

We're choking on information to the point of exhaustion, from electronic billboards, cell phones, radio, cable, satellite TV with ticker-tape headlines, and even plasma screens in elevators. A current *New York Times* Sunday edition probably contains more information than the average person was ever exposed to during their lifetime just one hundred years ago. Faced with too much information, we can become desensitized, indecisive, and frustrated.

Some concerns about this new technology, however, appear to be myths more than actual risks. For example, a popular urban legend has it that overuse of cell phones can cause brain tumors. A group of Danish epidemiologists systematically investigated this question and failed to confirm that cellular phone use had any effect on the incidence or size of brain tumors.

It is estimated that 75 percent of young adults and 20 percent of seniors use the Internet, with use among seniors jumping dramatically during the past decade. One of the greatest incentives for their Internet use is staying in touch with family members. Younger family members encourage their parents and grandparents to set up e-mail accounts, and the older folks love it. Several resources are available on the Internet to help seniors develop their Internet skills, including *www.generations online.com* and *www.seniornet.org.*

It is estimated that more than 60 percent of all e-mail users check their e-mail once a day and one third of users check it several times a day. The rise in popularity of instant messaging and hand-held Internet devices, such as the BlackBerry, have turned some people into virtual e-mail addicts — remaining immersed in online chatter for hours at a time. Though the quick and easy exchange of electronic information is efficient, too much technology use causes some people to disconnect from face-to-face human contact. E-mail tends to have an informal quality to it, which can lower our inhibitions when communicating. Without in-person visual cues, it is easier to misinterpret what gets said. Interoffice e-mails have become so problematic that many businesses are now legally obligated to monitor them.

Joyce and Brian carried the large, wrapped box into her parents' house, and the kids followed carrying a birthday cake and card. Joyce's mom, Ellen, was seventy today, and they all gathered around as she opened her present — a brand-new personal computer. Ellen smiled, a little disappointed. "You guys, really, you shouldn't have spent so much. I'll never learn to use this thing. And Daddy won't touch it — unless it's made of chocolate." Grandpa chuckled — she got that right. He was still figuring out how to use the remote control for the new TV they gave him last Christmas.

Ignoring her protests, Joyce told Brian to set the computer up in the den. "Don't worry, Mom, you're going to love it. You can e-mail the kids, see pictures of them, find new recipes, play bridge, all kinds of things. And we already signed you up for an online service."

With Joyce's help, Ellen learned how to use the computer, and started e-mailing with the kids one or twice a week. She shared photographs of her grandchildren with friends over the Web, and she liked trading cooking tips and recipes in a chat room that Joyce helped her find.

Two weeks later, Joyce slammed down the telephone receiver as Brian came home from work. "Whoa, what's going on?" Joyce went back to making dinner. "My folks' line has been busy for three hours!" Brian gave her a kiss. "It's probably just off the hook, honey. I'm sure everything's fine."

Another month went by and the kids hadn't seen their grandparents in weeks. Joyce called her mom about getting together. "But Sunday is Father's Day and we *always* come over." She listened. "Let me speak to Daddy." She paused. "Okay, fine. We'll be there Sunday at four. Bye."

When they arrived at the folks' place on Sunday, Grandpa was watching a ball game in the living room. The house was a mess — dishes, glasses, soda cans, and unfolded laundry were everywhere, and even Grandpa himself hadn't shaved.

Ellen was in the den, on the computer. Joyce approached her. "Mom?" "Not now!" Ellen hissed. "I'm up $500!" Joyce, horrified, saw that her mother was playing Internet poker.

Joyce and Brian sent the kids outside to play and had a serious talk with the folks. Apparently, Ellen had begun Internet gambling some weeks ago, and unbeknownst to Grandpa, she had developed a little "habit"— to the tune of a $3,500 loss. Unfortunately, other losses — her relationships with her husband, friends, and family — were just becoming apparent. Ellen was embarrassed and not quite sure how it had taken hold of her so quickly. She promised to stop the gambling and give up her Internet use until she could get some help for her new "problem."

Ellen went to see a therapist and realized that she had to completely lock out all gambling Internet sites if she wanted to keep the computer, because she had become addicted. He encouraged her to join a twelve-step program for gamblers. Her husband, friends, and family kept an eye on her and encouraged her to keep off the gambling sites. And it wasn't really hard to do — she was far too busy now bidding for really great things on e-Bay. She hadn't mentioned that to her therapist yet.

Computers were designed to enhance our daily lives, not to overtake them. Just as we can control the foods we eat, we can monitor and limit the amount of information we take in, preventing it from bombarding us and eroding the limited time we have to spend with important people in our lives. The following are some simple steps we can take to reduce the fatigue, confusion, and stress of too much technology and information.

- *Protect your address.* Anyone who uses e-mail or the Internet knows how easy it is to wind up on those mass-market spam e-mail lists. If you find yourself getting lots of junk e-mail, scan your messages and quickly discard those that are not important. You can remove yourself from junk e-mail lists by contacting the Internet provider of the sender (*postmaster@ provider-name.com*). Also, take a few minutes to download a spam filter, as well as to install spyware and virus protection software on your computer. Maintaining an unlisted telephone number will also cut down on those intrusive solicitation calls during dinner hour.

- *Just say no to newsgroups.* Unless you prefer this format for news updates, try declining newsgroup invitations in order to save time and cut down on data redundancy. Chances are you're getting the same information from newspapers, magazines, or the TV news.

- *Don't get lost on the Web.* With an estimated two billion Web pages out there, it's easy to become overwhelmed by information. Mastering some basic search techniques (see *www.meta crawler.com*) can help reduce a possible ten thousand entries to a reasonable ten.

- *Cut down on paper.* Judicious use of the printer can make a key bit of information more accessible, but paper clutter can pile up in no time at all. Any papers you don't need should be filed in the recycle bin.

- *Limit phone time.* Turn off your cell phone and hold calls during important meetings. If you must be available to some people at all times, try getting a pager and limit the access to it.
- *Get organized.* Use a file system to sort information coming in from that going out. Keep your "in" and "out" files in a convenient place on a desk or tabletop.
- *Quash junk mail.* If you contact the Direct Marketing Association (1120 Avenue of the Americas, New York, NY 10036-6700, 212-768-7277; *www. the-dma.org*), you can have your address taken off those annoying lists that lead to piles of junk mail.

TV Addiction

Television, as a tool for disseminating information, has transformed our environments — influencing our behaviors, tastes, activities, and even our beverage choices. It is among the most significant of technological tools in shaping social and political life. But one can get too much of a good thing. On average, Americans spend approximately three hours each day watching

TV — more time than any other activity, except for work and sleep. Add up the total number of hours spent in front of the tube over a lifetime, and by age seventy-five it comes to *nine years*.

One reason people are drawn to watching television is that it appears to trigger an instinctive orienting response first described by Dr. Ivan Pavlov, famous for his work with dogs in the area of conditioned response. We instinctively react to the TV's novel and sudden stimuli: heart rate slows, brain blood vessels dilate, and blood flows away from major muscles. This physiological reaction helps the brain focus on the mental stimulus. Television programs typically have rapid cuts and edits, which can stimulate and maintain our attention. However, when these cuts become too frequent, they can shift our orienting response into overdrive — we continue to watch, but experience fatigue, rather than mental stimulation.

Dr. Robert Kubey of Rutgers University and Dr. Mihaly Csikszentmihalyi of Claremont Graduate University have found that prolonged TV exposure may pose hidden hazards. By systematically monitoring mood and mental states during television viewing, they found that people feel relaxed and passive while watching TV, but their level of mental stimulation is lower compared with other activities such as reading.

The researchers also found that when people stop watching television, their sense of relaxation rapidly declines, and they feel less alert. Concentration abilities diminish, and many report a sense of depletion — as if the energy has been "sucked out of them" following a TV marathon. The more people watch TV, the less they seem to enjoy it. TV addicts are quicker to experience boredom and have more difficulties with attention. They also have a greater risk for being overweight than nonaddicts.

The scientific evidence is not strong enough to start banning television altogether, and many people derive pleasure, receive information, and get other benefits from their TV viewing. Since heavy watching does have a negative impact on our psychological state, there are some simple steps we can take to better control the TV habit.

- Try planning to watch specific shows of interest with family or friends, rather than getting into the habit of just lying around for hours, channel surfing solo.

- Make a list ranking the shows you enjoy watching each week and attempt to cut out one or more at the bottom of your list.
- Consider rearranging the furniture so that the TV is not the most prominent fixture in the room. Don't let your television shape your everyday experience: Control the remote, don't let the remote control you.
- Give books a chance. Plan or set aside a reading time, perhaps before going to bed.
- Consider other activities during your usual television-watching timeslot. Try playing a game with your mate, family, or friends — see if you're still the Mahjong Maven or the King of Scrabble.

Nine-to-Five Ergonomics

Many of us spend a large proportion of time sitting at a desk. The safety and esthetics of the space around our desk affects our productivity and quality longevity. *Ergonomics* is the science of designing objects, systems, and environments so that the job fits the person. An ergonomically designed work area takes into account anatomy, physiology, and psychology, so that the environment is comfortable, safe, and efficient for its users. Proper light, posture, and positioning will minimize work-related injuries, such as back and neck pain, hand injury, eye strain, and headache.

Because a computer monitor may cause eye strain or fatigue, screen images need to appear stable and free of distortion, flicker, or jitter. Typical ergonomic challenges involve awkward body postures, excessive repetitive movements and force, and contact stress, all of which can lead to pain, numbness, tingling, stiffness, or loss of strength. Such subtle changes as lowering your arm height or elevating your foot position may help you to avoid common work-related injuries. To ensure that your workstation is ergonomically safe, check the International Ergonomics Association Web site at *http://www.iea.cc*.

Even subtle environmental influences, such as color, can have an impact on our mood and productivity. Office workers have been found to prefer red-painted offices over white ones, and studies show that productivity is significantly greater in red offices. Other experiments indicate that memory and attention are influenced by color, as well.

Thermostat settings are also important. Many workers have heated arguments on workplace temperature settings. A recent study by Dr. Alan Hedge and associates at Cornell University found that workers at a large insurance company were more productive when the office temperature was increased from sixty-eight degrees Fahrenheit to the mid-seventies. Work output improved by 150 percent, and errors declined by 44 percent.

Workplace noise pollution can also reduce productivity and, when extreme, can permanently impair hearing. A person's risk depends on both the duration and volume level (measured in decibels, or db) of the sound. Normal conversation (60 db) or a ringing telephone (80 db) are in the safe range, but exposure beyond eight hours to a motorcycle or hair dryer (85 db), ambulance siren (140 db), or jet engine at takeoff (140 db) can put one at risk for hearing loss. If you are concerned about the noise level at your job, you might consider wearing hearing protectors — earplugs or earmuffs — or limiting the amount of time you spend exposed to the noise.

You Are What You Breathe

One of the advantages of living in a congested city is being able to *see* the air we breathe. Who knows what they're breathing in that clear country air? Seriously, polluted air poses many health hazards — it aggravates preexisting lung conditions such as asthma, and it can elevate blood pressure. Particularly smoggy days have been linked to increased mortality rates in U.S cities, and recent research has found that smog exposure when people are young may shorten life expectancy.

Toxic air exposure from sitting in traffic can nearly triple the risk for a heart attack. A recent study of more than nine hundred heart attack victims found that patients spent more time commuting the very day they suffered their heart attacks than on previous days. The risk was three times greater if they had been in a car or on public transportation during the hour before the attack, and four times greater if they had been on a bicycle. The good news is that when cities successfully reduce pollution, rates of cardiovascular illness decline.

Though most city dwellers cannot completely avoid breathing smoggy air, they can take steps to reduce their exposure.

One strategy is to try to work longer hours four days a week in order to eliminate one day of commuting from their work week. Closing windows and car vents will reduce exposure to outside air in heavily congested areas. Also, try to stay indoors during midday peak pollution hours, and reserve jogging, bike riding, and other outdoor activities to those times of day when air pollution is at a low point, usually early evening and morning hours.

Indoor air has its hazards, as well. Prolonged exposure to indoor dust and molds may cause or aggravate allergies or asthma. Just walking around your house or sitting down on a comfy sofa can kick up dust and mold spores, sometimes causing as much air pollution to enter one's lungs as smoking a cigarette.

Although not all forms of mold are dangerous, recent high-profile lawsuits have focused attention on the hidden dangers of some forms of household molds. Mold can not only exacerbate respiratory problems, but the unexpected physical and financial difficulties often lead to stress-related symptoms, including anxiety and depression.

Many insurance companies have stopped their coverage of mold damage after paying out billions of dollars for contaminations from toxic molds such as *Stachybotrys chartarum*. This kind of indoor mold can grow anywhere there is moisture and air — tiles, carpets, furniture, drywall, crawl spaces, and air ducts. The mold colonies sometimes look like slimy splotches and have a musty odor.

The Institute of Medicine recently warned of the public health dangers posed by excessive dampness in buildings and the mold that it causes. To maintain a safe indoor air environment, keep in mind the following:

- *Inspect before you buy.* House and apartment hunting can be an emotional experience. Many people tend to go with their gut feelings about a home, which can cloud practical considerations. Invest the time and money in proper inspections to ensure that the space is environmentally safe.
- *Fix leaks.* Be vigilant about water leaks. A leaky faucet or pipe can pose a health threat, since any moisture accumulation could create a breeding site for toxic mold. Also, make sure that your home has adequate waterproofing and drainage to prevent moisture from accumulating.

- *Bite the dust.* If you are dust-sensitive, consider losing the wall-to-wall carpets, and other dust and spore collectors such as venetian blinds. Make sure you dust furniture at regular intervals with a damp cloth, and keep floors clean with a moistened mop.
- *HEPA filters.* These air systems filter out extremely small particles that worsen asthma and allergy symptoms. When purchasing a portable HEPA (high-efficiency particulate air) filter, choose one with capabilities that match the size of your room. You may need to buy more than one for several rooms or consider a central HEPA filtration system for your entire house, apartment, or workplace. Some units reduce air contamination by adding ozone to the room air, which attacks the cellular structure of bacteria and fungi.

If you feel your workplace may have mold contamination, discuss your concerns with your employer. For more information about mold or other contaminations in the workplace, check out the U.S. Department of Labor's Occupational Safety and Health Administration (OSHA) Web site (*www.osha.gov*).

Cigarettes: No Butts About It

When I was a kid, many of my friends thought that smoking was cool — they wanted to look like the Marlboro Man. Most people, even many doctors, were unaware of the health hazards of smoking. Fortunately, those hazards are much better appreciated today.

Smoking not only increases our risk for cancer, strokes, and heart disease, it even makes us *look* older. Drs. Darrick Antell and Eva Taczanoski of Columbia University studied the aging effects of smoking in thirty-four sets of identical twins age forty-five to seventy-five years. They found that the depth and severity of wrinkles, amount of excess skin, quality of skin texture, and amount of gray hair varied according to smoking history — the nonsmoking twin consistently looked younger. One twin who had smoked a pack of cigarettes every day for forty years had approximately 50 percent more gray hair than his twin brother who had never smoked. Smoking also appeared to have a much greater influence on appearance than sun exposure, exercise, diet, or alcohol use.

Once someone gets hooked on cigarettes, it can be tough to quit, but the benefits emerge rapidly after quitting. The body's carbon monoxide levels drop dramatically, and within a week, the risk of dying from a heart attack declines. Five years later, that person's heart attack risk is similar to that of someone who never smoked. Intensive counseling and educational programs, as well as nicotine patches and gum, are often effective. The antidepressant bupropion (marketed as Wellbutrin) is sometimes used to assist people in quitting smoking. Because alcohol has been found to enhance the pleasurable effects of nicotine, avoiding it may help smokers quit. Internet sites are available to help people quit, as well (*www.quitnet.com*; *www.ashline.org*).

The government recently recognized the importance of smoking cessation programs by approving Medicare funding to help seniors quit smoking. The eleven-million-dollar annual cost of the Medicare program will be offset by the savings from fewer hospitalizations and health problems related to smoking.

Sunbathers Beware

Almost everyone has heard about the health risks of sunbathing; however, the sunlight that falls on our skin remains our main source of vitamin D, and scientists at Wake Forest University Baptist Medical Center recently found that exposure to ultraviolet light actually makes tanners feel more relaxed, motivating them to keep coming back for more tanning. The investigators believe that when exposed to UV light, the body secretes natural chemical endorphins, which are linked to both pain relief and feelings of euphoria.

This mood elevation may explain why people continue to tan, despite the overwhelming evidence of health risks. The sun's ultraviolet rays can damage and prematurely age the skin, cause cataracts, and suppress immune function. Prolonged unprotected sun exposure can lead to melanoma, a highly lethal cancer, if not detected and removed before it spreads.

If you do go in the sun, cover sensitive areas, wear a hat, and use a sunscreen with a Sun Protection Factor, or SPF, of fifteen or greater. The American Academy of Dermatology recommends reapplying sunscreen about every two to three hours. Also, keep in mind that ultraviolet rays will penetrate clouds and reflect off sand, water, and even concrete, so cover up and use sunscreen even on cloudy days. Try to avoid exposure during midday (generally between 10 a.m. and 4 p.m.).

Wear sunglasses that protect your eyes from ultraviolet rays. Also, check that your medications — particularly antibiotics and acne medicines — do not increase sun sensitivity. Stay away from artificial tanning devices, and examine your skin at regular intervals to make sure that there are no unusual changes. Finally, if a tan-skinned appearance is important to you, consider one of the many sunless self-tanning products available at drugstores and makeup counters.

Staying Behind the Wheel

Because we're living longer, we're seeing a larger number of older adults behind the wheel. By the year 2020, an estimated 40 million Americans age sixty-five and older will be licensed drivers. Most teenagers experience their first driver's license as a pivotal point of maturation — a time when they truly begin to feel independent and adult. The idea of relinquishing that privilege at some point is a prospect that most of us dread.

Yet as some people age, they experience

a decline in reflexes, coordination, and mental acuity, which can challenge driving safety. Arthritis may limit neck flexibility, visual impairments can make it harder to spot road hazards, and as people get older they are more likely to take medicines that may interfere with mental abilities, reaction time, or memory of addresses.

Protecting environmental safety includes being realistic about the fact that some older adults pose a danger when behind the wheel. Warning signs that someone may need to recheck their driving skills include multiple accidents and/or tickets, a tendency to drive too slowly or too closely behind other cars, and a nervousness or tenuousness when making turns or other driving decisions. If in doubt, check with your local motor vehicle department or the American Automobile Association for resources to help seniors stay safe on the road. The AARP also offers a Driver Safety Program class (call 1-888-227-7669 for more information).

An easy way to start minimizing the risk of accidents is to reduce the time one spends behind the wheel. Not only has the amount of time spent driving been correlated with stress levels, it is also associated with becoming overweight. A recent study found that for every additional half hour in the car, the risk for obesity increases by 3 percent. Consider walking or riding a bicycle instead of taking your usual cruise in the sedan.

Homes That Age Gracefully

As we live longer, our environmental needs often change. Perhaps we retire or start working from home; our children may move out or our parents may move in. We may decide to sell the big family house and move to a seaside condo, or closer to friends, theater, restaurants, museums, work, and other urban attractions. Perhaps we're looking for a home with fewer steps, wider doorways, guest rooms, or just more privacy. The "empty nest" may be just the excuse we need to spread our wings and explore a new environment or alter the one we have to maximize our space and our enjoyment of it.

Making sure that our home environment fits in with our changing needs throughout life is an important quality longevity goal. The trend today is toward openness and serenity in our living spaces, using fewer rooms and enjoying less clutter around us.

If you have the means, simply tearing down walls to create larger spaces or adding walls to divide up separate rooms can often alter your home to meet your requirements.

If older parents are no longer able to live on their own, they may face the tough decision of either moving in with adult children, finding in-home care for themselves, selecting an assisted living facility, or choosing another option. If parent care becomes a reality for your family, consider the advantages and disadvantages of several housing choices:

- *Long-distance parent care.* Many parents prefer to live in their own, familiar home and neighborhood so they can continue getting the emotional and practical support of friends and community. This is offset, however, by the impractical drawback of family members living some distance away. Help with even minor tasks like a ride or simple errand may require searching for others to pitch in. A parent's illness or accident means the adult child may have to hop on a plane, which adds additional stress, cost, and inconvenience to family life.

- *Under the same roof.* If you have the room, an older parent may want to move in. Respecting each other's privacy while involving the parent in everyday family life helps with the transition. Live-in parents can often be helpful with babysitting or tutoring.
- *Assisted living and life-care communities.* Assisted living promotes the resident's independence while providing assistance with meals, support services, social activities, and twenty-four-hour supervision. Life-care communities offer different levels of care, ranging from independent housing to skilled nursing care. Many offer contracts guaranteeing lifetime shelter and care.
- *Nursing homes.* These provide the most intense level of care, including meals, skilled nursing, rehabilitation, medical services, personal care, and recreation. New, smaller homes with more domestic settings have a closer sense of community, and many traditional institutions are remodeling to create a more homelike environment. The AARP offers a checklist to help families choose a nursing home (*www.aarp.org/life/housingchoices/*).

An Ounce of Prevention

Facing new challenges and taking some risks can be exciting and adrenaline-boosting, while offering up new experiences and adventures. However, recklessness can shorten our life expectancy and should be avoided. Simple measures such as fastening seat belts, wearing helmets, and stowing or removing firearms from the house save lives every day.

As we go through the various stages of our lives, the challenges of keeping our environments safe will change. With young children in the house, the number one indoor danger is falling down stairs. Stairs can become an environmental danger for elderly people as well. Use of medications, visual impairments, and arthritis can also increase the risk of falling for older people. Ensuring proper lighting, avoiding clutter, and safely securing throw rugs are helpful preventive measures. Here are some additional suggestions for maintaining safety at home as we get older:

- *Install handrails*. These are relatively inexpensive alterations that can help people who are unsteady on their feet. Be sure to have at least one handrail on all stairways and steps, and ensure that they are securely attached.

- *Secure steps*. Check that stairs are in good shape and that they are slip resistant. Try adding a strip along the edge of each step in a contrasting color so it is easier to see, or use reflective antiskid treads.
- *Clear walkways*. Arrange to have leaves, snow, and ice removed on a regular basis. During winter months, be sure to use salt or sand to avoid ice accidents.
- *Grab bars in the bathroom*. Installing grab bars in the bathtub, shower, and by the toilet can help prevent household falls. In the tub, grab bars on a side wall and the back wall are helpful for getting in and out. For additional support in the shower, consider a bench for showering while seated.
- *Mats*. A rubber mat in the tub and a nonskid bath mat beside it will help prevent falls.

Conserving Our Environment

Many people are aware of the need to conserve our planet's rain forests, oceans, water supplies, wildlife, and other natural resources, especially as more countries move toward industrialization. Nearly 80 percent of Americans live in urban environments, where parks and green areas are welcome breaks from the pavement of our cities. In urban settings, these green public areas have been linked to extended longevity. Japanese scientists found an increased life expectancy of up to five years for older Tokyo citizens correlating to the space available for taking a stroll near their homes or apartments, as well as the proximity of parks and tree-lined streets.

Our ability to conserve energy, keep the environment green, recycle, and avoid wastefulness helps us feel good about ourselves, as well as our surroundings. Trees, plants, and flowers, whether they are indoors or outdoors, enhance our mental and physical well-being. Landscaping often becomes a focal point, adding texture and enlivening the environment.

Conservationists take advantage of natural cycles and use several waste products from one cycle to fuel another. Kitchen and bath water can be recycled into the yard, and kitchen and garden trimmings can be used as compost material. Edible landscaping is another option — a vegetable or herb garden is pleasing to the eye and can really come in handy when you need a sprig of rosemary or a few basil leaves to complete a culinary masterpiece.

Conserving resources and creating pleasant, clutter-free, and stress-free surroundings can help us achieve our quality longevity goals. Small changes in the way we design, build, and maintain our homes will save us money and energy, as well as increase our health and satisfaction. For example, technological advances have made it more efficient and less expensive to harness the sun's energy with solar paneling. Easy access to nontoxic house paint and natural wax and oils for floors and furniture can help keep our homes toxin-free. Installing low-flow faucets and dual-flush toilets helps conserve water. Buying appliances with a high-efficiency Energy Star rating by the Environmental Protection Agency (*www.energystar.gov*) can minimize energy consumption. And finally, in areas where rainwater is scarce, you might want to consider drought-tolerant landscaping using native plants.

Mastering Your Environment

- Bear in mind function and aesthetics when designing your home and work space. Try to control clutter and noise and arrange the bedroom in a way that enhances sleep and restfulness.
- Minimize your exposure to sun, smoke, mold, smog, and other airborne toxins.
- Stay safe on the road — let someone else drive if you can't handle it.
- Make your workplace safe and comfortable and consider ergonomic designs.
- Manage your technology to avoid information overload.
- If parent care becomes a reality, consider the advantages and disadvantages of various housing choices.
- Help conserve natural resources to protect your environment.

Essential 6

Body Fitness – Shape Up to Stay Young

My grandmother started walking five
miles a day when she was sixty. She's
ninety-three today and we don't know
where the hell she is.
— ELLEN DeGENERES

Alan F. was excited about his company's upcoming annual ski retreat.
For the past few years, a knee injury
and then a back sprain had kept him
in the ski lodge Jacuzzi, while his wife
enjoyed the slopes with assorted
handsome young ski instructors.
Months before this year's trip, Alan
began a strengthening and flexibility
program at his gym to make sure that
his back was strong and his knee
wouldn't give out. He also swam laps

---

and did a stretching routine every morning. Alan gradually got stronger and more limber, and felt like his old self.

Alan was definitely psyched as he and his wife arrived at the ski lodge — this was *his* year to show the other guys at the conference that he could still ski the black diamond slopes. As his wife unpacked in their suite, he decided to run down to the fitness center to get on the treadmill before dinner. She heard the door shut as he left, but a couple minutes later she heard him come back in again. "That was a fast workout," she called to him. "Ice! I need ice!" he hollered from the other room as he limped to the sofa and elevated his leg. In his enthusiasm to get to the gym, he had skipped the elevator and instead raced down the stairs two at a time. Missing a step, Alan had gone tumbling down the last three stairs. His right ankle was already starting to swell. By dinnertime, Alan had seen a doctor, who wrapped his badly sprained ankle, gave him a set of crutches, and banished his dreams of skiing for yet another year. Alan's wife offered to stay at the lodge and play chess with him the next day, but he wouldn't have it, insisting she take off for the slopes and perhaps get a lesson from one of the young instructors standing by. That night, when the other guys at the conference saw that Alan had already sprained his ankle, they figured he'd done it skiing — he didn't mention the treacherous, double-diamond stairway leading from his room to the gym.

Years ago, our ancestors didn't worry about getting enough exercise — they were too busy hunting and gathering to think about it. Today, our lifestyles tend to be more sedentary — we spend time sitting in front of computers, driving in cars, and watching our televisions, so many of us need to plan our daily physical exercise. Sticking with those fitness plans not only has a major impact on our health and youthfulness, but it also increases the number of years we can expect to live. Regular exercise adds quality to those extra years because it makes us feel better — physically and emotionally.

All forms of physical activity, whether it's walking, cycling, basketball, or dancing, appear to prolong healthy living. A study of more than sixteen thousand Harvard alumni, age thirty-five to seventy-four, found that regular physical activity can add at least a couple of years to life expectancy. They found that men who played tennis, swam, jogged, or took brisk walks had up to 33 percent lower death rates and a 41 percent lower risk of heart disease than their more sedentary colleagues. Studies of championship skiers and college athletes have found an increased lifespan of four or more years, as compared with the general population. Many sports and forms of exercise work both the mind *and* the body, and extend life as well as protect the brain.

We don't need to run a daily marathon to reap the benefits of exercise. Walking merely ten to fifteen minutes a day, or what adds up to approximately ninety minutes each week, significantly reduces the risk for developing Alzheimer's disease. Physically active people have lower rates of heart attacks, colon and breast cancer, diabetes, and depression, and these benefits accrue at almost any age. One study of more than four thousand volunteers found that physical fitness earlier in life was associated with better cardiac health later in life. Another recent study found that men taking up exercise, even after age sixty, can increase their life expectancy.

Becoming physically active on a routine basis may even boost your sex life. A study of approximately five hundred middle-aged men found that those who exercised regularly reported more frequent and satisfying sexual encounters than their less active counterparts. Another investigation found that the level of sexual activity of middle-aged expert swimmers was comparable to that of the average adult twenty years younger, *after* drying off.

Regular exercise fortifies muscles, tendons, and cartilage, and increases bone density — all important for keeping our bodies fit and young. The improved strength and balance we gain reduces the risk of falling and injury. Working out also gives us a sense of euphoria — sometimes referred to as a "runner's high" — by stimulating endorphins. Exercise boosts immune function, improves cardiac health, and increases circulation throughout the body. By helping to control body weight, exercise can lower the risk for diabetes, high blood pressure, and strokes.

Looking and Feeling Younger

Almost every magazine cover or television program reminds us that our culture emphasizes youth and beauty. And many people are motivated to remain physically active because it helps them look younger and more attractive. When someone makes a commitment to pursue a quality longevity program — eating the right foods, getting enough exercise and sleep, remaining involved and staying mentally active — they often shed pounds, feel an increase in strength and stamina, and appear younger and slimmer. They often start to get positive feedback from friends, family, and coworkers about how good they look, which leads to higher self-esteem, which further fuels their sense of youthfulness and attractiveness.

Youthful looks are often synonymous with beauty, and what we consider to be beautiful varies among cultures and has deep psychological roots. Historically, women have had much more pressure to appear young and attractive than men have had, although that is beginning to change. In Westernized societies, where there is little risk of seasonal lack of food, scientists have found that a woman's waist-to-hip ratio is a strong indicator of her attractiveness to men. This makes sense because waist size conveys information on her reproductive and health status.

Studies of self-perception of attractiveness find that women tend to select a relatively lean body image as the most desirable, attractive, and healthy one. Although this can be taken to the extreme in women who develop eating disorders, dissatisfaction with body size and a wish to be thinner generally motivates women to eat healthier diets. As a woman ages, she lets up a bit on what she sets as her ideal body weight. Systematic studies have found that over the age of thirty, a woman will rate her ideal figure as significantly larger than that perceived as most attractive to men.

When a person perceives beauty, it triggers a predetermined physiological response in the brain. Dr. Itzhak Aharon and colleagues at the Harvard Medical School in Boston found that when a volunteer views a beautiful face, the brain activates a specific circuit involving the neurotransmitter dopamine. This is the same neural circuitry that controls eating, sexual appetite, making money, or seeking drugs. When dopamine is released in the brain, people experience a sense of pleasure that can be reinforced with repetition. This may explain why some people become obsessed with appearance and youthful looks in much the way that others become obsessed with food or addicted to drugs.

A sensible interest in maintaining an attractive appearance is a healthy and reasonable quality longevity goal. Feeling fit and attractive helps us to feel positive about ourselves and to remain socially connected. The Longevity Fitness Routine can improve our health and life expectancy, as well as provide the added benefit of making us look as good as we feel. Of course, many factors beyond physical appearance will influence our sense of attractiveness, including personality, accomplishments, self-confidence, mood, attitude, and external input. Many people have benefited from medical and surgical treatments in their pursuit of beauty and youthfulness (see Essential 8).

Pace Yourself

Baby boomers have come a long way from the physical education classes many recall from high school, when they had to run around a track, touch their toes, climb the ropes, and work out in ways that later in life might injure more than strengthen. Today we have numerous fitness regimens to choose from, and it is often best to sample several exercise techniques to discover what works best for each of us, paying particular attention not just to our health, but also to our enjoyment during workouts.

People with an ongoing medical condition should check with their doctor before starting any exercise program. Also, working out with a friend or in a group is a great way to get both physical *and* social. You can increase your stamina through mutual encouragement while you chat about other things on your mind, which can reduce stress while it helps pass the time.

Although building up our exercise stamina gradually is best for avoiding injury, it is also important to push ourselves to the next level whenever we're ready, in order to gain the full benefits from our

Harry A., a seventy-year-old retired entrepreneur, was excited about his new workout routine. After a session with his trainer, he was determined to avoid the injuries he typically suffered whenever he took up an exercise program or sport. His tennis days were over after his amazing backhand tweaked his lower back. After three months of abdominal crunches and hamstring stretches, he was back on the golf course, until his upper back protested following an awesome 250-yard drive. Who would've thought that you needed to warm up before golf? His physical therapist recommended Pilates, which got him flexible enough to try the new elliptical machine his wife gave him for his seventieth birthday. The physical therapist had warned him to start out easy and build up his endurance gradually. Harry kept that advice in mind as he carefully mounted the elliptical machine, adjusted his heart-rate monitor strap, focused on his posture and breathing, and began to pedal. He pushed in all the right buttons and got the machine going at the right pace. As he pedaled, Harry kept murmuring to himself: "I will *not* overdo it . . . I *will* pace myself . . . I *will* stop when the timer goes off." He gradually increased his speed, kept his breathing steady, and he began to feel a little sweat break out. Whew boy, he was getting tired, but Harry kept pedaling, and then boom — he could feel the endorphin boost kick in! In fact, before he knew it, the timer-buzzer went off and he had finished his workout. Yes! He had made it through his first session with no injuries at all! He looked up at the timer — three minutes had elapsed. Tomorrow he would *really* go for it and bump the timer up to four minutes.

workouts. So-called weekend warriors — people who exercise only on weekends or once a week — may have a higher risk for injury and often don't get enough of a benefit from their exercise for it to be longevity-promoting.

Longevity Fitness Basics

To get our bodies in optimal shape so we can live healthier longer, our exercise routines should cover three fitness categories: *cardiovascular conditioning, balance/flexibility,* and *strength training.* Many exercises, including some of those described later in the Longevity Fitness Routine, provide benefits in more than one of these categories. When we do a series of strength-training exercises, we are also getting a certain degree of cardiovascular workout. Some exercise techniques, such as yoga or Pilates, have benefits in all three categories.

Depending on your goals and your baseline fitness level, you may want to emphasize one category more than the others, although all three are vital. If a person wants to lose weight, then increasing the duration and frequency of his or her cardiovascular conditioning workouts can help by burning more calories. Those with injuries might want to give extra focus to strength training, especially to the muscles around and supporting the injured area. Concentrating on balance and flexibility is crucial for everyone who wants to remain free of pain and avoid future injuries.

Cardiovascular Conditioning

Any continuous exercise we do to raise our heart rate will boost our cardiovascular fitness, and as more oxygen enters the bloodstream we get what is known as the aerobic effect. Regular cardiovascular workouts — running, cycling, aerobics, basketball, hiking, stair-stepping, rowing — will improve the efficiency of the heart, lungs, and circulatory system so that they can get more nutrients and oxygen to the muscles and other tissues. Such exercise routines also burn calories and help to keep weight down, lower blood pressure, strengthen immune system function, and reduce stress, as well as lower the risk for diabetes, dementia, and other age-related illnesses.

How much cardiovascular conditioning each person needs varies, depending on his or her age and general health. Although research generally shows greater cardiac benefit with longer exercise sessions, even brief but regular workouts are longevity-promoting. A recent study found that three ten-minute cardiovascular workout sessions — such as brisk walks — throughout the day provided as much benefit in lowering risk for heart disease as a single thirty-minute session.

Calculating Your Target Heart Rate

Your maximum heart rate can be calculated by subtracting your age from 220. A 50-year-old man would subtract 50 from 220, leaving 170 — his maximum rate. Seventy percent of 170 is 119; and 90 percent of 170 is 153. So during his cardiovascular workout session, this man should aim for a heart rate of somewhere between 119 and 153.

Heart-rate meters, which are easily strapped around the chest and send moment-to-moment heart-rate information to a wristwatch receiver, are a convenient way to monitor your cardiovascular workouts as you build up to the higher end of your target heart rate. The information is also helpful in keeping you from surpassing your target rate and working harder than you need to in order to achieve optimal results.

We can get the most from our cardiovascular exercise by maintaining our target heart rate. To find this target rate, many experts suggest that the average person aim for somewhere between 70 and 90 percent of their maximum heart rate (see box).

Most fitness trainers recommend a warm-up phase before a cardiovascular workout, in order to increase body temperature and loosen joints. By also increasing the pulse rate slightly, it prepares the heart for a more vigorous workout. Warm-up phases usually include stretching and breathing exercises that may last from five to ten minutes. The actual workout phase can last anywhere from ten to sixty minutes, depending on your fitness level and your particular goal, such as increasing cardiovascular health, building up endurance, or losing weight.

Longer and more frequent cardiovascular workouts burn more calories and make it easier to lose weight; however, it's best to build up gradually to avoid soreness and injuries. Also, try not to exercise right after a large meal, when a good deal of the body's blood supply goes to the stomach and intestines to help digestion, and blood flow to other organs is down. Whenever possible, look for opportunities throughout the day when you can add an extra pop of cardiovascular work, such as skipping the elevator and taking the stairs, or briskly walking to do a nearby errand instead of hopping in the car.

Each cardiovascular workout should be followed by a five- to ten-minute cool-down phase that helps to gradually bring the body's physiology back to its resting level, allowing the heart to adjust back to a slower, nonexercising rate of blood flow. Stretching your muscles after exercising will help avoid soreness and increase your flexibility.

Consider the following types of cardiovascular exercise, and choose one or more activities that you enjoy and that fit in with your lifestyle needs. Try varying your exercise options to keep your workouts interesting.

Walking. A brisk walk is an ideal cardiovascular activity for people at any age. Walking requires no training or special equipment, carries minimal risk of injury, and is one of the easiest exercise routines to fit into a busy schedule. You can increase the aerobic challenge of your walks by lengthening the duration or distance covered; or you may want to challenge yourself by walking up and down hills.

Jogging. Jogging provides more of a cardiovascular challenge than walking, and many joggers seem to be addicted to a "runner's high" from endorphin hormone boosts they often get during their workout. You can jog almost anywhere and in almost any climate, and it requires very little special gear, other than proper running shoes. Unfortunately, knee and back injuries force some joggers to switch to exercises that are gentler on the joints.

Swimming. This sport uses nearly all the major muscle groups, so it does an excellent job of getting our hearts pumping. Because it is a non-weight-bearing exercise, it is ideal for people who have suffered joint injuries from higher impact cardiovascular workouts.

Cycling. Another non-weight-bearing exercise, cycling, can be done outdoors, so you can enjoy the scenery or run an errand, or indoors on a stationary bike, while you read or watch TV. Spinning classes have become very popular and involve a class full of stationary bikers riding to upbeat music and the encouragement of an instructor. To maximize performance and avoid knee strain, make sure to adjust your seat height so that your leg is not quite fully extended at the bottom of the downward pedal.

Racquet Sports. Tennis and racquetball offer the thrill and satisfaction of a contest, as well as the challenge of improving your skills. For younger adults, injuries are relatively rare, but after years of wear and tear on their joints, some older adults choose to segue to lower-impact alternatives.

Dancing. Dancing not only offers a cardiovascular workout, it also improves balance and flexibility. Dancing has even been associated with a lower risk for developing Alzheimer's disease, perhaps because of the mental challenge one gets from learning and following new steps.

Aerobics Classes. Some people prefer working out in a group instead of going it alone, and aerobics classes are a fun way to get motivated through the encouragement of classmates and the instructor. Fast-paced aerobics classes provide a cardiovascular workout as well as training in motor skills and coordination. Many people alternate between aerobics classes and spinning classes (see above) to keep things lively.

Workout Equipment. Since most of us are not out getting our cardiovascular exercise working the fields, technology has caught up with our need for convenient and targeted workout equipment. Treadmills, stationary bicycles, rowing machines, and many other types of equipment make it easier to read or watch the news while getting in your daily cardiovascular exercise. One can also adjust the resistance and elevation of many machines in order to gradually build up endurance and avoid injury.

Step or stair-climbing machines not only burn calories efficiently, but they help give definition to the muscles of your lower body. However, because they tend to put stress on the knee joints, many people have moved on to the newer elliptical equipment, which glides the leg joints through an oval or elliptical movement. For people with knee problems, stationary bikes are another sensible alternative to treadmills or stair machines.

Housework and Gardening. Rhythmic tasks such as sweeping, mopping, raking, or hoeing provide an efficient cardiovascular workout, but if you don't do them routinely, be sure to warm up properly before working at too fast a pace, in order to avoid injuries. Basic chores can burn lots of calories — ten minutes of lawn mowing eats up about seventy-five calories; spend the same amount of time hedging and/or planting seeds, and you'll burn up about fifty calories. In addition to the health benefits, you get the chores done and save money by not hiring help.

Balance/Flexibility

Adding regular stretching and balance training to our fitness goals helps us maintain or regain better balance and coordination, and makes us less prone to injuries from falls. It also increases the flexibility of our muscles, which can improve our daily performance in everything — even tasks such as lifting, bending, or running to catch a bus. Stretching also helps keep our muscles from getting tight, which tends to improve posture and minimize aches and pains.

Balance is the body's ability to right itself. This capacity to remain stable on our feet involves *proprioception,* a mechanism that sends messages from the brain to the body and back, letting us know how to react and with how much tension in each muscle group. This system is generally automatic, but it can be enhanced through exercise and training.

Exercises to increase flexibility through stretching and other movements are key to the Longevity Fitness Routine. Not only does stretching reduce stress, decrease muscle soreness, and increase performance, it also helps us to relax during and after a workout. Although not all studies have confirmed that stretching exercises prevent injury, many do show benefits for specific muscle groups, such as the hamstrings behind the thighs, and the triceps muscles at the back of the arms. Traditionally, stretching is done as a warm-up to increase blood flow prior to a workout, and as a cool-down after a cardiovascular or strengthening session to increase flexibility while the muscles and tendons are still warm.

Stretching along with strengthening is important for maintaining *range of motion,* or the ability of a joint to bend and straighten. In healthy joints, movement increases blood flow, providing oxygen, nutrients, and lubrication to the joints, thus allowing smooth, pain-free movement. When joints move less, they become stiff and painful, which then discourages further movement. Balance and flexibility exercises encourage healthy movement, and help us to avoid pain and stiffness.

Although balance and flexibility exercises can involve fancy equipment, many of the best exercises require nothing more than a simple willingness to learn the movements. Just standing on one leg, walking heel-to-toe, or reaching your arms to the sky can be effective balancing and stretching exercises. The following are a variety of fitness approaches that improve balance and flexibility.

Tai Chi. This is an exercise that incorporates a series of slow and smooth movements that help reduce stress and promote relaxation (see Essential 4). Qi Gong is a related series of movements with less complicated stepping patterns. These movements are designed to stretch and lengthen muscles, ligaments, and tendons gently, increase breathing capacity, and loosen joints. They are especially helpful in improving balance and flexibility. A recent study found that tai chi exercises done three times a week for twelve weeks resulted in significant improvement in strength, mobility, and flexibility in older adults.

Yoga. Yoga's sequence of poses and breathing exercises not only helps us to relax (see Essential 4) but also improves balance and flexibility. The challenge of many yoga poses is to stay well aligned, which strengthens the muscles required for greatest stability.

Pilates. This exercise system focuses on flexibility, balance, and coordination, while increasing muscle strength and tone. Originally designed to help dancers recover from and avoid injuries, the exercises are performed in a specific order and require a small number of repetitions. The focus is on strengthening core muscles, which include the muscles of the stomach, lower back, buttocks, and inner thighs. Pilates also emphasizes control and form. Many exercises are basic enough to be done on a mat, while others require the assistance of an instructor and special Pilates machines. A basic mat program can be learned and performed at home with teaching aids such as videos or books.

Stability Balls. Also known as Swiss balls or exercise fitness balls, these items are becoming increasingly popular for home workouts, since they are relatively inexpensive and versatile. They introduce instability into any given exercise movement, which challenges us to work additional muscle groups beyond what the exercise was originally intended to work. Learning to do the exercises while balancing on the ball strengthens our muscles and increases our stability in everyday situations. Recent research found that stability balls are particularly effective in augmenting core strength and balance.

Balance Boards. These devices consist of boards atop cylinders or domes. Standing on the board and trying to maintain balance challenges our ability to remain stable. With practice, we can learn to do exercises on these boards, which can improve balance, coordination, strength, and range of motion. A recent study found that balance-board training significantly reduced the risk of ankle sprain, the most common sports injury.

Strength Training

Weight lifting and resistance training help increase the size and strength of muscles and fortify bones. Denser bones lower the risk for osteoporosis, making them less likely to fracture. Strength-building exercises also protect our joints, which can decrease pain from arthritis. These exercises also help stabilize blood sugar levels, which makes diabetes less likely. The lean body mass that forms as a result of strength training raises metabolic rates, which helps burn more calories throughout the day and can be helpful for weight control.

Strength training is not just for bodybuilders, athletes, or action heroes. In fact, older people seem to benefit the most from weight or resistance training. Studies have found that older men who spend three months doing weight training may be able to double or triple the strength and size of the large muscles in their upper legs. Even residents in nursing homes have shown dramatic improvements in strength and bone density from weight training.

Having well-balanced muscle groups will reduce the risk of injuries that occur when one muscle group is weaker than its opposing muscle group. The best way to avoid such muscular imbalances is to make sure that when you train a specific muscle group, you train the opposing muscle group, as well. For example, if you do several reps of biceps training for the muscle at the front of your arm, you would also want to work the opposing muscle, the triceps at the back of the arm, in order to remain balanced. It is also recommended that you start out by using a weight light enough to allow you to complete ten to fifteen repetitions of each exercise. As your strength increases, so should your weights.

Because strength training tears down muscle fiber, it is important to have adequate periods of rest between training sessions so muscles will repair and rebuild. We can do this by cross-training, or working out different muscle groups on alternate days, which allows for that kind of rest. You can train one group of muscles, such as your arms, shoulders, and chest on one day, and another group, your thighs, calves, and hamstrings, the following day. Many exercisers like to switch between cardiovascular workouts one day and strength-training sessions the next, while including a flexibility (stretching) and balance component in all their workouts. The following are some options to consider for your strength-training program.

Weight Machines. This equipment comes in many shapes and sizes and features pulleys that provide resistance throughout the weightlifting movement.

Weight machines are relatively easy to use and can be safer than free weights because they guide the weight-lifting motions and reinforce correct posture. Targeting specific muscle groups can often be easier to do with these machines than with free weights, because correct form must be learned and sustained for free weights to work effectively.

Free Weights. Because they allow us to work our muscles from any angle, free weights offer more versatility than weight machines, which have a limited number of functions. Free weights are also less expensive and are the fastest way to increase muscle strength and size. They help develop control, balance, and coordination. Proper instruction on correct form will increase the effectiveness of free-weight workouts and help people avoid injury.

Resistance Bands. Used for strength training as well as stretching exercises, these bands come in varying degrees of elasticity, and can be used to work out both upper and lower body muscle groups. As you build strength, you can wrap the band around your hands to make it tighter, increasing the resistance, or swap up to a higher-resistance band. Available at most drugstores or sporting-goods outlets, these lightweight resistance bands allow you to take your workout equipment with you wherever you go.

Pain-Free Fitness

As our bodies get older, injuries generally take longer to heal — we can't always just "walk it out" as we might have in our twenties or thirties. A minor back sprain or knee tweak may mean a week or two on ice before we bounce back to the racquetball court. But if we're not physically conditioned, flexible, and strong, we may not bounce back for much, much longer.

Approximately four out of five Americans suffer from intermittent or chronic back pain at some point during their lives. Fortunately, most back sufferers find relief and improvement through targeted exercise. The usual risk factors for low-back pain are weak abdominal muscles and limited flexibility.

Toning your stomach muscles with sit-ups, crunches, or other abdominal exercises helps to strengthen and protect your back and its surrounding muscles. By adding stretching exercises, your back and the muscles around it will become more flexible and elongated, protecting it from future injury and pain. The Pilates program is a great way to protect the back, with its focus on strengthening the "core" muscles — those around your trunk and pelvis — which support the spine and help to align the body correctly.

To work your body's core, engage your deepest abdominal muscle by coughing once. The muscle you feel contracting deep in your abdomen is your transversus abdominis. It isn't the only muscle that makes up your body's core, but by trying to keep this muscle contracted throughout the exercises, the rest of your core muscles get a workout, too.

In addition to the following Longevity Fitness Routine, which includes a series of stretching, strengthening, and toning exercises that protect the back, several other simple interventions can bring relief to back-pain sufferers. These include wearing low-heeled shoes; avoiding long periods of sitting by walking and stretching at regular intervals; bending your knees when lifting heavy objects; and sleeping on your side with a pillow between your knees. Overweight back sufferers may find that shedding a few pounds can help relieve some of the discomfort.

Many athletes and nonathletes alike suffer from knee problems, and this joint becomes more vulnerable with age. Strengthening the quadriceps muscles (front of the thigh), the inner and outer thigh muscles, and the smaller muscles and ligaments surrounding the kneecap can protect that area from injury and help keep the kneecap from sliding out of place. Several exercise-related knee problems can be easily corrected by wearing the proper footwear or shoe inserts. Running or power-walking on hard surfaces such as concrete may contribute to knee problems, and joggers tend to prefer softer dirt and gravel roads to run on. If you should experience knee pain while exercising, stop and apply ice as soon as possible. If the discomfort does not improve, consult your doctor.

Longevity Fitness Routine

You don't have to join a gym or buy any special clothing or high-tech equipment to begin an exercise routine that incorporates the three basic longevity fitness areas: cardiovascular conditioning, balance/flexibility, and strength training. All you need for your workout is a little time, a chair, and a bath towel. If you don't own any free weights you can start out by using sixteen-ounce soup cans instead, although once you build up your strength and endurance, you may wish to buy heavier dumbbells.

Cardiovascular Conditioning

If you are new to cardiovascular conditioning, try beginning with a brisk five-minute walk, then work up to ten minutes, then fifteen, and eventually twenty or more. It's a good idea to warm up before doing any type of sport or workout, and follow your cardiovascular or strengthening routine by stretching your muscles, to avoid soreness and increase flexibility. You can use some or all of the stretching exercises included in the Flexibility and Strengthening Workout below. You can do your cardiovascular conditioning on the same day as your strength training, or on alternate days, depending on your time and fitness level.

Flexibility and Strengthening Workout

Begin this routine slowly, doing as many repetitions as you feel comfortable doing. Gradually, you will build up strength and stamina, and be able to increase your number of repetitions and sets, as well as the amount of weight you are lifting.

Alternating Overhead Stretch. This flexibility exercise helps improve range of motion in your arms, shoulders, and chest, as well as release muscle tension in your back and the sides of your trunk. Stand with your knees bent and feet hip-width apart.

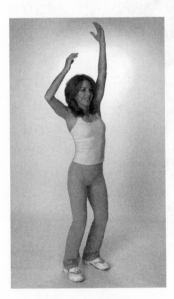

Raise both arms over your head and slowly reach for the ceiling, alternating your right and left arm. Keep your hips still and do twelve repetitions. Take a deep breath, and exhale as you bring your arms to your sides. Repeat the stretch two more times.

Alternating
Overhead Stretch

Side Stretch. This stretch works the sides of the trunk and the waist. Stand with feet shoulder-width apart, and keep your knees slightly bent. Raise your right hand overhead and reach over to your left side as far as you can, then hold the position and breathe for a count of five. Slowly bring your torso upright while exhaling. Raise your left arm overhead, reaching to the right side as far as you can. Hold and breathe for a count of five. Slowly return to upright. Repeat both sides.

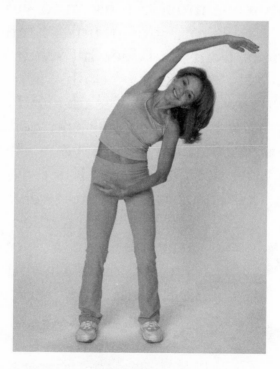

Side Stretch

Hip Stretch. The hip flexors help lift your leg in any position. Stretching the hip flexors helps to counter the prolonged hip flexion many of us experience by sitting for long periods of time. Stretching the muscles in front of your hips can help prevent "swayback" (a condition in which the spine is unnaturally arched backward).

Kneel on your left knee and extend your right leg in front of you, knee bent and foot flat on the floor. Shift your weight onto the bent right leg and press the right knee forward. Make sure the right knee does not extend past the right foot. Try to keep your pelvis tucked under and your abdominals pulled in. Feel the stretch through your left hip and thigh, as well as your right hamstring, as you breathe deeply for fifteen to thirty seconds. Relax, then repeat the stretch on the other side.

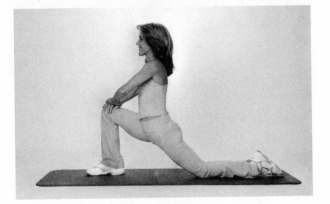

Hip Stretch

273

Quadriceps Stretch. Limber quadriceps muscles help us bend and straighten our legs, as well as lift and flex our knees. Steady yourself with your left hand on a chair back or wall, then bend your right leg behind you and grasp that ankle with your right hand. Keep your knees together and your standing leg slightly bent, as you gently pull your right foot closer toward your bottom. Feel the stretch through the front of your leg as you keep moving that foot back. Hold for a count of twelve and repeat on the other side. *Variation: For extra balance work, try doing this stretch without holding onto anything.*

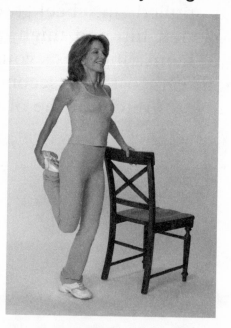

Quadriceps Stretch

Achilles Tendon Stretch. The Achilles tendon connects the leg muscles to the foot, allowing us to point our toes, rise on our toes, and walk. Correct stretching and warming up before a workout helps protect the Achilles tendon and its surrounding muscles.

Stand arm's length from a wall and place your hands flat against the wall in front of your shoulders. Lean forward and step your right leg straight back. Bend your forward knee and keep your right leg straight as you drop your right heel to the floor and push your chest forward. Feel the stretch through your right calf and hamstring muscles, as well as your Achilles tendon. Breathe and hold for a count of twelve, then repeat on the other side.

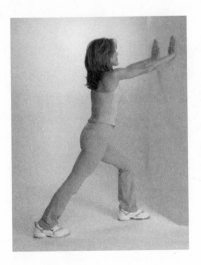

Achilles Tendon
Stretch

Forward Leg Lifts. The next few exercises strengthen the muscles in the front, back, and side of the leg, protecting the knees, hips, and pelvis. Holding on to a chair back or wall with your left hand, slowly lift your right leg forward, keeping it straight with the toes pointed. Your standing leg should be slightly bent to protect your back from strain. Pause for a second with your leg in the up position and then slowly lower it. After ten repetitions, hold your right leg in the up position. Now bend your knee in, very slightly, and then straighten it, keeping the toes pointed. Do this ten times, then switch legs and repeat the series. *Variation: To work on your balance, try doing the exercises without holding on to anything.*

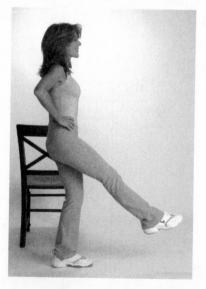

Forward Leg Lifts

Hip Abduction. Stand and hold on to a chair or wall with your left hand, keeping your left leg slightly bent, as you raise your *straight* right leg out to the side, foot flexed. Hold for a count of three, and then lower the leg. Do ten repetitions, keeping your hips and body straight during the exercise. Switch sides and repeat with the other leg. Work up to two sets.

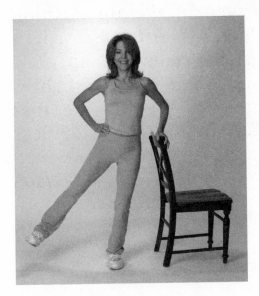

Hip Abduction

Hip Extension. Place both hands on the back of a chair. Hold your abdominal muscles tight and don't arch your back as you push your right leg straight behind you, until you feel a squeeze in the back of the thigh and buttocks area. Hold for a count of three, and release. Repeat ten times and then switch legs. *Variation: Try doing this* exercise with the working leg bent at the knee, but after each push back, don't release the leg any farther forward than the standing leg.

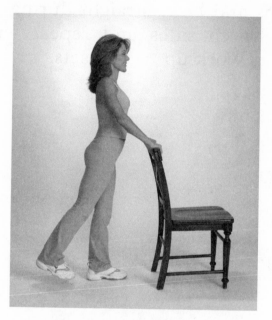

Hip Extension

Chair Squat. This is a toner for the thighs, hips, and buttocks. Stand in front of a chair with your feet slightly more than hip-width apart, your toes pointed forward, and your arms crossed. Bend at your hips and lower your bottom to the chair. The moment you touch it, push up to standing. Repeat ten times. Gradually build up to twenty repetitions. *Variation: When you feel ready, try doing this exercise without the chair.*

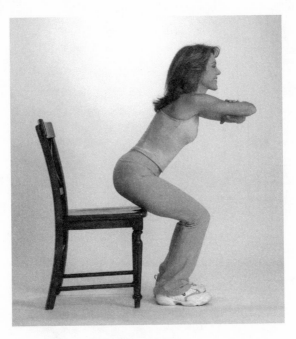

Chair Squat

Calf Strengthener. Stand on the balls of your feet on a first stair step. Raise your heels as high as you can, tightening your calf muscle. Pause for a moment, then slowly lower your heels until they're below the step and you feel a stretch in your calf muscle. Do ten repetitions. Build up to two to three sets.

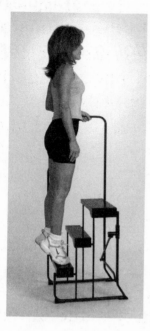

Calf
Strengthener
(Fig. A)

Calf
Strengthener
(Fig. B)

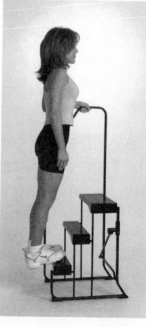

Biceps Curl. This exercise is a great way to strengthen the muscles in the front part of the upper arm. Stand upright with feet shoulder-width apart and knees slightly bent. Hold a set of dumbbells at your thighs, with your palms facing forward and your elbows anchored against your sides. Keep your back straight and abdominal muscles tight. Slowly raise both dumbbells toward your shoulders, making sure your elbows do not move, and do not rotate your wrists. Slowly lower to starting position, but don't fully extend your arms. Repeat twelve times. Gradually build up to three sets.

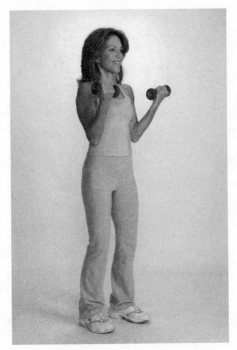

Biceps Curl

Upright Rows. The next two exercises benefit the upper back and shoulders. Stand with your feet shoulder-width apart and knees slightly bent. Hold a dumbbell in each hand in front of your thighs, palms facing in. Inhale as you raise both dumbbells up to just under your chin, with your elbows bent at shoulder height. Hold there a moment and then slowly exhale as you lower your arms to the starting position. Keep the dumbbells close in to your body throughout the exercise. Repeat ten to twelve times and gradually build up to two sets.

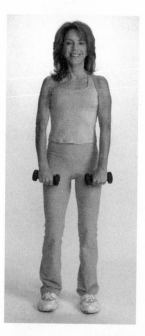 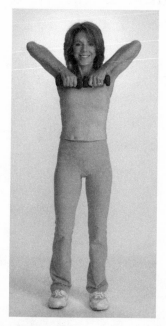

Upright Rows (Fig. A)   Upright Rows (Fig. B)

Lateral Lift. Stand upright with feet shoulder-width apart and knees slightly bent. Hold the dumbbells at your sides, with your palms facing each other. Raise both arms to the sides until they're shoulder height, and keep your elbows slightly bent. Pause for a moment and then slowly return to the beginning position. Repeat twelve times. Build up to three sets.

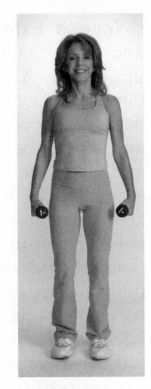

Lateral Lift
(Fig. A)

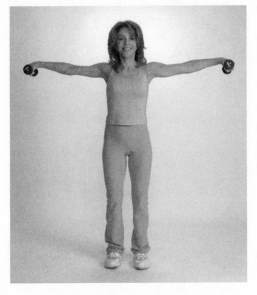

Lateral Lift
(Fig. B)

Triceps Extension. This will strengthen and tone the muscles in the back of the upper arm. Hold a dumbbell in your right hand and place your left hand on a chair back. With your feet shoulder-width apart and knees bent, keep your back straight and lean forward, bringing your right elbow back to shoulder height with the arm bent at a right angle. Slowly extend your arm from the elbow until the arm is straight and the head of the dumbbell is pointing up. Hold a moment and slowly return the weight to the starting position, keeping the upper arm and elbow still. Do ten to twelve repetitions on each arm. Build up to two sets.

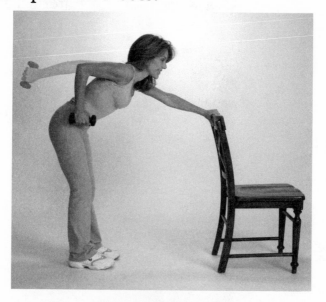

Triceps Extension

Overhead Press. This works the shoulders, the triceps, and the upper back, and helps develop overhead lifting strength. Stand upright with feet shoulder-width apart and knees slightly bent. Hold a dumbbell in each hand, out to your sides at shoulder height. Bend your arms to ninety-degree angles, with your palms facing forward. Be sure to keep your back straight and your head in line with your spine as you press the weights together straight up over your head, without locking your elbows. Hold a moment, then return to the starting position. Repeat ten times. Work up to two sets.

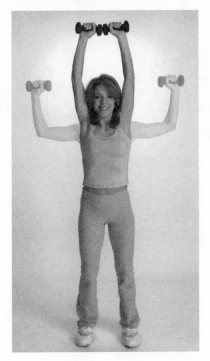

Overhead Press

Shoulder Stretch. You have worked your upper and lower body, so it is time for some more stretches. Reach one straight arm across your chest toward the other shoulder. With the opposite hand, grasp your elbow and pull your arm in as close to your body as possible. Hold for a count of ten, then release and stretch the other side for a count of ten.

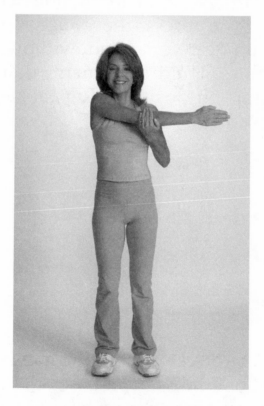

Shoulder Stretch

Upper Arm Stretch. Raise both arms overhead. Bend the right elbow, dropping the right hand behind your head. Hold the bent right elbow with your left hand and pull it down and back behind your head. Feel the stretch in your right triceps muscle and shoulder. Hold for a count of ten, and then repeat on other side.

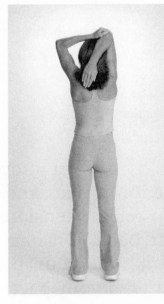

Upper Arm
Stretch

Chest Stretch. Clasp your hands behind your back. While keeping your chest high, lift your arms straight up behind you. Hold the stretch for fifteen seconds, then repeat. For a greater challenge, bend forward and raise your arms up higher.

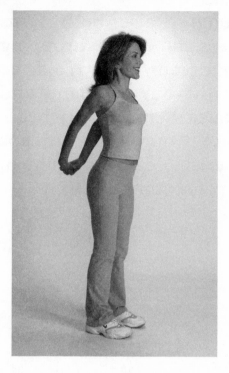

Chest Stretch

Cat Stretch. This is a yoga movement designed to relax the lower back and pelvic area. It can also help release tension in the shoulders and upper back. On hands and knees, exhale as you pull your belly in, drop your head, and arch your back up toward the ceiling as high as possible — like a cat stretching. Hold for a count of two. Now slowly inhale, raising your head to look upward, and lowering your back into a scooped or bowl position for the opposite stretch. Repeat four to five times, keeping the motions fluid.

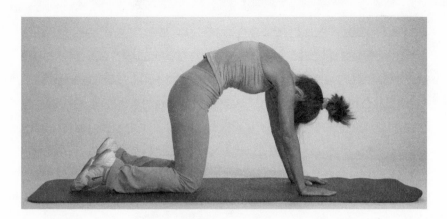

Cat Stretch (Fig. A)

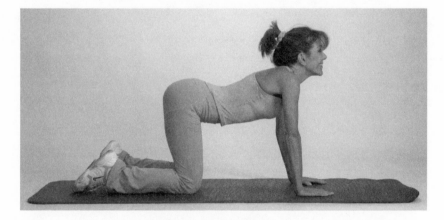

Cat Stretch (Fig. B)

Hamstring Stretch. Hamstring muscles in the back of the thigh work in opposition to the quadriceps in the front; however, they lag behind in strength and flexibility. Without proper stretching, they may be prone to injury and "pulls" from sudden movements. Lie on your back with your legs extended. Bring in one knee and wrap a towel around the arch of that foot. Holding the towel with both hands, gently straighten that leg toward the ceiling as much as possible. Use the towel to keep pulling the leg toward your nose. Hold for three to five deep breaths, then switch legs.

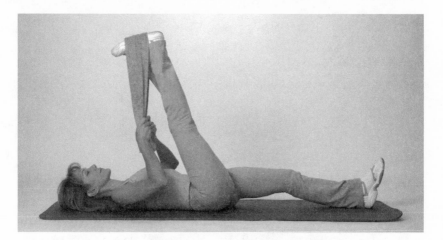

Hamstring Stretch

Abdominal Crunch. No strengthening routine is complete without working the abdominals, or core. Lie on your back with your knees bent, feet flat on the floor. Lace your fingers behind your head, keeping your elbows pointed out. Take a deep breath. As you exhale, pulling your navel down toward your spine, raise your upper torso off the floor and push your lower back into the floor. Focus on using your lower abdominal muscles without straining your neck. Hold for a moment and then release slowly. Complete a set of ten, but as soon as you are able, build up to five or more sets.

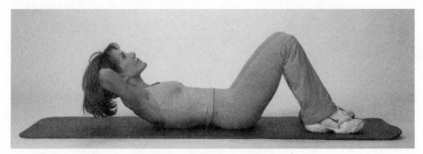

Abdominal Crunch

Abdominal Side Toning. This exercise for toning the lateral abdominal muscles is sometimes called the "bicycle." Lie on your back with hands clasped behind your head. Raise your knees directly above your hips with calves parallel to the ground. Take a deep breath. As you exhale, lift your head, torso, and *left* elbow toward your *right* knee, while pushing your *left* leg out straight. Hold for one count, then switch to the other side, lifting your head, torso, and *right* elbow toward your *left* knee, and pushing your *right* leg out straight. Be sure to pull your navel in toward your spine with each exhale and contraction. Do a set

291

of ten repetitions on each side, increasing the number of sets over time.

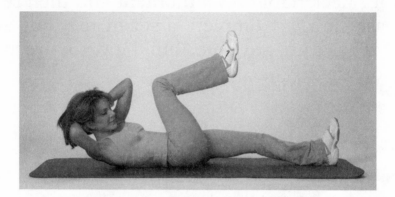

Abdominal Side Toning

Pelvic Tilt. This exercise strengthens the muscles in your buttocks, hamstrings, and abdominals, while it gently stretches the lower back. Lie on your back with your knees bent and feet shoulder-width apart on the floor. First, tighten your stomach muscles, then raise your buttocks off the floor slightly, tightening them. Be sure to keep your middle-to-lower back on the floor. Hold for a moment, then release. Repeat twelve to twenty times. *Variation: To notch it up a bit, raise your buttocks up about six inches from the floor while keeping your stomach and buttocks tight. Hold for a count of three and repeat twelve times.*

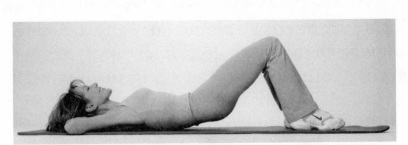

Pelvic Tilt

Back Leg Lift. Lie on your stomach with your legs straight and your hands folded under your cheek or chin. Tighten your stomach muscles, then lift your right leg two to three inches off the floor, tightening your buttocks. Hold it there a moment and lower it, and repeat the movement with your left leg. Do ten repetitions on each side. By keeping your stomach and your buttocks muscles tightened, and not lifting too high, you will protect your lower back. *Variation: Bend the lifting leg.*

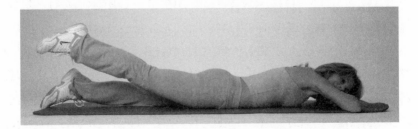

Back Leg Lift

Hip Twist. Lie on your back with your legs extended straight out on the floor. Slowly bend your left knee and bring it across your body to the right, until you feel a stretch in the lower back and hip area. Hold for a count of twelve. Return to starting position and repeat with the other leg.

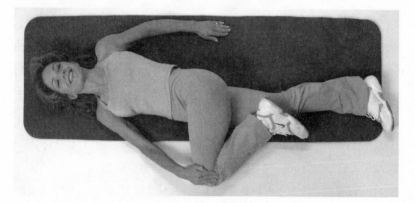

Hip Twist

Upper-Body Floor Stretch. Lie on your stomach with your palms on the floor, under your shoulders. Keeping your pelvis and thighs on the floor, slowly push your shoulders up until your arms are as straight as possible. Feel the stretch through your chest, shoulders, and back. Hold for a count of five, and then lower to the floor. Repeat two or three times.

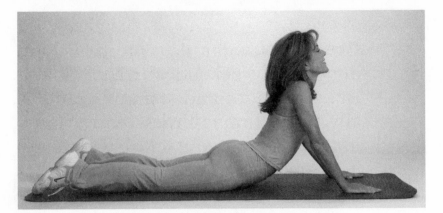

Upper-Body Floor Stretch

The Longevity Fitness Basics

- Sample different types of cardio-vascular exercise methods and choose one or more that you find fun and challenging. Sports and exercise protect your body *and* your mind.
- Exercise with a friend — getting physical *and* social reduces stress and keeps you connected to others.
- Divide your routine among the three basic Longevity Fitness areas:
  - Cardiovascular conditioning
  - Balance and flexibility
  - Strength training

- Exercise several days a week — don't be a weekend warrior.
- Build strength and stamina gradually to maximize fitness and avoid injury — push yourself to the next level only when you're ready.
- If you have an ongoing medical condition, be sure to check with your doctor before starting any exercise program.

Essential 7

The Longevity Diet

All you need is love. But a little chocolate
now and then doesn't hurt.
— CHARLES M. SCHULZ

You're halfway through a long business trip,
exhausted after visiting five cities in three
days. You almost missed your last connection and couldn't grab anything to eat at
the airport. It's midnight when you finally
check into your hotel room, too tired to
even call room service. Hell, maybe skipping a meal will help you lose those six
pounds that have crept on. You get ready
for bed and scan the room for some bottled
water, when you spot it — the *minibar*. You
steel yourself and head toward it with de-
termination: You're just getting a cold
bottle of water and you're out of there — no
chips, no cookies, and absolutely, for *damn*
sure, you are *no way* checking out the
candy shelf. Right — there's peanut
M&M's, chocolate-covered mints, a KitKat

bar, and a giant Snickers. The Snickers only has 170 calories per serving . . . *That's not bad* . . . You fold back the wrapper — just enough to have a couple of bites, as you flip on the TV. The entire bar is long gone before you glance around and realize you never got that water . . .

For as much time as we spend thinking, talking, and reading about food, many people still make the wrong choices about what they eat. Despite the greater attention placed on diets today, for health and weight loss, many still wonder *how much* to eat and *which* foods are healthy. Lots of people continue to ask the basic question: Can food that tastes good still be good for me? The answer is yes.

What we eat directly impacts our health and life expectancy by affecting our risk for heart disease, cancer, and other age-related illnesses. A large-scale, ten-year study found that people living a healthy lifestyle and eating a diet rich in antioxidant fruits and vegetables, olive oil and other monosaturated fats, as well as poultry and fish, had a 50 percent greater likelihood of living longer than study volunteers eating a less healthy diet.

Food also greatly affects our appearance and mental state. People often feel better about themselves when they look healthy and trim, and this has kept millions of people on various diets for decades — going up and down on the scale and wreaking havoc on their bodies. One of the biggest problems with many of today's popular diets is that they are hard to stick with for more than a few weeks or months, so people seldom get to enjoy the long-term health benefits. They tend to gain back all the weight they lost — and more. Often these diets fail because they leave people feeling not just bored, but deprived — whether it's a craving for carbohydrates, an urge to supplement calories to ease hunger pangs, or a desire to break down and splurge on a slice of chocolate cake or other favorite food.

Enter the Longevity Diet, which allows you to enjoy the foods you love (including that chocolate cake on occasion), trains you to add a variety of delicious and healthy foods, and emphasizes mindful awareness, so you know when you have had enough. Just as fitness experts put emphasis on cross-training our bodies — combining different forms of exercise in consecutive workout sessions in order to maximize results and minimize boredom — the Longevity Diet teaches us to cross-train our meals, allowing us to break free of the repetition and boredom of many of today's popular food plans.

Cross-Train Your Diet for Longevity

Every day you will enjoy foods from the three major food groups that are scientifically associated with longer, healthier living:

- *Antioxidant fruits and vegetables* — Rich in vitamins, minerals, and phytonutrients, they taste great, fight disease, and add endless variety to our menus.
- *Proteins, lean meats, and healthy fats* — Supplying essential amino acids that maintain and repair the body's cells, they satisfy hunger the longest. Ocean-caught (wild) fish and nuts are particularly good sources of omega-3 fats, which protect not only the heart, but the brain, as well.
- *Whole grains, legumes, and other carbohydrates* — Packed with fiber and cancer-fighting nutrients, these carbohydrates provide immediate energy and keep the digestive system on track.

The *cross-training* component helps your body maintain a balance of these three food groups, and keeps your diet interesting and appealing by shifting the emphasis among the groups throughout the day. Using your imagination, think of meals as major motion pictures *starring* one of the three food groups. No single food group can star in all three movies (meals) in any given day. If you are trying to lose weight, protein — with its ability to provide essential nutrients and satisfy hunger the longest — should *star* in two of your meals each day.

If a fresh grilled salmon steak is the *star* of tonight's dinner performance, then steamed broccoli, wild rice, and a dinner salad with olive oil vinaigrette dressing might all play minor roles. And, of course, there is always a healthy dessert after dinner. Earlier in the day, you cross-trained your other meals as well: Perhaps oatmeal gave whole grains the starring role at breakfast, backed up by skim milk (protein) and sliced melon as supporting characters. Lunch showcased a crispy Chinese chicken salad, filled with colorful vegetables and orange slices in starring roles, with a small portion of chicken and sesame oil dressing playing bit parts.

Integral to the Longevity Diet are the midmorning and midafternoon snacks. Besides providing the energy we need to carry us between meals, these snacks ensure that our blood sugar remains steady throughout the day, which not only keeps us from feeling hungry but lowers our risk of developing diabetes and other diseases. We integrate cross-training into our snacks by combining the quick and tasty energy boost we get from carbohydrate-containing whole grains, fruits, or crunchy vegetables together with the sustained gratification of an ounce or two of protein, such as yogurt, string cheese, or perhaps a handful of almonds.

For those of us (hello!) who like a little nibble at night while reading or watching a movie, the diet also includes the option of having a third snack later in the evening — or, you can always save your after-dinner dessert to enjoy as your *nighttime snack*. For a more restful sleep as well as for weight management, try to limit these later snacks to something light and healthful. Good choices include fresh fruit, frozen fruit-juice bars, fresh or frozen yogurt, air-popped popcorn, and many other delicious and healthy alternatives.

The Longevity Diet not only promotes

longer life but lets us toast to it with a glass of wine or other alcoholic beverage each day. Scientific evidence shows that drinking in moderation may protect the heart, lower risk for diabetes, and boost immunity and brain fitness. Scientists have found that on average, people who drink a glass of wine every day have less body fat and narrower waistlines than heavier drinkers or people who don't drink at all. Other research has shown that a daily glass of wine may help protect us against developing ulcers, gastritis, and stomach cancers.

So, you may be wondering, when do we get to eat the chocolate cake? Is now too soon? Cake is usually pretty loaded with sugar and fat, but at the end of a cross-training diet day, perhaps one that has been somewhat low in carbohydrates and fats, an occasional portion-conscious serving of cake at dessert time is fine. Tomorrow, go back to mixed berries or a scoop of sorbet for dessert. It's all good, and you won't feel deprived — you've stayed on your diet and you have nothing to feel guilty about. You've had your cake and eaten it, too!

Because the diet is designed to last for the long haul, it includes the food category

I call *cheat eats*. These are any foods you love, crave, have to have and can't believe could be allowed on *any* diet, anywhere. For some, it's key lime pie; others may pine for a delicate foie gras; or perhaps it's deep-dish pizza with three cheeses that rings your bell. Okay, so those are my top three cheat eats — and I have been able to routinely work them into my program just fine. Including cheat eats in your diet has a scientific rationale: Evidence linking healthy diet choices to longevity has shown that you can include an occasional treat.

If your goal is to lose weight, you should consider putting cheat eats on hold, and increasing your exercise program — the old adage of "more calories out than in" still holds when it comes to shedding pounds. After an initial weight-loss period, a portion-controlled amount of your favorite cheat eat is a reasonable Saturday night dividend for a week well invested in the Longevity Diet. Later, we'll learn how to adjust the diet to lose weight quickly.

It is vitally important to remain hydrated throughout the day by drinking at least eight glasses of water. Not only will this help minimize hunger between meals and snacks, but it has been scientifically shown to increase metabolism, allowing our bodies to burn calories more quickly. A recent study found that after volunteers drank seventeen ounces of water, their metabolic rates increased by 30 percent, and the increases lasted nearly an hour. Try starting each new day by drinking a cool glass of water. It refreshes and cleanses the body, while helping to relieve any dehydration effects that may have occurred while sleeping.

Avoiding excess salt in our food helps us control our blood pressure, which lowers the risk for strokes, heart attacks, and kidney disease. Besides weaning ourselves off the salt shaker, we need to keep an eye on canned and frozen foods, prepared meals, and fast food, which usually has high salt levels.

A key to the success of the Longevity Diet is developing mindful awareness of how our bodies feel before, during, and after eating. Although dining can be one of life's greatest pleasures, many people living today's high-pressure, multitasking lifestyle have allowed eating to become little more than a habit, and certainly less satisfying than it could be. Some people tend to eat mindlessly while working, watching TV, talking on the phone, or during any number of other distractions or activities.

Although meal time is a great opportunity to converse with family and friends, it is still vitally important to focus attention on:

1. How hungry we actually are before we begin eating, in order to gauge what portion size we really should take.
2. The moment-to-moment taste experience we have while eating, which allows us to slow down and savor our meals.
3. The increasing sense of fullness in our stomachs as we dine, and an awareness of when we are sated and have had enough.

Mindful eating not only helps us maintain an awareness of when we have had enough food, but also when we have had enough of a specific taste. Usually, after four or five bites of a particular food, taste buds become desensitized to that food's flavor. That is why even if someone cannot possibly eat another bite of grilled chicken, they may still have room for chocolate soufflé. Developing an awareness of this taste-specific satiety can help control binging and steer people away from unwanted calories.

Training yourself to use this and other mindful awareness eating techniques will not only help you *enjoy* meals more, you will most likely eat less and make healthier choices. You may notice the unique flavor of lemon juice on certain fresh vegetables, or a particular olive-oil vinaigrette dressing that you didn't realize you liked so much — both of which will help you eat more nutritiously. As you become more aware of how you feel before, during, and after eating — full, tired, energized, bloated — portion control will become easier, because you will have learned just how much food your body needs to feel good, as well as what foods make you feel energized and healthy. Also, stopping eating at the first sign of satiety is a great way to lose unwanted pounds without even trying, as well as maintain your target weight.

The Healthy Longevity Food Groups

To begin the Longevity Diet, familiarize yourself with the three major quality longevity food groups and the many food choices available in each of them. Each group has a list that includes several food suggestions, some of which you may already enjoy often, and some of which you may be less familiar with. Experimenting with various foods from the lists is a great way to expand your palate and increase your menu repertoire. I also encourage you to add other favorite healthy foods to your lists to help personalize your diet and keep it working for you for years to come.

Antioxidant Fruits and Vegetables

Just as metal gets rusty from being exposed to moist air, our bodies are vulnerable to oxidants, known as *free radicals*. We can't avoid free radicals, because they're everywhere — in our food, water, and air, and they also come from within us, as the by-products of our own metabolism. Many experts believe free radicals are the true culprits of aging. Our bodies are constantly under attack by free radicals and these attacks, collectively called oxidative stress, promote aging and diseases such as cancer, cataracts, arthritis, Alzheimer's, and heart disease.

We *can* fight back against free radicals by eating foods containing antioxidants such as vitamins A, E, and C; beans, broccoli, and dark leafy greens, such as spinach; and colorful fruits, such as blueberries, strawberries, and apples. Eating tomatoes, which contain the potent antioxidant lycopene, may also lower the risk for prostate cancer. We can get additional antioxidant vitamins by taking supplements (see Essential 8). I also recommend taking a multivitamin as well as a 500 mg (milligram) vitamin C tablet daily.

The box on pages 310–311 contains a list of some healthy antioxidant fruits and vegetables, which will help you plan your Longevity Diet meals and snacks.

Proteins, Lean Meats, and Healthy Fats

This food group gives us long-lasting appetite satisfaction while helping us to achieve and maintain our ideal body weight. Healthy proteins and fats also help us avoid age-related illnesses such as Alzheimer's and heart disease. Proteins, made up of amino acids, are the major structural component of all the body's cells and the enzymes that keep those cells functioning. Of the twenty vital amino acids our bodies need to function, nine of them — the *essential* amino acids —

Antioxidant Fruits and Vegetables

Fruits
Apricots
Avocados
Berries:
    blackberries,
    blueberries,
    cranberries,
    raspberries,
    strawberries
Cherries
Citrus: grapefruit,
    oranges
    tangerines,
    tangelos, lemons,
    limes
Dried fruits:
    apricots, prunes,
    raisins
Frozen juice bars
Grapes
Kiwi
Mangos
Melons:
    cantaloupe,
    honeydew
Nectarines

Papayas
Peaches
Pears
Pineapples
Plums
Tomatoes:
    Tomato juice,
    V-8, tomato
    sauce

Vegetables
Alfalfa sprouts
Asparagus
Beets
Bell peppers
Broccoli florets
Brussels sprouts
Carrots
Cauliflower
Celery
Corn
Cucumbers
Eggplant
Garlic
Green, leafy
    vegetables:

Vegetables (*cont.*)	Kale
cabbage,	Mushrooms
lettuce,	Onions
spinach,	Winter squash
Swiss chard	Zucchinis
Juices: from any	
vegetable	

cannot be synthesized by our bodies and must be gotten through our diet.

Animal proteins such as fish, poultry, meat, eggs, milk, yogurt, and cheese supply these nine essential amino acids, and are therefore considered *complete* proteins. Plant proteins such as nuts, seeds, legumes, and grains are often called *incomplete* proteins because they can be deficient in one or more of the essential amino acids. Soybeans, a type of legume, are unique because they contain all of the amino acids needed to make a complete protein, just like meat. They also contain isoflavones, a plant-based compound that may reduce the risk of some types of cancer. Many foods are made from soybeans, including tofu. Another way to get soy into our diet is through soy protein isolate powder, which can be mixed into a smoothie with fruit, or stirred into oat-meal. People on vegan diets can get adequate complete proteins by combining their sources of incomplete proteins, making sure they get all of the essential amino acids each day.

Milk and other dairy products are high in calcium and not only strengthen bones but also lower the risk of developing colon cancer. A recent analysis of ten large studies found that people who drank more than one eight-ounce glass of milk each day were significantly less likely to develop colon cancer than those who drank less than two glasses per week. Other studies suggest that increased calcium, particularly from lowfat and nonfat dairy foods, may not only help people lose weight, but may assist baby boomers in controlling the expanding waistlines that sometimes accompany middle age.

Many protein-rich foods contain fat, which is often mistakenly regarded as a dietary taboo — just check out the numerous food labels highlighting fat-free this or lowfat that on the container. Many people don't realize that there are some health benefits to eating a certain amount of fat, as long as it's the *right type* of fat. Scientific evidence has shown that foods high in omega-3 fats, such as fish, olive oil, and soy products, reduce the risk for cardiovascular disease, stroke, and Alzheimer's disease.

A study recently published in the journal *Nature* found that olive oil contains a natural form of the common anti-inflammatory drug ibuprofen (marketed as Advil or Motrin), which could explain why eating olive oil may lower the risk of cancer, heart disease, and Alzheimer's disease. Our UCLA research team has found that ibuprofen and another common anti-inflammatory drug, naproxen sodium (marketed as Aleve), have the ability to actually dissolve the abnormal protein plaques that are thought to cause Alzheimer's disease.

We want to avoid foods high in saturated fats, trans fats, and omega-6 fats, including many cuts of beef, poultry fat, butter, cream, whole milk, tropical oils (e.g., palm, coconut), and many frozen and canned foods (check the labeling for contents). Trans fats are often found in commercially baked goods (e.g., packaged cookies, cakes, and crackers), which also tend to contain high amounts of white sugar and flour. These unhealthy fats are known to raise "bad" LDL cholesterol levels, which increase the risk for heart disease and other ailments.

Eating foods containing small amounts of healthy fats helps our bodies absorb essential vitamins and protects our cell membranes. It also helps to satisfy our hunger so we consume fewer calories overall. It is recommended that we limit added fat to no more than six teaspoons for an average two-thousand-calorie day. However, if you are a small or inactive person, you will burn fewer calories each day and should consider consuming less fat and fewer calories. A recent study found that restaurant diners who dipped their bread in olive oil (omega-3) actually ate less total bread and took in fewer calories than diners who used butter (omega-6). I'm not encouraging the consumption of mass quantities of bread and oil; but a limited amount of olive or walnut oil for a salad or a bit of sesame oil in a stir-fry makes a tasty and healthy addition to a meal.

The American Heart Association recommends eating fish twice a week in order to get enough omega-3 fats. Fish-eaters tend to have lower rates of arthritis and may have a lower risk for depression and some cancers. Wild salmon, halibut, light tuna, cod, flounder, sole, sea bass, shrimp, lobster, scallops, and crab are excellent choices. Farmed fish should be avoided, since it has more total fat than wild, and the additional fat is largely omega-6. But eating too much fish may lead to increased body levels of mercury, which can cause fatigue, hair loss, and other symptoms. Larger fish such as shark and swordfish tend to have higher mercury levels per ounce than smaller fish such as salmon or sole, which may be wiser choices.

Use the following list of proteins, lean meats, and healthy fats to help plan your meals and snacks.

Proteins, Lean Meats, and Healthy Fats

Beef (lean cuts)
Chicken breast
Cheese — nonfat or lowfat cottage, cream (light), goat, mozzarella, ricotta, Swiss
Eggs (egg whites preferred)
Fish: anchovy, bluefish, halibut, herring, mackerel, salmon, sardines, sea bass, trout, tuna, whitefish
Milk: lowfat or nonfat (skim), soy milk (lowfat)
Nuts: walnuts, peanuts (actually a legume), almonds

Peanut butter	powder, soy
Seeds and oils:	meat
canola, flaxseed,	substitutes, soy
olive, sesame,	cereals, tofu
sunflower,	Turkey breast
walnut	Yogurt: high-
Soy proteins: soy	quality lowfat or
protein isolate	nonfat

Whole Grains, Legumes and Other Carbohydrates

Studies have found that whole-grain and high-fiber foods help control weight gain, lower blood pressure, prevent strokes, and reduce the risk for diabetes and heart disease. Carbohydrates are the body's main source of energy, and this food group's multitude of choices are some of the most delicious and satisfying foods on the Longevity Diet. Steaming brown-rice risotto with seafood, a crust of fresh whole-grain bread, and a crisp vegetable salad is a meal that sounds good to me on any diet.

Whole grains, unlike many processed ones, contain vitamins, fiber, minerals, phytochemicals, plant proteins, and other healthful ingredients. They are absorbed by the body much more slowly

The Glycemic Index System

All carbohydrates are made up of sugar molecules. After we eat and digest them, these sugars, known as glucose, end up in our blood system. A method for classifying carbohydrates in which 0 refers to the healthiest carbohydrate and 100 the unhealthiest is known as the glycemic index, or GI. The GI measures how fast and how far blood sugar rises after we eat a food that contains carbohydrates. The carbohydrate's underlying structure is what influences its GI rating and determines how easily it can be digested. "Instant" foods are digested and absorbed into the bloodstream very quickly and thus have a high GI rating, much like a piece of white bread, which has a high GI score, and causes blood sugar to spike rapidly when eaten. Munch on some brown rice (low GI rating), on the other hand, and you'll digest more slowly, causing a lower and gentler change in blood sugar. Also, carbohydrate foods with added fat or acid (vinegar, lemon juice) are absorbed into the bloodstream more gradually. High-GI diets are not considered longevity-promoting, since they increase the risk for diabetes and heart disease. The table on pages 319–320 gives examples of GI ratings for common foods.

than processed foods are. Whole-wheat bread, brown or wild rice, oatmeal, whole-grain pasta, and even popcorn are common sources of whole grains.

The fiber component of whole-grain carbohydrates cannot be broken down by the digestive system, so it moves through and keeps everything moving along with it in a healthful way. This is partially why eating fiber-rich whole grains and other high-fiber foods protect against constipation, hemorrhoids, and diverticulosis. High-fiber whole grains also lower our risk for cancer of the colon, rectum, stomach, pancreas, endometrium, ovary, and prostate. When food manufacturers process carbohydrate products, they remove much of the fiber, which increases the food's glycemic index (see box). Processing also removes many vitamins, minerals, and phytonutrients.

How Much Common Foods Spike Blood Sugar

Minimal (*Glycemic Index <40*)

Apples
Apricots, dried
Cherries
Fettuccine
Lentils

Lima beans
Nonfat yogurt
Peanuts
Skim milk
Soybeans

Low (*Glycemic Index 40–54*)

Baked beans
Bran cereal
Canned chickpeas
Cooked carrots
Grapes
Oranges

Orange juice
Oatmeal
Spaghetti
Unsweetened
    apple juice

Moderate (*Glycemic Index 55–70*)

Banana
Brown rice
Natural muesli
    cereal

Oat-bran cereal
Pineapples
Whole wheat
    bread

High (Glycemic Index 71–84)

Bagels	Pretzels
Cocoa Puffs	Puffed-wheat
Cheerios	cereal
Cornflakes	Total cereal
French fries	Vanilla wafers
Jelly beans	

Maximal (Glycemic Index >85)

Dried dates	Instant mashed
French	potatoes
baguettes	Instant rice

An easy way to get whole grains into your diet is to add them to recipes you already make without whole grains. Try adding wild rice or pearl barley to your next soup, stew, or casserole; add whole oats to cookies and other desserts; and if you like to bake, try replacing half the amount of white flour with whole-grain flour. Not only will the food taste great, you'll know that everyone eating it is getting a little longevity boost. You can also switch from white breads to 100 percent whole wheat, from refined cold cereals to whole-grain cereals, and from soda crackers to whole-grain wheat and rye crackers.

Whole-grain foods, including everything from a tasty array of whole-wheat pastas to long-grain rice pilaf mixes, are no longer specialty items for the very health-conscious shoppers with hours of time on their hands to seek them out. They are readily available, mass-marketed items accessible to everyone willing to take a few moments to notice what they're buying and eating. It is easy to shop and eat well, and the longevity benefits are tremendous.

The following list contains suggestions to help ensure that you get this basic healthy food group into your Longevity Diet.

Whole Grains, Legumes, and Other Carbohydrates

Barley: pearl, pot, or Scotch
Beans: black, cannellini, chickpeas (garbanzos), green, haricot, kidney, lima, pinto, soybeans
Bran: muffins, cereals, raw flakes
Breads: whole-wheat, multi-grain, rye, oat
Buckwheat: pancakes, kasha, muffins

Cereals:
  whole-grain,
  whole-wheat,
  wheat-berry,
  oat, bran, wheat
  germ, puffed
  rice, kasha
Crackers (whole
  grain)
Lentils: soup, dip
Oats: oatmeal,
  oatmeal cookies,
  oat cereals
Pasta: (whole-grain)
linguini,
  spaghetti,
  rigatoni,
  macaroni
Peas: Chinese,
  split, black-eyed
Popcorn
  (unbuttered)
Rice: brown, wild
Tortillas (corn)
Tortilla chips
  (baked)
Whole-wheat
  couscous

Michele R. had always been tall and thin. In the sixth grade, the boys teased her and called her "Beanstalk." In college, those same boys practically killed themselves to get a date with her. Never a fan of real exercise, Michele enjoyed an occasional game of tennis and maybe a walk on the beach, and *all* her girlfriends hated her for being able to eat whatever she wanted and never gain an ounce.

But after age forty-six, things began to change. Usually full of energy, Michele started feeling tired a lot — especially after eating. And although she had gained only a pound or two since high school, her clothes didn't seem to fit her in the same way — pants and skirts felt tighter in the waist, tops seemed snug, and she just couldn't wait to change into her sweats at the end of the day. It got to the point that Michele felt so exhausted after dinner, she could hardly keep her eyes open or carry on a conversation. Because she attributed these changes to getting older, Michele finally contacted me at the UCLA Center on Aging and came into the clinic to discuss her tiredness and other symptoms she was experiencing.

After an in-depth discussion, it became clear that Michele had been eating a diet high in carbohydrates — many of them with a high glycemic index — and very little meat and other proteins. This diet was likely causing her blood sugar levels to spike sharply as she ate, and then come crashing down quickly afterward — leaving her feeling tired and depleted. Not only was this blood-glucose roller coaster bad for her heart and longevity, it was leading to weight gain around the abdomen, which was setting her up to develop insulin resistance and possibly adult-onset diabetes. Also, since the protein in her diet was insufficient, Michele may not have been getting enough essential amino acids, which make up the body's cells and the enzymes that keep those cells functioning.

I suggested that Michele eat a combination of all three healthy food groups: fruits and vegetables; proteins, lean meats, and healthy fats; and whole grains — in correct and healthy portions throughout the day. I also mentioned that to remain healthy, strong, and young-looking — as well as to get those clothes to fit like they used to — she should be sure to exercise regularly.

Three Days on the Longevity Diet

The proven benefits of each of the three food groups overlap. Fish and nuts not only contain protein and omega-3 fats, they are also good sources of antioxidant vitamins; many whole grains possess potent antioxidants, as well as some protein, fiber, and other nutrients; olive and other vegetable oils contain not only omega-3 fats, but also vitamin E antioxidants. The Longevity Diet makes it easy to combine these food groups to stay fit, trim, and healthy for the long haul, while still indulging in those *cheat eats* we may want to pamper ourselves with once in a while.

To get a better idea of how the diet works, here are the first three days that Shirley I. followed. Although she dropped two pounds during her first couple of weeks on the diet, Shirley did not set out to lose weight. Her goal was to feel healthier and stronger, look better, and reap the quality longevity benefits.

Recipes for menu suggestions marked with an asterisk (*) can be found in Appendix 1.

DAY ONE

Shirley drank a fresh, cool glass of water upon waking up.

Breakfast

¾–1 cup whole-oat oatmeal topped with 1 teaspoon brown sugar
½ cup lowfat (or nonfat) milk
½ grapefruit
Cup of coffee
Vitamin supplements: 1 multivitamin and 1 vitamin C (500 mg)

(The oatmeal — whole grain — *stars* in this meal.)

Midmorning Snack

½ cup lowfat cottage cheese, plus 1 tablespoon raisins mixed in
½ banana
Sparkling juice (1 part fruit juice plus 2 parts soda water, served over ice)

Lunch

Chef salad with mixed greens and sliced vegetables, 2 ounces sliced chicken, 1 ounce sliced lowfat Swiss cheese, 1 sliced egg white, tossed with olive oil vinaigrette dressing

2 whole-grain crackers
Sliced pear
Iced tea

(The chef salad meal *costars* vegetables and protein.)

Afternoon Snack
1 cup tomato soup or juice
1 ounce roasted almonds
Soda water with lemon

Dinner
Iceberg lettuce wedge with Roquefort Dressing*
Grilled 6-ounce salmon filet with herbs and lemon slices
½ cup wild rice
Steamed broccoli
Strawberry Sorbet*
Glass of white wine, ice water

(Salmon filet gives protein the *starring* role.)

Nighttime Snack
Frozen nonfat yogurt

DAY TWO

A refreshing glass of water.

Breakfast

Raisin-Bran Muffins* spread with ricotta cheese and real-fruit jam

½ cup fresh blueberries (frozen are good, too!)

Coffee

Vitamin supplements

(Whole grains *star.*)

Midmorning Snack

Bag of raw vegetables: celery/red bell pepper/tomatoes

1 ounce string cheese

Lunch

3-ounce tuna sandwich on whole-wheat bread, with lettuce and tomato (light mayo)

Crisp apple

Soda water with lemon

(Vegetables/fruits and whole grains share star billing, backed by a small amount of protein from the tuna in this healthy cross-trained meal.)

Afternoon Snack

Peach slices topped with ⅓ cup cottage

cheese and a tablespoon of chopped almonds
Soda water with lemon

Dinner
6-ounce grilled chicken breast with herbs
Cheesy Pesto with Pasta* (side serving)
Steamed carrots
Apple Crumble à la Mode*
Glass of red wine, ice water

(Protein *stars.*)

Nighttime Snack
Frozen fruit-juice bar

DAY THREE
Wake-up water.

Breakfast
Vegetable omelet (use 1 whole egg plus 2
or 3 egg whites)
½ cup fresh or frozen blueberries
Coffee
Vitamin supplements: 1 multivitamin and
1 vitamin C (500 mg)

(Omelet — protein — *stars* in this meal.)

Midmorning Snack

½ cup nonfat plain or flavored yogurt with 1 tablespoon raisins

Tea (green has the most antioxidant value)

Lunch

Bowl of chicken soup (with white meat and vegetables)

Spinach salad with chopped apple and walnuts, vinaigrette dressing

Orange sections

Iced tea

(Fruits and vegetables *star.*)

Afternoon Snack

Raw vegetable sticks with 2 tablespoons of peanut butter (lowfat preferred)

Iced tea

Dinner

Tomato, avocado, and sweet onion salad; olive oil and vinegar

Mixed Seafood and Linguini* using ¾ cup whole-wheat linguini

Steamed asparagus spears

Cheat Eat: Slice of devil's food cake

Arnold Palmer on ice (½ iced tea and ½ lemonade)

(Seafood — protein — *stars* in this meal.)

Nighttime Snack
Sliced fresh apple with cinnamon

Losing Weight

Although many people lose pounds without even trying when they begin the Longevity Diet, others who wish to drop pounds more quickly can make some of the following modifications to the diet:

- Cut back on your carbohydrates and eat more lean and nonfat protein "starring" meals, along with vegetables, salad, and fruit for dessert.
- Cut out alcoholic beverages and *all* cheat eats.
- Limit your servings. Recent research shows that people eat less when they are served smaller portions.
- Remember to eat your healthy snacks between meals, so you don't get overly hungry and overeat later.
- Be sure to drink at least eight glasses of water a day.
- Increase your amount of exercise, especially the cardiovascular component.

Also, keep in mind that strength training helps build lean body mass, which raises your metabolism and helps you burn more calories and therefore lose more weight (see Essential 6).

This will serve as your *quick start* diet program, which should give you a greater sense of control, after which you can begin to add some more of the healthy whole grains, alcohol if you desire, and even the occasional cheat eat. You can stay on the weight reduction program as long as you need to, but unless you have more than ten pounds to lose, you should be able to transition to the regular Longevity Diet within four weeks and enjoy the benefits of a lifetime of delicious and healthy eating.

Getting Started

When preparing to begin the Longevity Diet, it's a good idea to take stock of your pantry and refrigerator, and make a shopping list of the foods you'll need for your first week of healthy longevity eating. Planning a few days' meals in advance will help.

By stocking up on some basics such as

fresh fruits, vegetables, and herbs, lean meats, fish, brown rice, olive oil, vinegar, whole-wheat bread and pasta, cheeses, eggs, nonfat yogurt, and milk, you will be ready to make just about any of the easy meals and recipes in this book, and many other delicious concoctions you come up with yourself.

Many people find it helpful to plan their cross-training meals and chart their progress using a daily food chart or diary. Make some copies of the following blank chart to help ensure that your meals and snacks include at least two of the three healthy food groups. Place an asterisk (*) next to the food that *stars* in each of your meals.

Day _____	Fruits/ Vegetables	Proteins/ Fats	Carbo- hydrates
Breakfast			
Snack			
Lunch			
Snack			
Dinner			
Snack			

Following the Longevity Diet

- Eat the foods you like the most from the following food groups. Each food group can *star* in up to two meals per day.
- Antioxidant fruits and vegetables
- Proteins, lean meats, and healthy fats
- Whole grains, legumes, and other carbohydrates
- Use mindful awareness to focus on how your body feels before, during, and after eating to help you gauge portion size and know when you've had enough.
- Occasionally indulge in a small portion of your favorite cheat eats.
- Drink at least eight glasses of water throughout the day.
- Enjoy two to three healthy between-meal snacks a day.
- Avoid excessive salts, bad fats, and high glycemic-index carbohydrates.
- If you wish to lose weight, cut back on carbohydrates, alcohol, and cheat eats until you reach your goal.

Essential 8

Modern Medicine for Feeling and Looking Younger

By medicine, life may be prolonged ...
— WILLIAM SHAKESPEARE

Medical breakthroughs in the last decade are promising to keep us alive and healthy longer than any generation before us. Within our lifetime, living past the age of one hundred may become commonplace. Modern medical technologies such as heart transplants and Lasik eye surgery have already become routine procedures. Complex neuroimaging techniques — windows into what used to be the hidden, secret workings of the body — have led to screening tests and new surgical methods that allow us to control and often beat major killers such as colon cancer and heart disease. More effective medicines with fewer side effects have added years to our lives. Soon, we may be able to manage Alzheimer's disease in the same way that we deal with high blood pressure today — through simple tests and preventive medicine.

This *Longevity Bible* Essential covers the newest medical techniques for *staying, feeling,* and *looking* young. We'll look at breakthrough interventions such as new cures for cancer, ways to fire up our libido, and the latest cosmetic innovations aimed at keeping us looking eternally youthful.

With the mapping of the human genome, we can now expect more targeted therapies that take into account an individual's specific genetic profile. Stem cells have the remarkable potential to develop into almost any cell type in the body, and scientists may eventually be able to grow these primitive cells to replace diseased ones, and even entire organs. Swedish scientists recently used adult human stem cells to generate functioning brain cells.

Nanotechnology is a new field that builds objects and substances one atom or molecule at a time. It is a form of molecular engineering that will lead to a manufacturing revolution. Scientists have already used nanotechnologies to build minute robots powered by the beat of a single heart cell. These could one day lead to micro-robotic heart muscles that would keep our hearts beating long beyond their previous capacity.

With obesity rapidly becoming one of the greatest health threats of the twenty-first century, scientists have developed an injectable hormone that literally switches off a person's appetite. In initial tests, it enabled people to lose over five pounds a month without trying. An implantable heart defibrillator is also being developed to provide an electric shock to the heart muscle to reset its rhythm in the event of a heart attack, which could save millions of lives each year.

Thanks to the latest in medical innovations, we should all start planning to look and feel younger — well into our eighties, nineties, and beyond. New treatments can make us *look* younger in a multitude of ways — from smoother skin to more hair — as well as *feel* younger, with greater mobility and improved joint function. We can now improve our quality of life by boosting our libidos and energy levels. With the wide array of medicines, treatments, and procedures becoming available, it is essential to become an informed consumer, choosing and monitoring your *medical portfolio* wisely — just as you would your financial portfolio. Knowing how to effectively use new medical technologies is a key to this quality longevity essential.

Living Longer

Only a generation ago, cancer was almost always fatal. Now there is not only earlier detection, but there are also more effective treatments and sometimes cures. Cancer and heart disease, however, are still the leading causes of death in the United States. In the most common form of heart disease, the coronary arteries — vessels that supply blood and nutrients to heart muscles — become clogged from the buildup of fatty plaque over time. For people with severe blockage of coronary arteries, bypass surgery or angioplasty can be lifesaving. In bypass surgery, the diseased coronary arteries are replaced by healthy blood vessels from the leg, arm, or chest. A less invasive alternative for some patients is angioplasty. In this procedure, the cardiologist inserts a balloon-tipped catheter into a large blood vessel in the arm or leg and guides it to the blocked coronary artery, where it is inflated to stretch the artery. A wire mesh tube, or *stent,* is left in place to keep the artery open.

With proper treatment, chronic and fatal conditions such as high blood pressure or high cholesterol pose less of a risk. In a study of patients with only mild elevations in blood pressure, treatment with anti-hypertensive drugs increased life expectancy by two to three years. Other studies have found that lowering blood pressure by only five points reduces the risk of stroke by an estimated 34 percent and heart disease by 21 percent.

A recent study found that taking a statin (cholesterol-lowering) drug within the first twenty-four hours after a heart attack can decrease the risk of death by 50 percent. Scientists have also found that statin drugs can reduce deaths from advanced heart failure by as much as 55 percent. By lowering blood cholesterol levels, statins keep fatty deposits from building up and eventually blocking circulation. The drugs may also protect the heart by reducing inflammation, which plays a role in heart failure.

Over the past decade, the total death rate from cancer has dropped by more than 12 percent in the United States. The greatest declines — accounting for over fifty-five thousand lives saved — were found in prostate and lung cancer in men, breast cancer in women, and colon cancer in both sexes. Earlier detection of prostate cancer is now possible through prostate-specific antigen (PSA) screening, a simple blood test.

A new cancer treatment, androgen blockade, can essentially beat cancer long enough for some patients to live normally and eventually die from unrelated causes. Better treatments for breast cancer, such as the drug tamoxifen and other chemo-therapies, are improving survival rates, along with widespread use of mammography for early detection. And invasive interventions are not always necessary to save lives. Recent reports published in the *New England Journal of Medicine* found that lumpectomy followed by radiation can be just as effective as complete mastectomy.

Colorectal cancer is the second leading cause of cancer deaths. If diagnosed early through colonoscopy, it is often curable with surgery. Risk for the disease increases after age fifty, particularly for those with a family history. Less than a third of Americans over age fifty have had a colonoscopy.

Although the preparation can be uncomfortable, this detection procedure takes only about a half hour and can be a lifesaver.

Feeling Younger

Besides extending life expectancy, medical interventions — drugs, surgeries, and alternative treatments — can improve our quality of life. Many patients are taking advantage of new technologies that allow them to monitor their own symptoms electronically. Wireless armbands can now take blood-sugar readings and beam them directly to physicians. "Smart" scales can wire your weight to the clinic and display back to you your doctor's follow-up questions and answers.

Managing Medicines

Numerous medications have become available to treat symptoms of severe diseases, as well as common and annoying age-related complaints. However, when we take too many drugs, we may get into trouble with side effects. Managing medicines can

When Nancy G. finally got to her mother's apartment, she knew they were already late for her mom's doctor's appointment. She frantically searched for Mom's daily blood-pressure chart — it was on the counter, hiding behind the insulin injection kit. Nancy called out to Mom to make sure she got her medications together — the doctor had specifically asked her to bring all her drugs to the appointment so he could make sure that her medicines weren't worsening her memory. When her mother came into the kitchen carrying two large shopping bags, Nancy once again felt frustrated by her mom's forgetfulness. "Mother, I told you that we don't have time to get to the mall today and return those gifts." But when Nancy looked *inside* the bags, she saw they were entirely filled with medicine bottles, samples, and prescriptions from various doctors. And these were just the drugs her mom was *currently* taking.

be a challenge — especially for older people, who tend to take more medicines throughout the day.

The average older person takes more than a half dozen prescription medicines at any one time, and the more medicines a person takes, the greater the possibility for side effects to occur. A recent study found that one out of every four older adults receives at least one inappropriate or unnecessary medicine. Also, many people still use older medicines they began taking several years ago that are often less safe than newer drugs developed for the same purpose.

As we get older, the receptors throughout our bodies become more sensitive to the effects of drugs, increasing the possibility of side effects at much lower doses. Also, our bodies become less efficient in breaking down and eliminating medicines, so that over time we may accumulate higher blood levels of drugs. This can lead to new or increased side effects, as well as interactions with other drugs that we hadn't experienced in the past. Even over-the-counter and herbal remedies, which many people consider safe, can sometimes have undesirable or dangerous side effects. For instance, someone taking ginkgo, aspirin, and vitamin E together

Alan F.'s wife kept nagging him to go back to the doctor for his routine checkup but he just didn't have the time — the hotel business had gotten so dog-eat-dog lately and there were so many young upstarts vying to secure management jobs like his. Besides, last time the doctor had put him on blood-pressure pills that made him so sleepy he'd hardly been able to keep his eyes open past 9 p.m. He knew his wife thought he just didn't want to be intimate with her anymore, but it wasn't true. He was simply too exhausted every night to deal with it. Unfortunately, Alan's growing marital stress at home, on top of the stress he had at work all day, wasn't doing his blood pressure any favors — even *with* the medication. Alan was beginning to feel depressed and considered asking his doctor about trying an antidepressant. But then he read that they could have negative sexual performance side effects, and that was the last thing he needed.

When Alan finally did go in for his

exam and explain all this, his physician switched him to a different blood-pressure medicine. The doctor told Alan to call sooner about any drug side effects that might arise when starting a new treatment. In fact, the doctor noted that the first blood-pressure medicine Alan had taken was occasionally associated with decreased libido. Alan wondered if he could get a doctor's note about that to give his wife.

With the new medicine change, Alan's energy and enthusiasm returned, along with his libido, and soon his depression lifted. The doctor had even given him some Viagra samples to try, but Alan didn't need them. His renewed vitality improved his outlook at work, as well. Alan's wife seemed happier, too, for some reason.

might experience unexpected bruising and excessive bleeding. Due to the changes in our bodies, doctors caring for older individuals often prescribe drugs in low doses initially and then slowly increase them as needed, to minimize any potential negative reactions.

Many medications have anticholinergic side effects, meaning that they oppose the actions of drugs prescribed for memory loss, thereby worsening memory. Over-the-counter antihistamines such as Benadryl can have this effect, particularly on older people. Drugs prescribed for anxiety — such as Xanax, Valium, or Librium — are frequently overused and can cause sedation and memory impairment, as well as an increased risk of falling. Drugs used to regulate heart rate or treat high blood pressure can make blood vessels less taut and decrease the heart's ability to pump blood. Since our vascular tone diminishes as we age anyway, medicines that aggravate this problem can lead to falls, head trauma, and other complications, so they should be taken with care.

When discussing possible drug interactions with your doctor, be sure to mention any over-the-counter medicines you take, as well as supplements and foods you eat that may increase or decrease the effects of your medicines. Some drugs interact with grapefruit juice, which can increase the medicine's effects and the risk for side effects. Be sure you truly need a particular drug, and that your doctor is aware of all the medicines you currently take. This is especially important if you are under the care of more than one doctor. Pharmacists can be helpful in answering questions regarding drug interactions, as well. For more information on specific drug interactions check the Web site *www.druginteractioncenter.org*.

It is important *not* to stop taking prescribed medications on your own. Researchers at the University of Michigan found that when middle-aged and older people stop their prescription medicines without consulting their doctors, 32 percent experience a serious decline in health.

The U.S. Food and Drug Administration (FDA) provides an Internet guide (*www.fda.gov/oc/buyonline/default.htm*) describing the risks of buying medicines and related products on the Internet. Dangers are everywhere on the Web, including contaminated or counterfeit products, incorrect dosages, expired medicines, illegal uses of medicines, and other problems. The guide helps consumers with clues for differentiating fake Internet sites from legitimate ones. Several points to keep in mind include finding out whether or not the online pharmacy is licensed and provides access to a registered pharmacist, being cautious of sites based in foreign countries, avoiding online pharmacy sites that let you get medicines without a doctor's prescription, and making sure the site provides an actual street address and phone number — an e-mail address is not enough.

Blood Pressure — Staying Low

Hypertension affects approximately 60 percent of the population, a 10 percent increase in just the past decade. Under high pressure, stiffened blood vessels can rupture, and may cause cerebrovascular disease involving blood leakage into the brain tissue, and eventual stroke. A stroke is often defined as the death of brain cells, resulting in a loss of physical or mental function, or both. When tissue death occurs in the heart, it pumps less effectively, which can cause heart failure or death.

Contrary to popular belief, people cannot tell if their blood pressure is high, and most patients with high blood pressure have no symptoms. Yet high blood pressure is easily detected with a blood-pressure cuff and stethoscope at your doctor's office or with a home device, and it's effectively treated with a variety of antihypertensive medicines. The most effective strategy combines medicine and lifestyle changes — avoiding cigarettes and overeating and getting enough exercise are crucial, as well as staying away from the salt shaker. Regular exercise and a healthy diet can sometimes even eliminate the need for medicines.

A new study suggests that what was previously considered normal blood pressure may not be so normal. The current guidelines set normal systolic blood pressure (when the heart is contracting) at less than 140 millimeters, and the diastolic (when the heart is relaxed) at less than 90. In this new study, patients had normal blood pressure, but were still at risk for heart problems. Those who received antihypertensive drugs had mild drops in blood pressure and a 30 percent decline in heart attacks, strokes, or hospitalizations for chest pain.

Keeping Bones Strong

More than ten million Americans, mostly women, suffer from osteoporosis, which essentially means that the bones get porous, brittle, and weak. Hip fractures are a major risk when bones weaken, and each year the number of women suffering from hip fractures exceeds the combined number who get heart attacks, strokes, and breast cancer. Age, estrogen deficiency, family history, and smoking are risk factors, and diagnosis is made using a special bone density scan called a DEXA (dual energy X-ray absorptiometry) scan, which is recommended for all women over age sixty-five, regardless of their risk.

To keep bones healthy, the National Academy of Sciences and the National Osteoporosis Foundation recommend daily calcium intakes of 1,000 to 1,200 milligrams for adult men and women, preferably from food, but also from supplements, if necessary. Between four hundred and eight hundred international units (IUs) of Vitamin D also are needed to help the body to absorb calcium.

Several medicines are available to treat osteoporosis, once it is diagnosed, which can greatly reduce the risk for bone fractures. Estrogen replacement therapy has been shown to significantly decrease this risk, and the bisphosphonates alendronate (Fosamax) and risedronate (Actonel) can substantially reduce the risk of both hip and spine fractures.

Calcitonin (Miacalcin) can be taken either by injection or through nose spray and is effective in increasing bone density, but mainly in the spine. It has been found to reduce pain from compression fractures of the spine. Selective estrogen receptor modulators augment bone strength without negative effects on the breasts or the uterus, but they can increase the risk of strokes.

Lifestyle has a large impact on hip-fracture risk. Routine weight-bearing, stretching, and strengthening exercises (see Essential 6) will improve muscle and bone strength, as well as balance. Seniors who begin a weight-lifting regimen not only help to keep their bones young and strong, but can actually improve bone density and eventually feel ten or more years younger. A recent study of forty-six pairs of identical twins found that moderate alcohol intake was associated with greater bone density, which reduces the risk for fractures.

Preventing and Controlling Diabetes

Approximately eighteen million Americans suffer from diabetes. Their bodies have trouble metabolizing sugar or glucose, and often pills or insulin injections are needed to get sugar from the blood into the body's cells to maintain the chemical reactions that sustain consciousness and life. Diet, weight control, and exercise are the most effective strategies for preventing and controlling this condition, but if oral medications are needed to lower blood-sugar levels, several are safe and effective. Sulfonylurea drugs stimulate the pancreas to produce and release more insulin. Another option is to use newer drugs known as meglitinides, which work quickly and can be safer.

Pharmaceutical companies have been pushing to develop drugs to prevent diabetes symptoms before people develop the full-blown disease. Metformin, marketed as Glucophage, as well as rosiglitazone (Avandia), treat diabetes symptoms, and studies show that such drugs may help prevent the disease in some people at risk. A recent report from the journal *Lancet* found that a group of overweight patients at risk for diabetes did significantly better than the placebo group, on a new drug known as rimonabant, which was effective in helping them to lose weight, improve insulin response, and lower blood cholesterol.

Cholesterol Busting

For many people, blood cholesterol levels creep upward over the years and, if untreated, may result in heart disease and stroke. Risk factors for developing high cholesterol include diabetes, smoking, high blood pressure, lack of exercise, and obesity. Quitting smoking, losing weight, dieting, and getting regular exercise all contribute to lower cholesterol levels.

For years, doctors have been telling us to control our cholesterol levels, especially the LDL, or "bad" cholesterol. A new report from the National Cholesterol Education Program updates earlier guidelines setting LDL goals for high-risk people to 70 (down from 100). These new levels mean that an estimated forty million Americans should be taking some action to lower their cholesterol, including taking statin drugs.

Recent research suggests that some patients should be on cholesterol-lowering drugs regardless of their blood cholesterol levels. The American College of Physicians recently recommended that all diabetics age fifty-five years or older should be on statin drugs, as should younger diabetics with other risk factors such as heart disease or high blood pressure. The guidelines stemmed from a review of studies finding that statin drugs reduced the rate of heart attacks and other cardiac problems by approximately 23 percent in diabetics with cardiac risks.

The power of statins appears to benefit other illnesses. In laboratory studies, statin drugs inhibit the growth of colon-cancer cells, and a recent study of nearly four thousand volunteers found that at least five years of statin use was associated with a 47 percent reduction in the risk of colorectal cancer. Although these studies are encouraging, doctors are not yet recommending statins as preventive treatments for cancer until additional investigations confirm these initial findings. Other research suggests that statins may delay the onset of Alzheimer's disease or delay its progression.

Keep Your Joints Moving

Osteoarthritis is the most common form of arthritis and can be a debilitating progressive disease. There is no cure, but treatments have advanced considerably in recent years. The big push in therapy has been to augment treatments that reduce pain and increase mobility with therapies that interfere with the actual disease progression. Most current treatment strategies include medicines along with physical therapy, exercise, weight management, and, as a last resort, surgery.

Nonsteroidal anti-inflammatory drugs (NSAIDs) relieve pain and fight inflammation and are available over the counter or by prescription. Examples include ibuprofen (Advil, Motrin, and others) and naproxen sodium (Aleve). These drugs do have potential side effects, such as bleeding, ulcers, and liver and kidney damage. Newer anti-inflammatory drugs known as COX-2 inhibitors (e.g., Celebrex, Bextra, and Vioxx) were originally thought to be safer as far as causing stomach bleeding, but potential cardiac side effects led manufacturers to take several of them off the market.

Over-the-counter Tylenol (acetaminophen) can reduce pain as effectively as NSAIDs, but taking more than the recommended dose may damage the liver. Another approach involves the use of lidocaine patches that are applied to areas of pain, such as the back or the knee. A recent study presented at the American Pain Society found that such patches were as effective as the anti-inflammatory drug Celebrex. The lidocaine, which is similar to the novocaine injected to numb the gums during dental procedures, inhibits pain signals to the brain but does not cause numbness. The only potential side effect from the patches is minor skin irritation.

Surgical techniques for joint replacement — most often the knee or hip — have advanced considerably, and these are now often outpatient procedures that allow people to get back on their feet quickly. The surgeon removes the damaged joint and replaces it with a plastic or metal prosthesis. Many patients resume normal levels of activity and enjoy improved mobility and pain reduction.

Alzheimer's Disease Prevention and Treatment

Alzheimer's disease afflicts approximately five million Americans, and millions more suffer from mild cognitive impairment, which puts them at risk for developing the disease. Family members and friends also suffer as they watch patients gradually lose their memory and other cognitive functions. Recent research has shown that lifestyle choices can significantly lower the risk for developing the disease. Innovative medicines and vaccines that might delay its onset are under investigation.

Most of the currently available drugs to improve memory and other cognitive symptoms do so by enhancing the brain's level of acetylcholine, the chemical neurotransmitter that facilitates the passage of nerve impulses across synapses. The brains of Alzheimer's patients have a deficiency of acetylcholine, which can result from either impaired production or excess breakdown by enzymes called cholinesterases. Drugs such as Aricept, Exelon, and Razadyne inhibit these enzymes, so they are called "cholinesterase inhibitors."

Memantine, marketed as Namenda, works on the brain's NMDA (N-methyl-D-aspartate) receptors by blocking the chemical glutamate, which overstimulates these receptors, allowing too much calcium to enter cells, leading to cell destruction. Namenda has been approved for patients with moderate to severe Alzheimer's disease, but many clinicians find it effective in milder stages, as well. The drug is safe when used with a cholinesterase inhibitor drug such as Aricept, and initial studies show that the combination provides a greater benefit than using only one drug.

Dosing of Commonly Used Drugs for Dementia

Drug	Start Dose	Highest Dose
Donepezil (Aricept)	5 mg, once a day	10 mg, once a day
Rivastigmine (Exelon)	1.5 mg, twice a day	6 mg, twice a day
Galantamine (Razadyne ER)	8 mg, once a day	24 mg, once a day
Memantine (Namenda)	5 mg, once a day	10 mg, twice a day

Alzheimer's patients who take these drugs need fewer medications for treating depression and behavior problems. They also remain at home and out of nursing homes longer than patients who do not take the medicines. These drugs not only improve memory and thinking, but can also reduce agitation and depression and can help with related illnesses, including vascular and Lewy Body Dementia. At UCLA, we are testing these drugs to see if they slow down brain aging in healthy people and possibly prevent Alzheimer's disease.

Scientists have found that the earlier the disease is recognized and treated, the better the outcome. In September 2004, the Centers for Medicare and Medicaid Services approved the use of positron emission tomography (PET) scans for Medicare reimbursement to assist doctors in better diagnosing Alzheimer's disease, in part so that the disease can be recognized and treated earlier. A recent study indicated that when Aricept was used in patients with mild cognitive impairment, it delayed the onset of Alzheimer's disease, as compared with a placebo.

At UCLA, our approach to Alzheimer's disease is to protect the brain before damage sets in — using several of the *Longevity Bible* Essentials. Our initial studies found that healthy volunteers ages thirty-five to seventy who spent just two weeks on a healthy lifestyle program, combining body fitness, mental aerobics, healthy diet, and stress reduction, experienced significant improvement in brain efficiency in a key memory center where Alzheimer's disease often strikes. In some people, memory scores improved by over 200 percent — in just fourteen days — as if volunteers had subtracted two decades from their brain age.

Our scientific team at UCLA has developed a new way to use the PET scanner so that the physical evidence of Alzheimer's disease, the abnormal amyloid protein build-up, can be measured in the living patient, as opposed to the traditional method whereby Alzheimer's could be proven only after a patient died, through autopsy. Our research group has been able to spot these abnormal proteins using the new amyloid-PET scanner in people with only mild cognitive impairment, years before they are likely to develop Alzheimer's disease. This will allow doctors to initiate prevention strategies as soon as possible. Many companies are developing drugs and vaccines designed to disrupt the buildup of the amyloid proteins that begin accumulating in the brain's memory centers early in adulthood and may lead to Alzheimer's disease.

Avoiding the Blues

An estimated 15 percent of the population develops a clinical depression at some point in their lives. When left untreated, patients experience not just emotional symptoms of sadness, loss of interest, and guilt, but also have physical symptoms, including weight loss, fatigue, and insomnia. Depressed people also tend to experience more physical pain. Professional treatment of the depression can alleviate both the physical and emotional symptoms. Many depressions involve more than one trigger or cause, with overlapping psychological and biological factors contributing. Regardless of the specific cause, patients who receive psychotherapy, antidepressant drugs, or both usually improve, even if their symptoms are severe.

One feature of depression — decreased ability to concentrate — seems to become more prominent as we age. Middle-aged and older people tend to emphasize these concentration difficulties and their depressions are often colored by memory complaints. Unfortunately, many people still consider depression to be a sign of character weakness, so they avoid seeking professional help or taking antidepressants.

What those people often don't realize is that untreated depression can increase a person's risk for serious physical illness or even death, as well as raise the risk for suicide. The life-expectancy rate for patients whose depressions are properly treated and improved is twice that of those who do not receive adequate care.

Although all types of antidepressant drugs have been effective in relieving some symptoms of depression, the improved side effect profiles of the newer antidepressants, such as fluoxetine (Prozac), sertraline (Zoloft), citalopram (Celexa), or paroxetine (Paxil), to mention a few, have caused them to become preferred treatments over older medicines such as amitriptyline (Elavil) or imipramine (Tofranil). These older medicines can potentially worsen memory performance because of their anticholinergic side effects. Some also cause blood pressure drops that can cause people to fall when they get up too quickly.

It is best to start low and go slowly with antidepressant medicines, particularly when treating older people. Many primary-care physicians can treat depression quite effectively using antidepressants, but for a complicated and more severe depression, the expertise of a psychiatrist may be needed. A psychiatrist with additional geriatric training can offer the most sophisticated care for some depressed older patients.

Protecting Vision

As we age, vision tends to decline, and it often gets harder to read small print, whether it's in a newspaper or on a pillbox. To accommodate the millions of baby boomers with lower visual acuity, several publishers are now increasing the height and print size of their mass-market paperbacks. If you can't find your favorite novel with the right font size, corrective lenses are available in a variety of shapes and sizes.

Eye disease is also more likely as we age, but preventive measures — including sunglasses to block damaging ultraviolet light, getting enough antioxidant fruits and vegetables, or taking supplements such as vitamins A, C, and E — greatly reduce risks. Because diabetes and hypertension can lead to eye disease, a healthy diet and regular exercise are effective prevention strategies. Also, regular eye exams, including checks of eye pressure, are essential.

Approximately 50 percent of older adults get *cataracts* that cloud vision from damage to the lens. Vision often improves following cataract surgery to replace the cloudy lens with a clear plastic one. Laser or conventional surgery also may benefit *macular degeneration,* a common eye disorder in older people that causes hazy vision and a central blind spot from the breakdown of light-sensitive cells in the central part of the eye's retina.

Glaucoma causes vision loss in approximately three million Americans. Excess fluid elevates eye pressure and damages the optic nerve, a bundle of nerve fibers at the back of the eye. With early detection, treatment, and monitoring, blind spots and eventual blindness usually can be prevented. One of the most prescribed eye drops for lowering eye pressure is a prostaglandin analogue known as latanoprost (Xalatan). Research has found that after two years of treatment with Xalatan, only 7 percent of patients require additional glaucoma medicine or need to switch to another medicine. Other commonly used alternatives are bimatoprost (Lumigan), travoprost (Travatan), and timolol (Timoptic). If eyedrops alone don't bring down eye pressure, an oral medication may be added, such as a carbonic anhydrase inhibitor. Laser treatments and conventional surgery are other options that may be necessary to lower eye pressure.

Hearing Well

The blaring rock concerts some of us enjoyed in our youth were lots of fun, but the exposure to those high decibel levels can catch up with us eventually. Approximately one third or more of older adults have some degree of hearing loss, and exposure to loud noises is one of the most common contributing factors. It is best to avoid exposure to extreme sounds by either using ear protection or just not going there. Although hearing aids can help many forms of hearing loss, only about one out of every five people who could benefit actually use them. A doctor who specializes in hearing can help guide you to the best intervention. The wide range of hearing aids available include cochlear implants, small devices that are surgically implanted under the skin, behind the ear. A recent study found that such implants significantly improve not just the comprehension of speech, but overall quality of life, as well.

Libido Boosters

Individuals differ in their sexual needs and desires throughout life. As people age, the hormone testosterone declines in both men and women, which may diminish sexual desire. Also, physical illnesses, depression, hormonal changes associated with menopause, and some medications can reduce sex drive. Chronic pain can also limit sexual activity, so careful timing of pain medicines can make sex more enjoyable and satisfying. Despite such age-related changes, several treatments are safe and effective and help millions to continue to have fulfilling sex throughout their lives.

Female Enhancers. After menopause, hormonal changes may diminish sex drive in women, but many women find they can get a libido boost with estrogen replacement therapy. Although it isn't clear that estrogen replacement has a direct effect on libido, it has been shown to help those who experience pain associated with intercourse. Because of concern about long-term side effects from estrogen pills or patches, many have turned to locally applied estrogen creams. These creams also help reduce vaginal dryness, which often hinders post-menopausal sex drive. Sexual activity itself increases vaginal blood flow, which stimulates lubrication.

Testosterone is usually thought of as a male sex hormone, but women also have small amounts in their bodies, produced primarily by their ovaries. After menopause, testosterone levels will decline, which can lower the drive for sex. Although not yet approved by the FDA, the testosterone patch has been found to improve sexual desire in women with low libido. In a recent controlled study, the testosterone patch increased sexual desire and satisfaction in women who had had their ovaries surgically removed. The patch is usually applied to the lower stomach area and is changed twice each week.

Male Enhancers. You've probably seen the TV ads showing a middle-aged couple walking hand-in-hand on the beach, or a man and woman relaxing in a hot tub for two. With the introduction of Cialis and Levitra, Viagra no longer has the corner on the erectile dysfunction market. The clinical impression is that all three drugs are similar in effectiveness, though Cialis claims to last about thirty-six hours — you can't be *too* ready if the time is right —

compared to about four hours for the others.

Doctors who prescribe these drugs should first check for high blood pressure, diabetes, and other medical conditions. These medicines should not be used more than once daily, and should never be used in combination with nitroglycerine, because it can be lethal. Recent rare reports of sudden vision loss in some men who took Viagra have led the manufacturer to change its labeling, but whether the drug directly causes this side effect has not been substantiated.

Supplements and Hormones

People of all ages spend billions each year on dietary supplements. Despite the numerous dramatic promises of a better sex life, a more muscular physique, or a cure for a variety of illnesses, the safety and the effectiveness of many of these products often fall short of the claims. As we get older, we are more inclined to use supplements: The majority of people age sixty and older currently take some kind of supplement.

False claims have been a problem for

many years. Back in 1994, the Dietary Supplement and Health Education Act set forth the only standards for manufacturers, who are responsible for the truthfulness of label claims. Manufacturers must have evidence that supports their claims, but the FDA provides no guidelines for validating that evidence, nor does it require manufacturers to submit that evidence.

Of course, many of the claims are enticing. The supplement called conjugated linoleic acid, or CLA, has been touted as effective for weight loss and muscle building, and as a preventive treatment for heart disease, cancer, and diabetes. Although some initial studies were interesting, there is no definitive evidence to back the claims. Also, many herbal sex aids sold in magazines and on the Internet are, at best, ineffective and, at worst, dangerous.

To prove that a supplement really works for a specific illness or condition, scientists need to complete a "double-blind" clinical trial. To do this, they need to compare their supplement to an inactive placebo, and make sure neither the investigators nor the study subjects are aware of which pill is the active compound and which is the placebo. Most supplements don't get this kind of supportive evidence, so be cautious.

When deciding on which form or brand of supplement to take, consumers need accurate information about the level of evidence on the supplement's safety, effectiveness, and dosage. A knowledgeable pharmacist or physician can often help. Other resources include the National Center for Complementary and Alternative Medicine (*nccam.nih.gov*) and the Natural Medicines Comprehensive Database (*www.naturaldatabase.com*). Dietary supplements are available in most food and drug stores nationwide.

Vitamins. Because of vitamin E's ability to neutralize free radicals — unstable molecules that may damage the genetic material of healthy cells — it has been studied and used to help prevent such age-related conditions as heart disease, cancer, and Alzheimer's. This fat-soluble vitamin boosts the immune system and helps keep eyes and skin healthy. The average individual gets about 10 to 15 IUs of vitamin E each day from their diet. For patients with Alzheimer's disease, one previous study found that 2000 IUs of daily vitamin E delayed functional decline.

Recently, the Women's Health Study did

not find that 600 IUs of daily vitamin E prevented heart attacks, stroke, or cancers of the lungs, breast, or colon. It *did* find, however, that vitamin E increased the risk of heart attack in women over age sixty-five. Another recent study from Johns Hopkins University School of Medicine found that people taking 400 IUs or more of vitamin E each day had a higher death rate than those on placebo. Because the deaths generally occurred in study subjects who also suffered from chronic diseases, the results may not apply to healthy people. Although many other studies have found vitamin E to be safe, this controversial Johns Hopkins study has left many doctors waiting for further evidence before routinely recommending high doses of vitamin E. People who want to play it safe can stop taking vitamin E for the time being, or drop their daily dose to less than 400 IUs.

Vitamin C is an antioxidant that can be taken safely at 500 to 1,000 mg daily. Like other antioxidant vitamins, it may not only protect brain health, but may also defend against some forms of cancer and diabetes, as well as increase immune defenses against colds and viruses. The Longevity Diet (see Essential 7) recommends a daily

500 mg vitamin C supplement.

Coenzyme Q_{10} is an antioxidant that has been used to treat age-related memory loss and to slow the progression of Alzheimer's and Parkinson's disease, although definitive scientific evidence of its effectiveness is limited. Coenzyme Q_{10} should be taken with caution, because it can interact with medicines used to treat heart failure, diabetes, and kidney or liver problems.

A daily multivitamin is a good idea because, as we age, our bodies lose their ability to absorb many vitamins and nutrients. Vitamin B_{12} absorption is a particular challenge: 20 percent of people age sixty and older, and 40 percent of those over age eighty, lose some of their ability to absorb vitamin B_{12}. The antioxidant B vitamin folate, or folic acid, protects us from developing strokes and heart disease. Some studies have shown that when Alzheimer's victims are treated with high doses of vitamin B_{12} or folate, their memory abilities improve. A large-scale seven-year study found that high doses of vitamins C and E, beta carotene, and zinc caused a 25 percent slowing in the progressive visual loss associated with macular degeneration. If the estimated eight million Americans over age fifty-five who are at risk for this disease took this combination of vitamins, 300,000 fewer individuals would lose their vision in the next five years. The Longevity Diet (see Essential 7) recommends a daily multivitamin.

It's important to avoid the potential toxic effects of unnecessary vitamin megadoses. This may be a particular problem with vitamins A, D, E, and K, which get stored in fat and can hang around in our bodies for weeks, months, or longer. If you're unsure about how much of any vitamin to take, check with your doctor or pharmacist.

Curcumin. This yellow spice found in curry powder also gives mustard its bright yellow color. Curcumin has been used for many years as an herbal remedy in India. Laboratory studies have demonstrated its anti-inflammatory and antioxidant effects, which may protect brain cells and help prevent cancer. Evidence suggests its potential benefits for colorectal, breast, prostate, and lung cancer. India — where curried food is so popular — has one of the world's lowest rates of Alzheimer's disease. The frequency of the disease in adults in India ages seventy to seventy-nine years is more than four times less than the frequency in the United States for the same age group. Curcumin is currently under study as a treatment for mild memory loss and Alzheimer's disease.

Omega-3 Supplements. Because of their potential for reducing the risk of cardiovascular disease, stroke, and Alzheimer's disease, omega-3 fats, such as docosahexaenoic acid or DHA, are available as supplements. Omega-3 fats minimize inflammation that can damage brain and heart cells, and have an antioxidant effect that fights against free radicals, which can further injure cells. Recent studies suggest that omega-3-rich supplements may help a person's mood, as well as their memory. These supplements usually contain fish oil, which is sensitive to light and to air oxidation. Make sure that you purchase the supplements from an establishment that keeps them refrigerated, and buy small quantities so your supply stays fresh.

Ginkgo Biloba. This popular ancient herbal remedy is made from a leaf extract and is thought to improve memory ability by inhibiting oxidative cell damage and improving cerebral circulation. It has been used for mild forms of age-related memory loss, early Alzheimer's disease, and other dementias. A recent systematic study review concluded that ginkgo appears to be safe, and that the evidence for memory benefits is promising, although additional studies are recommended. Initial research has found ginkgo to be helpful for treating leg cramps caused by poor circulation, a condition known as intermittent claudication. Studies of its use for the eye disease macular degeneration and for tinnitus (ringing in the ears) have been inconclusive. Possible side effects include nausea, heartburn, headaches, dizziness, excessive bruising or bleeding, and low blood pressure. Because ginkgo biloba has anticoagulant properties, taking it along with aspirin and other blood-thinning drugs requires careful monitoring.

Glucosamine and Chondroitin. Glucosamine, derived from shellfish, and chondroitin sulfate, derived from cow cartilage, are the components of a popular supplement combination used as a treatment for arthritis sufferers. Systematic studies have found that a daily combination of 1500 mg of glucosamine and 1200 mg of chondroitin sulfate not only reduces arthritis symptoms just as well as nonsteroidal anti-inflammatory drugs, but also may slow joint deterioration. The most common side effects are intestinal gas and softened stools. People with diabetes should check their blood-sugar levels more frequently when taking this supplement. The combination can interact with other medicines such as aspirin, which thin the blood. Those allergic to shellfish should consult with their doctor before taking glucosamine.

Echinacea. This herbal preparation comes from the same plant family as sunflowers and daisies. In the 1960s, it became a popular treatment for the common cold, in part because of laboratory studies suggesting that it may boost the immune system. In a recent study published in the *New England Journal of Medicine*, researchers found that echinacea was no different than a placebo in treating or preventing the symptoms of colds. Although echinacea advocates argue that the study doses were inadequate, the findings raise skepticism about whether echinacea has any effect on the common cold.

SAMe (S-adenosylmethionine). This naturally occurring compound plays a role in the immune system, maintains cell membranes, and helps produce and break down important brain chemical messengers. Research on SAMe suggests that it may be useful in the treatment of depression and arthritis. A recent study found that SAMe was as effective as traditional anti-inflammatory drugs in reducing pain and increasing mobility in patients with arthritis. Possible side effects include dry mouth, nausea, diarrhea, headache, and insomnia.

Policosanol. This supplement contains fatty alcohols derived from waxes of plants. Studies have found it to be effective in lowering the "bad" LDL cholesterol and raising levels of the "good" HDL cholesterol. Potential side effects include upset stomach, headache, and weight loss. Despite claims, no evidence supports the use of policosanol to boost energy or sexual performance.

Estrogen and Testosterone. Recent studies have left women confused about the pros and cons of taking hormone replacement therapy after menopause, and whether to take estrogen alone or estrogen plus a progestin. The Women's Health Initiative Study found that women age sixty-five and older taking different combinations of estrogen and a progestin (Premarin and Provera) had twice the likelihood of developing dementia than women who took a placebo. It is still possible that estrogen may protect the brain if taken in a different form, or earlier in life (right after menopause), but there is not yet enough evidence to recommend estrogen for dementia prevention.

Even though estrogen has not been found to prevent dementia, it does relieve menopausal symptoms. To help women make a more informed choice, the North American Menopause Society convened a panel of experts to help analyze the available research evidence and make recommendations. These experts concluded that estrogen (in pills or skin patches) should definitely be considered for younger women experiencing menopause, since estrogen helps relieve hot flashes, night sweats, and sleep disturbances caused by hot flashes. Estrogen is also an effective treatment for vaginal dryness, atrophy, or thinning, which can lead to irritation and infection. A vaginal estrogen cream, tablet, or ring is recommended for such symptoms.

Although estrogen increases the risk for uterine cancer, progestin protects against this risk. Women who have had their uterus removed don't need to take progestin when they use estrogen. Hormone therapy has been associated with increased risk for breast cancer, but more research is needed to determine the degree of risk at different ages. Hormone therapy does increase breast density, making it more difficult to detect abnormalities on mammograms, but ultrasound machines can be used, as well, to examine breasts for abnormal growths that might go undetected by mammograms in very dense breasts. Experts agree that if a woman decides to use hormone replacement therapy in order to relieve menopause symptoms, it is best to use the lowest dose she can, for the shortest amount of time. Also, her need for treatment should be reevaluated every year.

Approximately one out of five men sixty-five and older develop an abnormally low testosterone level; however, some men with normal levels augment their testosterone in an attempt to cure memory complaints, fatigue, low sex drive, and shrinking muscle mass. Although, in some cases, testosterone may improve these symptoms, it does pose risks — older men often have inactive cancer cells in their prostates, which excess testosterone could awaken.

DHEA (Dehydroepiandrosterone). Secreted by the body's adrenal gland, DHEA is a building block for estrogen and testosterone. Because DHEA declines with age, the theory is that one could extend life expectancy and avoid age-related health problems by keeping levels high. Some initial research suggests that DHEA may help treat depression in patients who do not respond well to conventional antidepressants. Its potential for protecting brain cells suggested promise for treating dementia and memory loss, but systematic studies have not backed this up. Recently, investigators found that when given to older people, DHEA can trim belly fat and help the body use insulin more effectively. The supplement does have its down side — DHEA can increase the risk of prostate cancer. Some athletes take DHEA to build strength and bulk before big events — despite its ban by organizations such as the National Football League and the International Olympic Committee.

Growth Hormone Stimulants. These natural products, also known as growth hormone "releasers," are thought to trigger the release of chemical messengers that promise to build muscle mass, trim fat, increase energy, improve sex life, boost memory, restore hair growth and color, and strengthen the immune system. Companies marketing "hormone releaser" pills say their products are a cheaper, needle-free alternative to human growth hormone injections. The active ingredient is often arginine or another amino acid that signals the pituitary gland to release or secrete growth hormone. Although growth hormone levels decline with age, it is not known whether trying to maintain the levels that exist in young persons has any benefit. For now, muscle-building athletes and others who take these products should be cautious of potential side effects, and they should know that, so far, there is minimal evidence of any benefit.

Looking Better

Remaining young-looking and attractive is an important quality longevity goal for many people. However, being comfortable in our own skin is what truly counts; and often this means aging gracefully and celebrating every well-deserved line and wrinkle. Some people choose to adamantly fight the physical signs of aging, and maintain their youthful appearance as long as possible.

When we feel that we look good, it boosts our self-esteem and confidence, which can lead to a more positive outlook, more fulfilling relationships, and other quality longevity benefits. There are a variety of approaches to looking young, ranging from face creams to surgeries.

Billions of dollars are spent every year on cosmetics to help people look younger by taking care of their skin and enhancing their appearance. Experts agree that the best way to minimize wrinkles is to avoid sun exposure, use moisturizers, and always wear sunscreen (see Essential 5). Many people, particularly women, use cosmetics to create a more youthful look (see box).

Using Makeup to Look Younger

Many people wear makeup, and experts agree it's best to apply moisturizer and sunscreen before foundation. At about middle-age and older, the face tends to take on a gray or yellowish cast, so cosmetologists advise choosing creamy foundations in beige or golden tones, and pumping up the color on the lips and cheeks — moving away from browns, and selecting more corals or rose-color tints. Avoiding powders if the skin is dry will keep the powder from settling into the lines and help give the skin a dewy appearance. However, applying a soft-shade blushing powder on the cheekbones going outward and slightly upward gives definition to the face.

Grooming eyebrows gives the illusion of lifted lids, and having more skin showing at the brow bone opens up the entire eye. Using a lash curler before applying mascara also makes eyes look more open.

Thinning and graying hair can be common as we age. Many hair experts suggest either overall color to cover gray or perhaps augmenting with golden or honey highlights to add dimension, brighten the face, and make hair look thicker. As women get older, they may find it more attractive to lighten and brighten their hair color, rather than darken it.

Cosmetic Medicine

Each year, millions of Americans choose to undergo medical treatments or surgical techniques to improve their appearance, and make themselves look younger and healthier. Although some individuals can go too far with plastic surgery, most cosmetic-medicine consumers are simply trying to look and feel better about themselves.

When considering cosmetic surgery, a person should be clear about his or her motivation. Pressure from friends, family, or a loved one is not the best reason to go forward. Cosmetic surgery is usually an elective procedure — something the patient *wants,* as opposed to *needs.* Also, it is important to be realistic about what any particular procedure can and cannot accomplish. Cosmetic surgery will not cure a clinical depression, although it may help you to look a lot more attractive when visiting the psychiatrist.

Choosing the right surgeon, perhaps one who specializes in the particular procedure you have chosen, is critical. A good strategy is to rely on recommendations from physicians and friends you trust. You can also check with the American Board of Plastic Surgery or the American Society of Plastic and Reconstructive Surgeons (888-475-2784 or *www.plasticsurgery.org*), although keep in mind that simply being a member of a professional society does not ensure a surgeon's quality.

Learn all you can about the procedure you will be having, and talk with the doctor about potential risks and benefits. Ask the specialist to show you photographic examples of his or her work — "before" and "after" — and be skeptical of guaranteed promises or extravagant claims.

The following section includes some of the more popular procedures that are currently available. They differ in cost, degree of invasiveness, recovery time, potential complications, and long-term outcomes, all of which should be discussed in advance with the doctor.

Surgical Techniques

Face Lifts. To get an idea of how your face might appear after a lift, look at yourself in a mirror while lying on your back. A face lift can smooth out wrinkles, loose skin, a sagging neck, and other aging changes. The procedure involves camouflaged incisions around the ears and usually some repositioning of the skin, as well as of the underlying tissue. A forehead or brow lift corrects drooping brows and smooths the horizontal lines and furrows that can make a person appear angry, sad, or tired. It restores a youthful, natural look to the upper third of the face. The incisions are hidden just behind the hairline.

These procedures can subtract years from someone's appearance, but there are occasional complications, including infection, bleeding, or a wide-eyed, unnatural appearance. However, in recent years, the aim has shifted toward more subtle results, rather than a drastic change in appearance, and less invasive "minilifts" have become popular. The results are less dramatic than complete face lifts, but the costs and risk of complications are lower. Minilifts and other minimally invasive procedures, such as endoscopic neck and midface lifts, are frequently used in younger patients who have reasons to justify doing a procedure, but who do not need a more comprehensive surgical intervention.

Breast Lifts. These procedures, often performed in an outpatient setting, reverse the natural sagging that occurs from age, pregnancy, breast feeding, and weight fluctuations. New techniques reduce visible scarring after the procedure, and most women are pleased with their outcome. Complications may include loss of sensation in the nipple, an unnatural appearance to the breast, and scarring.

Liposuction. This technique helps sculpt the body by removing unwanted fat from the abdomen, hips, buttocks, thighs, knees, upper arms, chin, cheeks, or neck. The surgeon injects fluid into the fat tissue and suctions out the fat along with the fluid. New methods, including ultrasound-assisted lipoplasty (UAL), the tumescent technique, and the super-wet technique, are helping plastic surgeons provide some patients with more precise results and quicker recovery times. Although it is not a substitute for dieting and exercise, liposuction can reduce stubborn areas of fat that don't respond to traditional weight-loss methods.

Liposuction, which usually requires general anesthesia, can have permanent effects if the patient is able to avoid future weight gain. Possible side effects include bleeding, infection, numbness, or a bumpy appearance to the area, if fat removal is uneven. An extremely rare and unfortunate complication is pulmonary embolism, which can cause death.

Eyelid Surgery. With age, the skin around the eyes loses elasticity and the resulting loose folds and creases can cause a puffy, tired look. Cosmetic eyelid surgery can remove the excess skin, bags, and fat from around the upper and lower eyelids. This outpatient procedure can yield long-lasting results, with patients typically appearing refreshed and rested. Complications may include eye irritation, dryness, bleeding, and loss of the natural shape of the eye from over-correction of excess skin.

Lasik Eye Surgery. Many people who want to stop wearing glasses opt for this outpatient procedure, a relatively quick and painless way to correct vision. The surgeon makes a thin flap on the surface of the cornea, lifts the flap, and reshapes the underlying cornea with a laser. Flattening the center of the cornea corrects nearsightedness. Farsighted people have a ring of tissue around the center of the cornea removed, in order to make the cornea steeper. For people with astigmatism, the oblong-shaped cornea is made more spherical.

Although most patients get twenty-twenty vision after the procedure, those with more serious myopia, farsightedness, or astigmatism may have less than optimal results. Temporary side effects may include eye dryness, or seeing imaginary halos or spots of light. Very rarely, patients may develop infection or permanent damage to their vision.

For some patients, conductive keratoplasty, a minimally invasive procedure that does not require incisions, is effective for the treatment of mild farsightedness. It uses electrical energy to reshape the cornea. It not only allows patients to see at a distance, but can also create blended vision, so they can forgo reading glasses, as well.

Surgical Hair Enhancement. Hair transplants involve taking tiny hair follicles from the back or side of the scalp and implanting them into balding areas, typically on the crown of the head or the front of the hairline. Another technique, known as scalp reduction, involves minimizing an area of bald skin on the head by surgically removing it and stretching hair-bearing scalp in its place. Both procedures can be combined to provide a natural-appearing hair line. Rare complications of surgical hair enhancements may include infection, scarring, or further hair loss.

Nonsurgical Treatments

Botox Injections. Those crow's-feet around the eyes and frown lines on the face that accrue over the years can now be smoothed out with Botox injections. Derived from the bacteria that cause botulism, Botox literally paralyzes the muscles for a period of four to six months. The recovery time from injections is brief and improvement is usually observed within two weeks. Potential side effects include drooping upper eyelids and less facial expression due to difficulty raising the eyebrows. Recent research suggests that Botox injections may stave off migraine head-aches.

Collagen Injections. Collagen is a natural protein that provides texture and soft-tissue support throughout the body. When small amounts are injected into collagen-weak areas, depressions in the surrounding skin are raised, and the area appears smoother. Although collagen injections can be effective in lessening wrinkles around the eyes, mouth, and nasolabial folds, the benefits last only a few months. A test injection, usually on the inside of the forearm, is necessary to determine if the patient is among the four percent of individuals allergic to the commonly used collagen derived from cows.

Cosmoderm and Cosmoplast, FDA-approved facial fillers, can be used without pretesting for allergic reactions. These purified human collagen treatments are bioengineered from living human cells. For lips, in particular, collagen treatment of some type is recommended as a preliminary trial before considering placement of a longer-lasting material, such as Restylane or fat injections.

Restylane Injections. Collagen has been

replaced by Restylane as the most popular filler. Restylane lasts at least twice as long — up to six to nine months — and requires no pretreatment skin test. Restylane is derived from synthetic hyaluronic acid, and allergic reactions occur in less than one percent of those injected. Since 1996, over one million patients have been treated in more than sixty countries.

Fat Injections. This outpatient procedure is often performed in conjunction with liposuction and is similar to injecting collagen, but has the advantage of not producing allergic reactions. The suctioned fat from an unwanted area of the body is reinjected to smooth out wrinkled areas or to augment lips.

Mesotherapy. Cellulite is the dimpled skin that can appear on the hips, thighs, and buttocks of people as they age. Mesotherapy involves injecting medicines and other substances into the layer of fat and connective tissue under the skin, known as the mesoderm, where the cellulite is located. The procedure is still being studied, so its effectiveness is not known and it has not been accepted by the established medical community. Possible complications include infection, irregular contouring, and scarring.

Microdermabrasion. This procedure involves gently sandblasting the face, usually by spraying tiny crystals and vacuuming the resulting debris. It helps repair facial skin damaged by the sun and aging, but the benefits last for only a few months. Microdermabrasion is basically painless and requires no recovery time, but it can cause mild swelling and redness for a day.

Laser Resurfacing. This method uses high energy laser light to vaporize the outer skin layers, which then grow back smoother and tighter. Laser resurfacing can smooth out deep wrinkles and fine lines around the mouth or eyes and can last for years. Initial recovery time is usually seven to ten days, during which crusting resolves. Possible complications include loss of skin pigmentation, scarring, and sun sensitivity. Some people have pink or red skin for up to six months after the treatment, which may require concealing makeup.

Fraxel Laser. This new technique, also

known as Fractional Resurfacing Technology, delivers laser light to only a fraction of the skin through a series of microscopic, closely spaced laser spots, while preserving normal healthy skin between the laser spots. This preservation of healthy skin results in rapid healing following the laser treatment. Fraxel laser can treat the entire face in approximately thirty minutes and requires three to five sessions spaced several weeks apart. It has been used effectively on the face, neck, chest, arms, and hands for photodamaged skin (brown spots), fine and moderate wrinkles, and acne scarring. The procedure involves minimal discomfort and causes only slight redness for a day or two, followed by bronzing of the skin for about a week.

Radio Wave Therapy. The FDA recently approved radio wave therapy as a non-surgical treatment for wrinkles. The technique, sometimes marketed as Thermage, involves a spray that cools the skin surface while radio waves are emitted and penetrate to deeper skin layers, particularly the collagen layer. There is some immediate tightening of the collagen fibers, which smooths the overlying skin. Eventually, new collagen grows from the heat stimulus of the radio waves, which further tightens the skin over a two- to six-month period.

Photofacial. Intense Pulsed Light Therapy, or IPL, can eliminate dark aging spots, sun freckles, and superficial capillaries, as well as diminish fine wrinkles and tighten pores in the skin. This form of photorejuvenation can be utilized as a treatment for rosacea, or simply to improve the tone and texture of the skin. It is FDA approved and usually requires four to six treatments. Patients looking to revitalize their appearance without any down time often choose this procedure.

Chemical Peels. This method improves the appearance of the skin on the face, neck, chest, and hands. A chemical solution is applied to the skin, causing it to peel off so that new, smoother, regenerated skin replaces the older, wrinkled skin. Chemical peels can improve fine lines under the eyes and around the mouth, mild scarring, and acne, as well as wrinkles from sun damage and aging. However, deeper wrinkles generally do not respond unless the clinician uses a more concentrated acid solution, which may result in skin or pigment loss and an unnatural change in skin texture. After a peel, the new skin is temporarily more sensitive to the sun. Superficial peels usually result in redness, followed by scaling for up to a week. Deeper peels may lead to swelling, blisters, and crusting for up to two weeks.

Skin Creams. The FDA regulates the safety of many skin-care products, but doesn't really concern itself with their effectiveness. Product brand names can often be deceptive, sometimes alluding to cosmetic surgery–like results — for example, the "mini-lift miracle cream" or the "botoxin-smoothie mask." Many of the latest products contain a small fragment of protein that is absorbed into the skin's top layer. These fragments are thought to stimulate collagen production, which smooths the skin. Some creams actually contain collagen, but these tend to be less effective, because collagen has to be injected in order for it to penetrate the skin. Other ingredients in many products, including actual DNA molecules or hyaluronic acid, have not been demonstrated to show benefits. These creams *do* help to moisturize the skin, which any effective skin cream or lotion can do.

Another cream ingredient is a vitamin A

derivative (e.g., Retin-A or Renova), which can tighten the skin and replace old skin with new skin. Noticeable improvement may take months, and potential side effects include temporary redness, scaling, burning, itching, and thinning of the skin over time.

Medicines for Hair Growth. Although baldness has become a cool look for some men, many still define their youthful self-image by how much hair they have on their head. Some women also experience hair loss as they get older. Two drugs are available for the treatment of balding: minoxidil, marketed as Rogaine, and finasteride, marketed as Propecia or Proscar. Both medicines help stave off future hair loss, and can sometimes stimulate the growth of new hair.

Rogaine is rubbed onto the scalp twice daily — the new hair may be thinner and shorter than previous hair, but it can blend in and help hide bald spots. It occasionally causes scalp irritation. Propecia is a prescription pill that is taken once daily and usually shows results within a few months. Rarely, it can decrease sex drive, and as with Rogaine, the benefits stop if the medicine is discontinued.

Keeping Your Smile Young. As we get older, our gums tend to recede, which exposes some of the roots of our teeth, making them more susceptible to infection and decay. Gum or periodontal disease becomes more common with age, afflicting approximately 50 percent of people fifty-five years and older. In addition to decay, it can cause tooth loss and bleeding, which allows bacteria to enter the bloodstream and contribute to inflammation throughout the body. This may be why gum disease increases the risk of heart disease or stroke. A recent study also found that gum disease early in life increases the risk for Alzheimer's disease late in life.

Although genetics plays a role in the risk for gum disease, proper brushing and flossing are the best defense, and can even offset a genetic risk. When brushing, use a brush with small and soft bristles. To help reduce decay, brush with a fluoride toothpaste and floss at least twice daily. Ask your dentist or dental hygienist to review your technique, and be sure to get your teeth cleaned at regular intervals. Avoid mouth dryness by taking small sips of water throughout the day. Also, brush or rinse after eating sweet or sticky foods such as raisins. A cosmetic dentist can also advise you on procedures to improve the appearance of your smile and teeth, such as whitening products and bonding.

Staying Young with Modern Medicine

- Medical breakthroughs are focusing on early detection and prevention of disease before damage sets in. Becoming informed consumers of new medical technologies and treatments helps us live longer, and look and feel younger.
- Don't hesitate to get help — screen early rather than late for illnesses such as osteoporosis, cancer, diabetes, and hypertension.
- Augment your medicine's benefits by exercising, eating right, eliminating stress, and embracing the other quality longevity essentials.
- Listen to your doctor's advice — taking the correct medicine in the right way can add healthy years to your life. Don't use more medicines than you need, and discuss side effects with your doctor.
- Libido boosters and sexual enhancers

---

for both men and women can help keep sex a vital part of life, well into old age.

- If you decide on a cosmetic treatment or procedure, make sure to review the pros and cons of the many options available.

Part 3

Putting It All Together

The secret of longevity is to keep breathing.

— SOPHIE TUCKER

People start getting proactive about their quality longevity at various stages of life, and for many different reasons. Some are like Nancy G., whose family history of Alzheimer's disease motivated her to take charge. Or Shirley I., whose memory slips encouraged her to get involved. Sometimes all it takes to motivate someone to pursue a *Longevity Bible* lifestyle is a little age reminder such as a new line in your face, or perhaps noticing how much older people look at your high school reunion.

Regardless of your reason for pursuing a longer, healthier, and more youthful life, you now have some knowledge of the Eight Essential areas where you *do* have some control. How much you need to emphasize each area will depend on your current strengths and needs, as well as the feasibility of making changes that fit in with your lifestyle. If your job involves a lot of travel, adhering to the Longevity Diet will be a challenge, but it is definitely achievable. If you are a long-distance runner, you probably don't need to worry about upgrading your level of physical activity. If you happen to be a rocket scientist, you may not need to spend too much time doing mental aerobics. This means you will have more time to concentrate on the other essential areas.

Working the Eight Essentials Together

When we work several of the Eight Essentials together, we benefit from the synergy of their combined effects. Your particular quality longevity challenges will determine the specifics of your *Longevity Bible* program, and the program itself will continually change as you achieve results in one area and then find yourself able to focus more on another area. Eating a healthy longevity diet as well as sharpening your mind can lead to a more positive attitude. This often benefits your relationships and may lead you to experience less stress in your life. As a result, you may be able to cut back on your relationship exercises and the amount of time you spend each day on stress reduction. This in turn can free up more time for improving your environment by decluttering some of the rooms in your apartment or house. You may also have more time to work out, which can help lower your blood pressure and reduce the need for medicines.

To help you individualize your quality longevity program, first review the following key points for achieving each of the Eight Essentials. Place a check mark next to the points you feel you need to emphasize as you begin your program. Then review the details of those essentials to fine-tune the strategies you've chosen.

Sharpen Your Mind

Regular mental activity will help keep the mind sharp, improve memory skills, and protect the brain from future decline. When combined with the other *Longevity Bible* Essential Strategies, it not only makes people feel happier and function more effectively, but it may also extend life expectancy.

❑ To get the most out of your mental workouts, apply the *P's and Q's* for Sharpening the Mind: 1) maintain *presence* and focus; 2) *persevere* in your endeavors to further sharpen your mind; 3) look for the *quality* and meaning of things; and 4) always *question* to learn more.

❑ Try different approaches to expanding your mental horizons, such as traveling to new destinations, learning a musical instrument, taking up ballroom dancing, or going back to school.

❑ Learn and practice the three basic memory techniques:
  - Look: Focus attention on what you want to remember
  - Snap: Imagine a mental snapshot of the information
  - Connect: Link the snapshots together in your mind's eye

❑ Practice more advanced memory strategies for remembering names and faces.

❑ Stay mentally active through puzzles, games, reading, and other stimulating hobbies, but be sure to train and not strain your brain — find the level of mental challenge that keeps you interested without frustrating or exhausting you.

Keep a Positive Outlook

A positive outlook helps us live longer and stay healthier. Optimists have fewer physical and emotional difficulties, experience less pain, enjoy higher energy levels, and are generally happier and calmer in their lives. Although genetics plays a role, scientific evidence shows that maintaining a positive attitude, like any other skill, can be learned.

❑ Make a conscious effort to be extroverted and energetic — happiness is contagious.
❑ Forgive yourself and others who wrong you — letting go of grudges lowers stress levels and fosters a positive outlook.
❑ Build self-esteem by making moral choices. Keep in mind your accom-

❑ plishments and successes to help rebut your inner self-critic.

❑ If you don't already have an active spiritual or religious life, consider getting involved in one, whether it's through meditation, organized religion, seeking harmony with nature, or any other method.

❑ Learn to be optimistic through simple, systematic approaches. Recognize what your negativity triggers are, and challenge any negative assumptions you are quick to make.

❑ Avoid pessimistic thinking by focusing on your strengths and setting achievable and realistic goals.

❑ Don't be a loner — ask others for support and get professional help if you need it.

Cultivate Healthy and Intimate Relationships

Staying socially connected not only bolsters physical and emotional well-being, it reduces stress levels and can add years to our lives. Empathy and other basic skills that help us stay connected to others can

- ❏ Stay connected and involved socially, whether you are single or in a couple. Try to spend time with a healthy crowd.
- ❏ Reduce relationship clutter by cutting loose unsatisfying or "toxic" friends and acquaintances.
- ❏ Develop and maintain your empathy skills. Listen to others, try to identify with their feelings, and let them know that you understand.
- ❏ If you are in an intimate relationship, make efforts to nurture it: Schedule time together, share feelings without criticizing, and stay in touch with friends and other couples. A healthy sex life adds to quality longevity.
- ❏ Having a pet may contribute to longer life expectancy. Pets can also be enjoyable, stress-reducing companions.
- ❏ Planning ahead for the emotional and practical challenges of parent care can make the role-reversal much less stressful for both older parents and their adult children, should the need arise.

be learned and improved upon, and even the most social among us can fine-tune his or her skills.

Promote Stress-Free Living

Chronic stress has been associated with an increased risk for cancer, high blood pressure, and heart disease, and may speed up the very aging of our cells by a decade or more. Stress impairs memory, and makes us look and feel older. Although we cannot control all of the outside factors that contribute to stress in our lives, we *can* have a major impact on how we react to stress, and minimize its influence on our health and longevity.

❑ Practice mindful awareness — staying in the moment and being aware of what is going on inside your body — through meditation, relaxation techniques, yoga, or other exercises you enjoy. Take stress release breaks throughout the day.
❑ Avoid multitasking by scheduling a regular time each day for completing

priority chores; try finishing one task before beginning another.

❑ Learn to say "no" when you need to.

❑ Modulate stress with healthy expressions of anger.

❑ Use humor to gain perspective on stressful situations.

❑ Get a good night's sleep every night. Take simple steps to beat insomnia without medication.

❑ Discover ways to limit stress on the job.

❑ Place emphasis on saving for the future.

❑ Reduce stress by decluttering your personal environment.

❑ Plan your strategy for dealing with stressful events you know about in advance.

Master Your Environment

Our environment has a major influence on how we feel and how long we live. Whether it's traffic, noise, smog, or other aspects of the environment at large, or more personal environmental issues such as clutter, aesthetics, or bedroom temperature, our quality longevity requires that we not only adapt to these influences, but learn to shape them to meet our individual tastes and needs. Consider the following personal solutions for environmental issues, and check off any that could be helpful for your longevity program.

❑ Bear in mind function and aesthetics when designing your home and work space. Control clutter and noise, and arrange the bedroom in a way that enhances sleep and restfulness.

❑ Minimize your exposure to sun, smoke, mold, smog, and other airborne toxins.

❑ Stay safe on the road — let someone else drive if you can't handle it.

❑ Make your workplace safe and comfortable: Consider ergonomic designs for comfort and safety.

❑ Manage your technology to avoid information overload.

❑ If parent care becomes a reality, consider the advantages and disadvantages of various housing choices.

❑ Help conserve natural resources and protect your environment.

Body Fitness — Shape Up to Stay Young

Physical activity, whether it's walking, cycling, playing tennis, or dancing, keeps us living longer, feeling healthier, and looking younger. Even a short, brisk ten-minute daily walk can reduce the risk of age-related diseases such as Alzheimer's. Physically active people also have lower rates of heart attacks, cancer, diabetes, and depression, and these benefits can be experienced at almost any age. The Longevity Fitness Routine promotes health and boosts energy levels.

❑ Sample different types of cardiovascular exercise methods and choose one or more that you find fun and challenging. Sports and exercise protect your body *and* your mind.

❑ Exercise with a friend — getting physical *and* social reduces stress and keeps you connected to others.

❑ Divide your routine among the three vital Longevity Fitness areas:
- Cardiovascular conditioning
- Balance and flexibility
- Strength training

- ❑ Exercise several days a week — don't be a weekend warrior.
- ❑ Build strength and stamina gradually to maximize fitness and avoid injury — push yourself to the next level only when you're ready.
- ❑ If you have an ongoing medical condition, be sure to check with your doctor before starting any exercise program.

The Longevity Diet

Diet directly impacts our health and life expectancy by affecting our risk for heart disease, cancer, and other age-related illnesses. It also influences our appearance and mental state. The Longevity Diet is based on the latest scientific evidence on foods that improve health and lengthen life, and it still allows us to occasionally get away with eating our favorite cheat eats without guilt. Learning to "cross-train" our eating among healthy food groups allows us to break free of the boredom and repetition of many of today's popular diets.

❏ Eat the foods you like the most from the following food groups every day. Each food group can *star* in up to two meals per day.
  - Antioxidant fruits and vegetables
  - Proteins, lean meats, and healthy fats
  - Whole grains, legumes, and other carbohydrates

❏ Use mindful awareness to focus on how your body feels before, during, and after eating, to help you gauge portion size and know when you've had enough.

❏ Occasionally indulge in a small portion of your favorite cheat eats.

❏ Drink at least eight glasses of water throughout the day.

❏ Enjoy two to three healthy between-meal snacks a day.

❏ Avoid excessive salts, bad fats, and high-glycemic carbohydrates.

❏ If you wish to lose weight, cut back on carbohydrates, alcohol, and cheat eats until you reach your goal.

Modern Medicine for Feeling and Looking Younger

Today's medical technology is keeping our generation living longer, as well as looking and feeling better than any generation before us. By combining a healthy lifestyle with new disease-detection methods, better medicines and vaccines, and novel surgical procedures, we can expect a significant increase in the number of years we live, as well as the health and youthfulness we enjoy during those years. With the range of treatments and procedures now available, it is essential to become an informed consumer, choosing and monitoring our own *medical portfolios* wisely.

❑ Medical breakthroughs are focusing on early detection and prevention of disease before damage sets in. Becoming informed consumers of new medical technologies and treatments helps us to live longer, and look and feel younger.

❑ Don't hesitate to get help — screen early rather than late for illnesses such as osteoporosis, cancer, diabetes, and hypertension.

❑ Augment your medicine's benefits by exercising, eating right, eliminating stress, and embracing the other quality longevity essentials.

❑ Listen to your doctor's advice — taking the correct medicine in the right way can add healthy years to your life. Don't use more medicines than you need, and discuss side effects with your doctor.

❑ Libido booster and sexual enhancers for both men and women can help keep sex a vital part of life, well into old age.

❑ If you decide on a cosmetic treatment or procedure, make sure to review the pros and cons of the many options available.

Getting With the Program

When beginning a *Longevity Bible* Program, many people find it helpful to set short-term and long-term goals for each of the Eight Essentials. After reviewing the checklists, Alan F. came up with the following list of goals:

419

GOALS

8 Essentials	Short-Term	Long-Term
Sharp Mind	1. Start doing daily crossword puzzles this week. 2. Take guitar lessons.	Lower risk for Alzheimer's.
Attitude	1. Inner-critic exercises twice this week. 2. Start going to church on Sundays.	Increase self-confidence.
Relationships	1. Try attentive-listening exercises. 2. Go away with girlfriend on weekend.	Eventually get married; feel closer to kids.
Stress-Free	1. Go to yoga classes. 2. Delegate tasks to reduce workload.	Feel less anxious.
Environment	1. Wear sunscreen. 2. Have mildew-smelling basement checked for toxic mold.	Reduce risk for cancer and other illnesses.

Body Fitness	1. Take a 10-minute walk after dinner. 2. Begin Longevity Fitness Routine.	Increase stamina; avoid injuries.
Diet	1. Cut back on red meat and salt. 2. Get more whole grains into diet.	Lose ten pounds and lower blood pressure.
Medicine	1. Take daily blood pressure medicine. 2. Get colonoscopy this month.	Lower blood pressure and detect treatable illnesses.

The synergy of the Eight Essentials helped Alan F. make quick gains in his quality longevity. With his increased confidence, he became less defensive and more comfortable about moving forward in his relationship with his girlfriend. He also started feeling closer to his son. The stress reduction from his yoga classes lowered his anxiety levels. This, along with his low-salt diet, made it possible for his doctor to reduce his blood pressure medicine. When Alan became more proactive by delegating some of his work tasks, he had more leisure time, which lowered his stress levels further and allowed him to spend more time with the people he cared about in his life.

Alan tried not to obsess over every detail of his longevity program. Within each of the Eight Essentials, he didn't focus on everything all at once, but started on the areas in which he felt he could use the most work. This allowed him to enjoy the benefits of his efforts as soon as possible. Once a person begins to achieve his or her short-term goals, that individual usually gains motivation to take on even greater challenges, which can further increase the quality and number of his or her years ahead.

In the Appendices that follow, you'll find additional resources for more help with the Eight Essentials. I've included some recipes you may want to try as you become familiar with the Longevity Diet, as well as more mental aerobics exercises to use for additional brain workouts.

None of us will live forever, but we *can* take greater control of how well and how long we live. Our genes don't have the final word on our quality longevity trajectory. Starting a *Longevity Bible* lifestyle today will help you live to enjoy the benefits for years to come.

Appendix 1

The Longevity Diet Recipes

Apple Crumble à la Mode

(makes 4–6 servings)

4 apples, peeled and thinly sliced
$1/4$ teaspoon cinnamon
$2/3$ cup whole-grain and oat granola
2 cups frozen vanilla yogurt or fat-free
vanilla ice cream

Preheat the oven to 350°F. Lightly coat a small baking dish with cooking spray and arrange the apples in the dish. Sprinkle them with the cinnamon and granola. Bake until the fruit is bubbling, about 30 minutes. Let cool 5 to 10 minutes. Scoop the frozen yogurt into bowls and top with baked apple crumble. Serve immediately.

Variation: Can also be prepared with berries, nectarines, peaches, pears, or plums.

Buttermilk Dressing, Lowfat

(makes 2 cups)

1 cup nonfat sour cream
1 cup reduced-fat buttermilk
2 tablespoons honey
2 tablespoons scallions, minced
Kosher salt and freshly cracked black
   pepper, to taste

In a small bowl, whisk together the sour cream, buttermilk, and honey. Fold in the scallions and season with salt and pepper.

Caramelized Onion Dip

1 tablespoon extra-virgin olive oil
½ sweet onion, finely chopped
1 tablespoon balsamic vinegar
1 cup nonfat sour cream
1 teaspoon garlic powder
1 teaspoon seasoning salt
Fresh sliced vegetables for dipping

Heat the olive oil and onion in a nonstick skillet, over medium heat. Sauté the onions until they begin to soften and caramelize, stirring occasionally, about 15 minutes.

Add the balsamic vinegar and continue to sauté until balsamic vinegar is nearly dry. Allow the onion to cool completely and fold into the sour cream. Add the garlic powder and seasoning salt, and mix well. Refrigerate for at least 30 minutes before serving. Serve with sliced vegetables for dipping.

Cheesy Pesto with Pasta

(makes 6–8 side servings)

- 1 package frozen chopped spinach, thawed and drained
- 4 cloves garlic, crushed
- 2/3 cup lowfat cottage cheese
- 2/3 cup fresh basil, chopped (or substitute 4 tablespoons dried)
- 1/2 cup parmesan cheese, grated
- 1/2 cup pine nuts
- 2 tablespoons olive oil
- 2/3 cup hot water
- 8 ounces whole-grain pasta (fusilli, spaghetti, or linguini)

In a food processor or blender, mix the spinach, garlic, cottage cheese, and basil. Separate a small amount of the parmesan cheese and pine nuts to sprinkle on top later, then add the rest to the mixture, along with the olive oil and water. Process until smooth, adding more water if needed. Toss warm pasta with desired amount of pesto sauce, and top with remaining parmesan cheese and pine nuts. Store leftover pesto in refrigerator or freezer.

Five-Minute Fat-Free Chilled Strawberry Soup

(makes 4 servings)

1 quart fresh strawberries, stems removed
12 ounces fat-free vanilla yogurt
A pinch or two of ground ginger
Juice of 1 orange
4–6 fresh mint leaves

Place ingredients in food processor or blender and puree until smooth. Chill and serve with a small dollop of yogurt and a mint sprig as garnish.

Fennel, Orange, and Red Onion Salad

(makes 4 servings)

2 large bulbs fennel, quartered and
   cored
1 bag designer baby arugula
1/2 red onion, thinly sliced
1 can unsweetened mandarin oranges
2–3 tablespoons extra-virgin olive oil
Salt and pepper, to taste

Thinly slice the fennel and place in a large
bowl with the arugula and red onion. Drain
the juice from the mandarin oranges into a
small bowl, and add the orange sections to the
fennel and arugula. Whisk the olive oil into
the reserved orange juice and season with salt
and pepper. Toss the dressing with the salad.

Green Beans with Lemon

(makes 4 servings)

1 pound fresh green beans, cleaned and
   trimmed
2 teaspoons fresh lemon juice
2 teaspoons finely chopped fresh flat-
   leaf parsley leaves

1 teaspoon freshly grated lemon zest
Salt and pepper, to taste

In a large saucepan of boiling salted water, cook beans until crisp-tender, about 3 to 4 minutes. Drain, then toss beans in a large bowl with lemon juice, parsley, and lemon zest. Season with salt and pepper.

Mixed Seafood and Linguini

(makes 4–6 servings)

8 ounces whole-wheat linguini
1 yellow pepper, cut into ½-inch pieces
½ cup onion, chopped
2 cloves garlic, crushed
½ teaspoon instant chicken bouillon powder
1 teaspoon dried basil
½ teaspoon dried oregano
2 tablespoons cornstarch
8 ounces scallops and 8 ounces shrimp (shelled)
2 large tomatoes, seeded and chopped
2 tablespoons fresh parsley, chopped
Freshly grated parmesan cheese
Freshly grated pepper, to taste

Cook the linguini and keep warm. In a large skillet, cook the yellow pepper, onion, garlic, bouillon, basil, and oregano, slowly adding one cup of water. Continue cooking until vegetables are tender, about 5 minutes. In a separate bowl, stir together the cornstarch and 2 tablespoons water, then add to vegetables. Cook until bubbling. Add shrimp and scallops and cook 3 to 4 minutes until seafood is done. Stir in tomatoes. Toss with linguini and sprinkle with parsley. Serve with grated parmesan cheese and pepper.

Raisin-Bran Muffins

(makes 12 muffins)

1 cup whole-bran cereal
1 cup nonfat milk
1 egg, slightly beaten
¼ cup canola oil
¼ cup sugar
½ teaspoon shredded lemon peel
¾ cup whole-wheat flour
¾ cup all-purpose flour
¼ teaspoon salt
2 teaspoons baking powder
¾ cup raisins

Preheat oven to 400°F. Combine cereal and milk and let moisten. Add egg, oil, sugar, and lemon peel. In a separate mixing bowl, stir flours, salt, and baking powder. Add cereal mixture to flour bowl, then stir raisins into batter. Spray a 12-cup muffin pan with nonstick cooking spray and fill each cup 2/3 full with batter. Bake 17 to 20 minutes, or until golden brown.

Roquefort Dressing

2 ounces Roquefort or blue cheese, crumbled
1 cup buttermilk (reduced fat)
3/4 teaspoon sherry vinegar
1/2 teaspoon walnut oil
Ground pepper to taste

In a food processor or blender, combine the cheese, buttermilk, vinegar, and oil. Process until smooth and creamy (about 1 minute), then transfer to a container and add pepper. Keeps in refrigerator up to 1 week.

Split Pea Soup, Lowfat

(makes 8 servings)

2 quarts low-sodium chicken or
  vegetable stock
2 cups dried split peas
1 cup chopped celery
1 finely chopped medium onion
1 bay leaf
10 sprigs fresh flat-leaf parsley
1 medium carrot, quartered
4 slices uncooked turkey bacon

In a large stockpot combine the chicken stock, peas, celery, onion, bay leaf, parsley, carrot, and uncooked turkey bacon. Bring to a boil, reduce heat, and simmer for 1 hour. Remove and discard the bay leaf and the turkey bacon. Reserve one cup of peas. In batches, process the soup in a blender until smooth. Add the reserved peas and serve immediately.

Strawberry Sorbet

(makes 4–6 servings)

2 pints fresh strawberries, hulled
1½ tablespoons honey
1 teaspoon orange liqueur (optional)

Freeze the strawberries on a cookie sheet, until solid. Put in food processor and process until the texture of cornmeal. Add honey and optional liqueur and process until firm. Serve immediately or transfer to a bowl and freeze for 1 day before serving.

Variation: Sorbet can also be made with peaches or pears: Cut fruit into chunks, then toss with 1 tablespoon lemon juice before freezing. Skip the liqueur.

White Bean Salad

16 ounces Great Northern beans
½ red bell pepper, diced
¼ cup scallions, thinly sliced
1 can white albacore tuna, drained
   (optional)
½ cup flat-leaf parsley, roughly chopped
1 tablespoon extra-virgin olive oil
Juice of 1 lemon

Toss all ingredients together in a large bowl. Season with salt and pepper, to taste.

Appendix 2

More Mental Aerobics to Tease Your Brain

1. With your nondominant hand (i.e., your left hand if you are right-handed), draw a simple three-dimensional cube. Start with a small square, then draw three diagonal lines and connect them like the figure on the right. Shade in the far side of it.

2. All of the vowels have been removed from the following proverb, and the remaining consonants are in the correct sequence broken up into groups of two to five letters. Replace the vowels and find the proverb:

FR NDNN DSF RN DNDD

3. Try to figure out the implied phrase below.

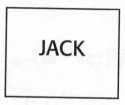

JACK

4. See how many words you can spell from the letters below. No letter may be used twice, and each word must have the letter "H" in it.

H	S	E	R	C	A	O

5. Starting with NOOK, change one letter at a time until you have the word BARN. Each change must be a proper word.

NOOK

· · · ·

· · · ·

· · · ·

BARN

6. Can you make the names of three U.S. capitals from the letters below? No letter may be used more than once.

PCKOXLN ASHV INSNI EJLEHAO

7. Which of the following words is the odd one out?

ELBAT AFOS PMAL LLAW RESSERD

8. When he has leisure time, Jim will read only certain kinds of material. He'll read *biographies,* but not *science fiction.* He likes the *sports page,* but not the *business section.* He'll review a *law journal,* but not a *mystery.* Based on this reading pattern, would he choose to read a *movie poster* or a *magazine?*

9. Figure out the missing number from the center square.

3	4	6
3		3
5	3	2

10. Mini-Crossword:

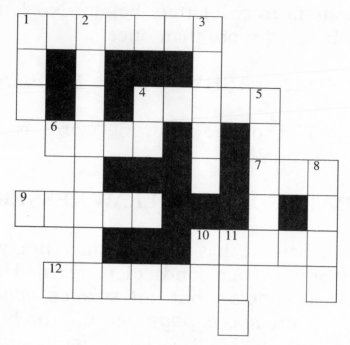

Clues

ACROSS
1. Social glue
4. Inactive potato
6. Brain teasers sharpen it
7. Cash source (abbrev.)
9. Omega-3 oil
10. Relating to birth
12. In need of relaxation

DOWN
1. Lasik target
2. Quality longevity outlook
3. The _____ and the Restless
4. _____-ROM
5. Blood pumper
8. Calcium booster
11. Visually creative work

11. Which of three numbered symbols below will complete the sequence?

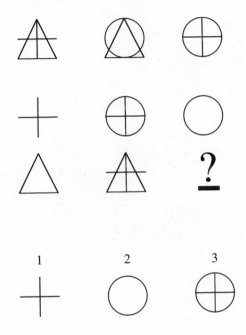

12. Figure out the message in the box below.

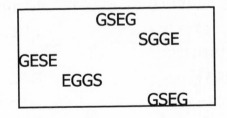

13. Which of three lettered symbols below will complete the sequence?

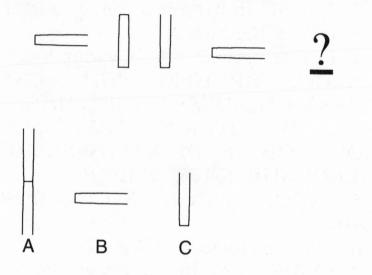

14. Try to fill in the box below so that you spell out the following words, either horizontally or vertically: AMEN, ENDS, LEND, MATE, MOLE, OMEN, TEND

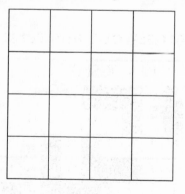

Answers to More Mental Aerobics

1. No correct answer.

2. A friend in need is a friend indeed.

3. Jack in the box.

4. I came up with the following words:
ARCH, ARCHES, ASH, CASH, CHASE, CHORE(S), CHOSE, HARE(S), HAS, HE, HEAR(S), HO, HOE(S), HOSE, OH, RAH, RASH, SEARCH, SHARE, SHE, SHOE, SHEAR

5. NOOK, NOON, BOON, BORN, BARN

6. Phoenix, Jackson, Nashville

7. **LLAW** — All the others are pieces of furniture spelled backward.

8. A *magazine*. Jim reads only material that has the letter "a" in it.

9. 4 — Each column adds up to the number 11.

10. Mini-crossword answers:

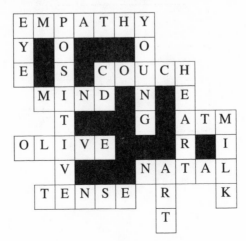

11. 1 — The last symbol in each column and row is always the same as the preceding two symbols minus any part that has been duplicated.

12. SCRAMBLED EGGS

13. A — This will spell the word "couch."

14.

M	O	L	E
A	M	E	N
T	E	N	D
E	N	D	S

Appendix 3

Additional Resources

Many organizations provide information on general health and other issues important to achieving quality longevity. Several national organizations also have local or state chapters. Check your telephone directory or Internet search engine for related organizations and Web sites.

AARP
6601 E Street NW
Washington, DC 20049
www.aarp.org

Nonprofit, nonpartisan organization dedicated to helping older Americans achieve lives of independence, dignity, and purpose.

888-687-2277

Academy of Molecular Imaging
Box 951735
Los Angeles, CA 90095-1735
www.ami-imaging.org

Provides leadership in research and clinical aspects of molecular imaging of the biological nature of disease. Their Web site includes a listing of local PET centers.

310-267-2614

Administration on Aging
Washington, DC 20201
www.aoa.gov

Provides information for older Americans and their families on opportunities and services to enrich their lives and support their independence.

202-619-0724

Aging Network Services
4400 East-West Highway,
Suite 907
Bethesda, MD 20814
www.agingnets.com

Nationwide network of private-practice geriatric social workers serving as care managers for seniors living at a distance from their families.

301-657-4329

Alliance of Information and Referral
  Systems
11240 Waples Mill Road
Suite 200
Fairfax, VA 22030
www.airs.org

Professional organization that provides human services information and referrals.

703-218-AIRS (2477)

Alzheimer Europe
145 Route de Thionville
L-2611 Luxembourg
www.alzheimer-europe.org

Organizes support for caregivers and raises awareness about dementia through cooperation among European Alzheimer's organizations.

352-29-79-70

Alzheimer's Association
225 N. Michigan Ave.,
Floor 17
Chicago, IL 60601
www.alz.org

National organization that provides information on Alzheimer's services, programs, publications, and local chapters.

800-272-3900

Alzheimer's Disease Education & Referral
  Center
P.O. Box 8250
Silver Springs, MD 20907-8250
www.alzheimers.org

National Institute on Aging service that distributes information and free materials on topics relevant to health professionals, patients and their families, and the general public.

800-438-4380

Alzheimer's Foundation of America
322 Eighth Avenue,
6th floor
New York, NY 10001
www.alzfdn.org

National nonprofit foundation supporting organizations that help lighten the burden and improve the quality of life of Alzheimer's patients and their caregivers.

866-AFA-8484
(866-232-8484)

American Academy of Neurology
1080 Montreal Avenue
St. Paul, MN 55116
www.aan.com

Professional organization that advances the art and science of neurology, thereby promoting the best possible care for patients with neurological disorders.

651-695-2717
800-879-1960

American Association for Geriatric
  Psychiatry
7910 Woodmont Avenue,
Suite 1050
Bethesda, MD 20814-3004
www.aagpgpa.org

Professional organization dedicated to enhancing the mental health and well-being of older adults, through education and research.

301-654-7850

American Diabetes Association
Attn: National Call Center
1701 North Beauregard Street
Alexandria, VA 22311
www.diabetes.org

America's leading nonprofit health organization, providing diabetes research, information, and advocacy.

1-800-DIABETES
(800-342-2383)

American Dietetic Association
120 South Riverside Plaza,
Suite 2000
Chicago, IL 60606-6995
www.eatright.org

Consumer nutrition hotline that provides information on finding a dietitian.

800-877-1600

American Geriatrics Society
The Empire State Building
350 Fifth Avenue,
Suite 801
New York, NY 10118
www.americangeriatrics.org

Professional association providing assistance in identifying local geriatric physician referrals.

212-308-1414

American Heart Association
7272 Greenville Avenue
Dallas, TX 75231
www.americanheart.org

Nonprofit health organization whose mission is to reduce disability and death from cardiovascular diseases and stroke.

800-242-8721

American Psychiatric Association
1000 Wilson Blvd.,
Suite 1825
Arlington, VA 22209
www.psych.org

Medical specialty society that works to ensure humane care and effective treatment for all people with mental disorders.

888-357-7924

American Psychological Association
750 First Street, NE
Washington, DC 20002
www.apa.org

Scientific and professional organization that represents psychology in the U.S. and aims to promote health, education, and human welfare.

800-374-2721

American Society on Aging
833 Market Street,
Suite 511
San Francisco, CA 94103
www.asaging.org

National organization concerned with physical, emotional, social, economic, and spiritual aspects of aging.

415-974-9600
800-537-9728

Children of Aging Parents
1609 Woodbourne Rd.,
#302-A
Levittown, PA 19057
www.caps4caregivers.org

National organization providing information and referrals for caregivers of older adults.

215-945-6900
800-227-7294

Dana Alliance for Brain Initiatives
745 Fifth Avenue,
Suite 900
New York, NY 10151
www.dana.org

Nonprofit organization committed to advancing public awareness about the progress and benefits of brain research.

Family Caregiver Alliance
180 Montgomery Street,
Suite 1100
San Francisco, CA 94104
www.caregiver.org

Resource center for families of adults with brain damage or dementia, which provides publications for caregivers and professionals.

415-434-3388
800-445-8106

Gerontological Society of America
1030 15th Street NW,
Suite 250
Washington, DC 20005
www.geron.org

National interdisciplinary organization on research and education in aging.

202-842-1275

Memory Fitness Institute
638 Camino De Los Mares,
Suite H130
San Clemente, CA 92673
www.memoryfitnessinstitute.org

Helps people of all ages to optimize their memory function and brain health, using state-of-the-art diagnostic, intervention, and prevention strategies.

(888) MEMFIT4

National Association of Area Agencies on
   Aging
1730 Rhode Island Avenue, NW,
Suite 1200
Washington, DC 20036
www.n4a.org

Umbrella organization for the 655 area agencies on aging. Helps older people and people with disabilities live with dignity and choices in their homes and communities for as long as possible.

202-872-0888

National Center for Complementary and
   Alternative Medicine,
National Institutes of Health
9000 Rockville Pike
Bethesda, MD 20829
www.nccam.nih.gov

Branch of the National Institutes of Health dedicated to exploring complementary and alternative healing practices in the context of rigorous science.

888-644-6226

National Consumer Law Center
77 Summer Street,
10th floor
Boston, MA 02110
www.consumerlaw.org

Nonprofit legal resource organization committed to making consumer law work for the interests of older adults and low-income individuals.

The National Council on the Aging
300 D Street, SW,
Suite 801
Washington, DC 20024
www.ncoa.org

National network of organizations and individuals dedicated to improving the health and independence of older persons and increasing their continuing contributions to communities, society, and future generations.

202-479-1200

National Institute of Mental Health,
Public Information and Communications
  Branch
6001 Executive Boulevard,
Room 8184, MSC 9663
Bethesda, MD 20892-9663
www.nimh.nih.gov

Part of the National Institutes of Health. Principal biomedical and behavioral research agency of the United States government.

866-615-6464

National Institute of Neurological
  Disorders and Stroke
P.O. Box 5801
Bethesda, MD 20824
www.ninds.nih.gov

National Institutes of Health agency that supports neuroscience research. Focuses on rapidly translating scientific discoveries into prevention, treatment, and cures, and provides resource support and information.

301-496-5751
800-352-9424

National Institute on Aging
Building 31, Room 5C27
31 Center Drive,
MSC 2292
Bethesda, MD 20892
www.nih.gov.nia

National Institutes of Health agency that supports research on aging and provides information about national Alzheimer's centers, and a free directory of organizations that serve older adults.

301-496-1752

National Osteoporosis Foundation
1232 22nd Street, NW
Washington, DC 20037-1292
www.nof.org

Nonprofit organization dedicated to preventing and curing osteoporosis. Supports numerous programs of awareness, education, advocacy, and research.

202-223-2226

National Stroke Association
9707 East Easter Lane
Englewood, CO 80112
www.stroke.org

Their mission is to reduce the incidence and impact of stroke disease and improve quality of patient care and outcomes.

800-787-6537

North American Menopause Society
P.O. Box 94527
Cleveland, OH 44101
www.menopause.org

Advocacy organization devoted to promoting women's health and quality of life
through an understanding of menopause.

440-442-7550

Older Women's League
1750 New York Avenue, NW
Suite 350
Washington, DC 20006
www.owl-national.org

Advocacy organization addressing family
and caregiver issues.

202-783-6686
800-825-3695

Safe Return Alzheimer's Association
225 North Michigan Avenue,
Floor 17
Chicago, IL 60601
www.alz.org

Joint program of the Alzheimer's Association and the National Center for Missing
Persons that provides patients with dementia with a bracelet showing the person's

name, the registered caregiver's name, and a toll-free number (800-572-1122) to aid in that person's return, if lost.

888-572-8566

SeniorNet
1171 Homestead Road,
Suite 280
Santa Clara, CA 95050
www.seniornet.com

National nonprofit organization that works to build a community of computer-using seniors.

408-615-0699

UCLA Center on Aging
10945 Le Conte Avenue,
Suite 3119
Los Angeles, CA 90095-6980
www.aging.ucla.edu

University center that works to enhance and extend productive and healthy life, through research and education on aging.

310-794-0676

U.S. Dept. of Veterans Affairs
810 Vermont Avenue, NW
Washington, DC 20420
www.va.gov

Provides information on VA programs, veterans benefits, VA facilities worldwide, and VA medical automation software.

800-827-1000

Bibliography

Agdeppa, E. D., Kepe, V., Petric, A., et al. In vitro detection of (S)-naproxen and ibuprofen binding to plaques in the Alzheimer's brain using the positron emission tomography molecular imaging probe 2-(1-{6-[(2-[^{18}F]fluoroethyl) (methyl)amino]-2-naphthyl}ethylidene) malononitrile. *Neuroscience* 117(2003): 723–30.

Age-Related Eye Disease Study (AREDS) Research Group. A randomized, placebo-controlled, clinical trial of high-dose supplementation with vitamins C and E and beta carotene for age-related cataract and vision loss: AREDS report no. 9. *Archives of Ophthalmology* 119 (2001):1439–52.

Aharon, I., Etcoff, N., Ariely, D., et al. Beautiful faces have variable reward value: fMRI and behavioral evidence. *Neuron* 32(2001):537–51.

Allen, K., Blascovich, J. Effects of music on cardiovascular reactivity among surgeons. *Journal of the American Medical Association* 272(1994):882–4.

Altena, T. S., Michaelson, J. L., Ball, S. D., Thomas, T. R. Single sessions of intermittent and continuous exercise and postprandial lipemia. *Medicine & Science in Sports & Exercise* 36(2004):1364–71.

Andersen, L. D., Remington, P., Trentham-Dietz, A., Reeves, M. Assessing a decade of progress in cancer control. *Oncologist* 7(2002):200–4.

Antell, D. E., Taczanowski, E. M. How environment and lifestyle choices influence the aging process. *Annals of Plastic Surgery* 43(1999):585–8.

Appel, L. J., Champagne, C. M., Harsha, D. W., et al. Effects of comprehensive lifestyle modification on blood pressure control: Main results of the PREMIER clinical trial. *Journal of the American Medical Association* 289(2003):2083–93.

Arterburn, D. E., Maciejewski, M. L., Tsevat, J. Impact of morbid obesity on medical expenditures in adults. *International Journal of Obesity and Related Metabolic Disorders* 29(2005):334–9.

Ball, K., Berch, D. B., Helmers, K. F., et al. Effects of cognitive training interventions with older adults: A randomized controlled trial. *Journal of the American*

Medical Association 288(2002):2271–81.

Barberger-Gateau, P., Letenneur, L., Deschamps, V., et al. Fish, meat, and risk of dementia: Cohort study. *British Medical Journal* 395(2002):932–33.

Bassuk, S. S., Glass, T. A., Berkman, L. F. Social disengagement and incident cognitive decline in community-dwelling elderly persons. *Annals of Internal Medicine* 131(1999):165–73.

Beauchamp, G. K., Keast, R. S., Morel, D., et al. Phytochemistry: Ibuprofen-like activity in extra-virgin olive oil. *Nature* 437(2005):45–6.

Bell, M. L., McDermott, A., Zeger, S. L., Samet, J. M., Dominici, F. Ozone and short-term mortality in 95 U.S. urban communities, 1987–2000. *Journal of the American Medical Association* 292(2004):2372–8.

Bennett, M. P., Zeller, J. M., Rosenberg, L., McCann, J. The effect of mirthful laughter on stress and natural killer cell activity. *Alternative Therapies in Health and Medicine* 9(2003):38–45.

Benson, H. *The Relaxation Response.* New York: Avon, 1975.

Berk, L. S., Tan, S. A., Fry, W. F., et al. Neuroendocrine and stress hormone changes during mirthful laughter. *Amer-*

ican *Journal of Medical Science* 298 (1989):390–6.

Berkowitz, L., Harmon-Jones, E. Toward an understanding of the determinants of anger. *Emotion* 4(2004):107–30.

Berman, B. M., Lao, L., Langenberg, P., et al. Effectiveness of acupuncture as adjunctive therapy in osteoarthritis of the knee: A randomized, controlled trial. *Annals of Internal Medicine* 141(2004):901–10.

Betts, L. R., Taylor, C. P., Sekuler, A. B., Bennett, P. J. Aging reduces center-surround antagonism in visual motion processing. *Neuron* 45(2005):361–6.

Bijlani, R. L., Vempati, R. P., Yadav, R. K., et al. A brief but comprehensive lifestyle education program based on yoga reduces risk factors for cardiovascular disease and diabetes mellitus. *Journal of Alternative and Complementary Medicine* 11(2005):267–74.

Birks J., Grimley Evans, J. Ginkgo biloba for cognitive impairment and dementia (Cochrane Review). The Cochrane Library, Issue 2, 2005. Chichester, U.K.: John Wiley & Sons, Ltd.

Block, J. D. *Sex Over 50*. Paramus, NJ: Reward Books, 1999.

Bone, H. G., Hosking, D., Devogelaer, J. P., et al. Ten years' experience with alendronate for osteoporosis in post-menopausal women. *New England Journal of Medicine* 350(2004):1172–4.

Bookheimer, S. Y., Strojwas, M. H., Cohen, M. S., et al. Brain activation in people at genetic risk for Alzheimer's disease. *New England Journal of Medicine* 343(2000):450–6.

Booth, A., Johnson, D. R., Granger, D. A. Testosterone and men's health. *Journal of Behavioral Medicine* 22(1999):1–19.

Boschmann, M., Steiniger, J., Hille, U., et al. Water-induced thermogenesis. *Journal of Clinical Endocrinology and Metabolism* 88(2003):6015–19.

Bowman, R. E., Beck, K. D., Luine, V. N. Chronic stress effects on memory: Sex differences in performance and monoaminergic activity. *Hormones and Behavior* 43(2003):48–59.

Boyd-Brewer, C., McCaffrey, R. Vibro-acoustic sound therapy improves pain management and more. *Holistic Nursing Practice* 18(2004):111–18.

Brand-Miller, J., Volwever, T. M. S., Colaguiri, S., Foster-Powell, K. *The Glucose Revolution.* New York: Marlow & Company, 1999.

Braunstein, G. D., Sundwall, D. A., Katz, M., et al. Safety and efficacy of a testosterone patch for the treatment of hypoactive sexual desire disorder in surgically menopausal women: a randomized, placebo-controlled trial. *Archives of Internal Medicine* 165(2005):1582–9.

Breiter, H. C., Aharon, I., Kahneman, D., Dale, A., Shizgal, P. Functional imaging of neural responses to expectancy and experience of monetary gains and losses. *Neuron* 30(2001):619–39.

Brickman, P., Coates, D., Janoff-Bulman, R. Lottery winners and accident victims: Is happiness relative? *Journal of Personality and Social Psychology* 36(1978):917–27.

Brinkhaus, B., Becker-Witt, C., Jena, S., et al. Acupuncture Randomized Trials (ART) in patients with chronic low back pain and osteoarthritis of the knee — design and protocols. *Forsch Komplementarmed Klass Naturheilkd* 10(2003): 185–91.

Brown, K. W., Ryan, R. M. The benefits of being present: Mindfulness and its role in psychological well-being. *Journal of Personality and Social Psychology* 84(2003):822–48.

Calle, E. E., Rodriguez, C., Walker-Thurmond, K., Thun, M. J. Overweight, obesity, and mortality from cancer in a prospectively studied cohort of U.S. adults. *New England Journal of Medicine* 348(2003):1625–38.

Carnethon, M. R., Gidding, S. S., Nehgme, R. et al. Cardiorespiratory fitness in young adulthood and the development of cardiovascular disease risk factors. *Journal of the American Medical Association* 290(2003):3092–100.

Carr, L., Iacoboni, M., Dubeau, M.-C., Mazziotta, J. C., Lenz, G. L. Neural mechanisms of empathy in humans: A relay from neural systems for imitation to limbic areas. *Proceedings of the National Academy of Sciences of the United States of America* 100(2003): 5497–5502.

Chafin, S., Roy, M., Gerin, W., Christenfeld, N. Music can facilitate blood pressure recovery from stress. *British Journal of Health and Psychology* 9(2004): 393–403.

Chainani-Wu, N. Safety and anti-inflammatory activity of curcumin: A component of turmeric (*Curcuma longa*). *Journal of Alternative and Complementary Medicine* 9(2003):161–8.

Chao, A., Thun, M. J., Connell, C. J., et al. Meat consumption and risk of colorectal cancer. *Journal of the American Medical*

Association 293(2005): 172–82.

Chapman, S. B., Weiner, M. F., Rackley, A., Hynan, L. S., Zientz, J. Effects of cognitive-communication stimulation for Alzheimer's disease patients treated with donepezil. *Journal of Speech, Language, and Hearing Research* 47(2004): 1149–63.

Charnetski, C. J., Brennan, F. X. Sexual frequency and salivary immunoglobulin A (IgA). *Psychological Reports* 94(2004): 839–44.

Chen, J. T., Wesley, R., Shamburek, R. D., Pucino, F., Csako, G. Meta-analysis of natural therapies for hyperlipidemia: Plant sterols and stanols versus policosanol. *Pharmacotherapy* 25(2005): 171–83.

Chlebowski, R. T., Wactawski-Wende, J., Ritenbaugh, C., et al. Estrogen plus progestin and colorectal cancer in postmenopausal women. *New England Journal of Medicine* 350(2004): 991–1004.

Choi, J. H., Moon, J. S., Song, R. Effects of Sun-style tai chi exercise on physical fitness and fall prevention in fall-prone older adults. *Journal of Advanced Nursing* 51(2005):150–7.

Christensen, H. C., Schüz, J., Kosteljanetz,

M., et al. Cellular telephone use and risk of acoustic neuroma. *American Journal of Epidemiology* 159(2004):277–83.

Clark, A., Seidler, A., Miller, M. Inverse association between sense of humor and coronary heart disease. *International Journal of Cardiology* 80(2001):87–8.

Clark, N. *Nancy Clark's Sports Nutrition Guidebook*, Third Edition. Champaign, IL: Human Kinetics Publishing, 2003.

Colcombe, S. J., Erickson, K. I., Raz, N., et al. Aerobic fitness reduces brain tissue loss in aging humans. *Journal of Gerontology: Biological Sciences and Medical Sciences* 58A(2003):176–80.

Contento, I. R., Basch, C., Zybert, P. Body image, weight, and food choices of Latina women and their young children. *Journal of Nutrition Education and Behavior* 35(2003):236–48.

Dahlberg, L. L., Ikeda, R. M., and Kresnow, M. Guns in the home and risk of a violent death in the home: Findings from a national study. *American Journal of Epidemiology* 160(2004):929–36.

Dallongeville, J., Marecaux, N., Ducimetiere, P., et al. Influence of alcohol consumption and various beverages on waist girth and waist-to-hip ratio in a sample of French men and women. *In-*

ternational *Journal of Obesity and Related Metabolic Disorders* 22(1998): 1178–83.

Davey Smith, G., Frankel, S., Yarnell, J. Sex and death: are they related? Findings from the Caerphilly Cohort Study. *British Medical Journal* 315(1997): 1641–4.

Davidson, R. J., Kabat-Zinn, J., Schumacher, J., et al. Alterations in brain and immune function produced by mindfulness meditation. *Psychosomatic Medicine* 65(2003):564–70.

de Castro, J. M. The time of day of food intake influences overall intake in humans. *The Journal of Nutrition* 134(2004): 104–11.

de Lorgeril, M., Salen, P., Martin, J.-L., et al. Mediterranean diet, traditional risk factors, and the rate of cardiovascular complications after myocardial infarction: Final report of the Lyon Diet Heart Study. *Circulation* 99(1999):779–85.

De Smet, P. Herbal remedies. *New England Journal of Medicine* 347(2002):2046–56.

Del Ser, T., Hachinski, V., Merskey, H., Munoz, D. G. An autopsy-verified study of the effect of education on degenerative dementia. *Brain* 122(1999):2309–19.

Dickey, R. A., Janick, J. J. Lifestyle modifications in the prevention and treatment of hypertension. *Endocrine Practice* 7(2001):392–9.

Doerksen, S., Shimamura, A. P. Source memory enhancement for emotional words. *Emotion* 1(2001):5–11.

Draganski, B., Gaser, C., Busch, V., et al. Neuroplasticity: Changes in grey matter induced by training. *Nature* 427(2004):311–12.

Eckman, P. *Emotions Revealed: Recognizing Faces and Feelings to Improve Communication and Emotional Life.* New York: Times Books, 2003.

Ehlenfeldt, M. K., Prior, R. L. Oxygen Radical Absorbance Capacity (ORAC) and phenolic and anthocyanin concentrations in fruit and leaf tissues of highbush blueberry. *Journal of Agriculture and Food Chemistry* 49(2001):2222–7.

Eng, P. M., Fitzmaurice, G., Kubzansky, L. D., Rimm, E. B., Kawachi, I. Anger expression and risk of stroke and coronary heart disease among male health professionals. *Psychosomatic Medicine* 65(2003):100–10.

Epel, E. S., Blackburn, E. H., Lin, J., et al. Accelerated telomere shortening in response to life stress. *Proceedings of the*

National Academy of Sciences of the United States of America. 101(2004): 17312–15.

Eriksson, J., Lindstrom, J., Tuomilehto, J. Potential for the prevention of type 2 diabetes. *British Medical Bulletin* 60(2001):183–99.

Evans, J. R. Ginkgo biloba extract for age-related macular degeneration (Cochrane Review). The Cochrane Library, Issue 4, 2005. Chichester, UK: John Wiley & Sons, Ltd.

Fairfield, K. M., Fletcher, R. H. Vitamins for chronic disease prevention in adults: Scientific review. *Journal of the American Medical Association* 287(2002): 3116–26.

Fajardo, M., Di Cesare, P. E. Disease-modifying therapies for osteoarthritis: Current status. *Drugs & Aging* 22(2005):141–61.

Fan, J., Liu, F., Wu, J., Dai, W. Visual perception of female physical attractiveness. *Proceedings of the Royal Society of London* 271(2004):347–52.

Feldman, H. A., Johannes, C. B., McKinlay, J. B., Longcope, C. Low dehydroepiandrosterone sulfate and heart disease in middle-aged men: Cross-sectional results from the Massachusetts Male Aging Study. *Annals of Epidemiology* 8(1998):217–28.

Feldman, S. R., Liguori, A., Kucenic, M., et al. Ultraviolet exposure is a reinforcing stimulus in frequent indoor tanners. *Journal of the American Academy of Dermatology* 51(2004):45–51.

Ferro, A. R., Kopperud, R. J., Hildemann, L. M. Source strengths for indoor human activities that resuspend particulate matter. *Environmental Science & Technology* 38(2004):1759–64.

Fonarow, G. C., Wright, R. S., Spencer, F. A., et al. Effect of statin use within the first 24 hours of admission for acute myocardial infarction on early morbidity and mortality. *American Journal of Cardiology* 96(2005):611–16.

Frank, L. D., Andresen, M. A., Schmid, T. L. Obesity relationships with community design, physical activity, and time spent in cars. *American Journal of Preventive Medicine* 27(2004):87–96.

Fraser, G. E., Shavlik, D. J. Ten years of life: Is it a matter of choice? *Archives of Internal Medicine* 161(2001):1645–52.

Gadek-Michalska, A., Bugajski, J. Repeated handling, restraint, or chronic crowding impair the hypothalamic-pituitary-adrenocortical response to acute restraint stress. *Journal of Physiological Pharmacology* 54(2003):449–59.

Gage, F. H. Neurogenesis in the adult brain. *Journal of Neuroscience* 22(2002): 612–13.

Gauderman, W. J., Avol, E., Gilliland, F., et al. The effect of air pollution on lung development from 10 to 18 years of age. *New England Journal of Medicine* 351(2004):1057–67.

Geday, J., Gjedde, A., Boldsen, A.-S., Kupers, R. Emotional valence modulates activity in the posterior fusiform gyrus and inferior medial prefrontal cortex in social perception. *NeuroImage* 18(2003): 675–84.

Gilewski, M. J., Zelinski, E. M., Schaie, K. W. The Memory Functioning Questionnaire for assessment of memory complaints in adulthood and old age. *Psychology and Aging* 5(1990):482–90.

Glass, T. A., de Leon, C. M., Marottoli, R. A., Berkman, L. F. Population based study of social and productive activities as predictors of survival among elderly Americans. *British Medical Journal* 319(1999):478–83.

Green, C. S., Bavelier, D. Action video game modifies visual selective attention. *Nature* 423(2003):534–7.

Greenblatt, D. Treatment of postmeno-pausal osteoporosis. *Pharmacotherapy* 25 (2005):574–84.

Gurung, R. A., Taylor, S. E., Seeman, T. E. Accounting for changes in social support among married older adults: Insights from the MacArthur Studies of Successful Aging. *Psychology and Aging* 18(2003): 487–96.

Hathcock, J. N. Vitamins and minerals: Efficacy and safety. *American Journal of Clinical Nutrition* 66(1997):427–37.

Hayashi, K., Hayashi, T., Iwanaga, S., et al. Laughter lowered the increase in post-prandial blood glucose. *Diabetes Care* 26(2003):1651–2.

He, F. J., MacGregor, G. A. Effect of modest salt reduction on blood pressure: A meta-analysis of randomized trials. Implications for public health. *Journal of Human Hypertension* 16(2002):761–70.

Heart Protection Study Collaborative Group. MRC/BHF Heart Protection Study of cholesterol lowering with simvastatin in 20,536 high-risk individuals: A randomized placebo-controlled trial. *Lancet* 360(2002):7–22.

Heber, D., Bowerman, S. *What Color Is Your Diet?* New York: Regan Books, 2001.

Heisler, M., Langa, K. M., Eby, E. L., et al. The health effects of restricting prescription medication use because of cost. *Medical Care* 42(2004):626–34.

Henwood, T. R., Taaffe, D. R. Improved physical performance in older adults undertaking a short-term programme of high-velocity resistance training. *Gerontology* 51(2005):108–15.

Hightower, J. M., Moore, D. Mercury levels in high-end consumers of fish. *Environmental Health Perspective* 111(2003):604–8.

Horwich, T. B., MacLellan, W. R., Fonarow, G. C. Statin therapy is associated with improved survival in ischemic and non-ischemic heart failure. *Journal of the American College of Cardiology* 43(2004):642–8.

Hui, K. K., Liu, J., Makris, N., et al. Acupuncture modulates the limbic system and subcortical gray structures of the human brain: Evidence from fMRI studies in normal subjects. *Human Brain Mapping* 9(2000):13–25.

Hummer, R. A., Rogers, R. G., Nam, C. B., Ellison, C. G. Religious involvement and U.S. adult mortality. *Demography* 36(1999):273–85.

Irwin, M. R., Pike, J. L., Cole, J. C.,

Oxman, M. N. Effects of a behavioral intervention, tai chi chih, on varicella-zoster virus specific immunity and health functioning in older adults. *Psychosomatic Medicine* 65(2003):824–30.

Järvinen, R., Knekt, P., Hakulinen, T., Aromaa, A. Prospective study on milk products, calcium, and cancers of the colon and rectum. *Journal of the National Cancer Institute* 55(2001):1000–7.

Johnson, S. M. The revolution in couple therapy: A practitioner-scientist perspective. *Journal of Marital and Family Therapy* 29(2003):365–84.

Joseph, J. A., Nadeau, D., Underwood, A. *The Color Code: A Revolutionary Eating Plan for Optimum Health.* New York: Hyperion, 2002.

Kabat-Zinn, J., Lipworth, L., Burney, R., Sellers, W. Four year follow-up of a meditation-based program for the self-regulation of chronic pain: Treatment outcomes and compliance. *Clinical Journal of Pain* 2(1986):159–73.

Kabat-Zinn, J., Massion, A. O., Kristeller, J., et al. Effectiveness of a meditation-based stress reduction program in the treatment of anxiety disorders. *American Journal of Psychiatry* 149(1992):936–43.

Kabat-Zinn, J., Wheeler, E., Light, T., et

al. Influence of a mindfulness-based stress reduction intervention on rates of skin clearing in patients with moderate to severe psoriasis undergoing phototherapy (UVB) and photochemotherapy (PUVA). *Psychosomatic Medicine* 60 (1998):625–32.

Kahn, R. L., Rowe, J. W. *Successful Aging*. New York: Pantheon, 1998.

Karlin, W. A., Brondolo, E., Schwartz, J. Workplace social support and ambulatory cardiovascular activity in New York City traffic agents. *Psychosomatic Medicine* 65(2003):167–76.

Karvonen, M. J. Sports and longevity. *Advances in Cardiology* 18(1976):243–8.

Kiecolt-Glaser, J. K., Preacher, K. J., MacCallum, R. C., et al. Chronic stress and age-related increases in the proinflammatory cytokine IL-6. *Proceedings of the National Academy of Sciences of the United States of America* 100(2003):9090–5.

Knoops, K. T. B., de Groot, L. C., Kromhout, D., et al. Mediterranean diet, lifestyle factors, and 10-year mortality in elderly European men and women. *Journal of the American Medical Association* 292(2004):1433–9.

Koenig, H. G., George, L. K., Titus, P.

Religion, spirituality, and health in medically ill hospitalized older patients. *Journal of the American Geriatrics Society* 52(2004):554–62.

Kousa, A., Moltchanova, E., Viik-Kajander, M., et al. Geochemistry of ground water and the incidence of acute myocardial infarction in Finland. *Journal of Epidemiology and Community Health* 58(2004):136–9.

Kubey, R., Csikszentmihalyi, M. Television addiction is no mere metaphor. *Scientific American* 286(2002):74–80.

Kwallek, N., Lewis, C. M. Effects of environmental colour on males and females: A red or white or green office. *Applied Ergonomics* 21(1990):275–8.

Law, M., Wald, N., Morris, J. Lowering blood pressure to prevent myocardial infarction and stroke: A new preventive strategy. *Health Technology Assessment* 7(2003):1–94.

Lazar, S. W., Bush, G., Gollub, R. L., et al. Functional brain mapping of the relaxation response and meditation. *Neuroreport* 11(2000):1581–5.

Lee, I. M., Cook, N. R. Gaziano, J. M., et al. Vitamin E in the primary prevention of cardiovascular disease and cancer: The Women's Health Study: A randomized controlled trial. *Journal of the American Medical Association* 294(2005):56–65.

Lee, I. M., Hsieh, C. C., Paffenbarger, R. S. Exercise intensity and longevity in men. *Journal of the American Medical Association* 273(1995):1179–84.

Lee, I. M., Sesso, H. D., Oguma, Y., Paffenbarger, R. S. Jr. The "weekend warrior" and risk of mortality. *American Journal of Epidemiology* 160(2004): 636–41.

Leetun, D. T., Ireland, M. L., Willson, J. D., Ballantyne, B. T., Davis, I. M. Core stability measures as risk factors for lower extremity injury in athletes. *Medicine & Science in Sports & Exercise* 36(2004):926–34.

Lim, G. P., Chu, T., Yang, F., Beech, W., Frautschy, S. A., Cole, G. M. The curry spice curcumin reduces oxidative damage and amyloid pathology in an Alzheimer transgenic mouse. *Journal of Neuroscience* 21(2001):8370–7.

Liu, S., Manson, J. E., Stampfer, M. J., et al. Whole-grain consumption and risk of ischemic stroke in women: A prospective study. *Journal of the American Medical Association* 284(2000):1534–40.

Liu-Ambrose, T., Khan, K. M., Eng, J. J., Janssen, P. A., Lord, S. R., McKay, H. A.

Resistance and agility training reduce fall risk in women aged 75 to 85 with low bone mass: A 6-month randomized, controlled trial. *Journal of the American Geriatrics Society* 52(2004):657–65.

Loewenstein, D. A., Acevedo, A., Czaja, S. J., Duara, R. Cognitive rehabilitation of mildly impaired Alzheimer disease patients on cholinesterase inhibitors. *American Journal of Geriatric Psychiatry* 12(2004):395–402.

Ma, Y., Bertone, E. R., Stanek, E. J., III, et al. Association between eating patterns and obesity in a free-living U.S. adult population. *American Journal of Epidemiology* 158(2003):85–92.

MacDonald, G. *Massage for the Hospital Patient and Medically Frail Client.* New York: Lippincott Williams & Wilkins, 2004.

Maguire, E. A., Valentine, E. R., Wilding, J. M., Kapur, N. Routes to remembering: The brains behind superior memory. *Nature Neuroscience* 6(2003):90–5.

Malliaropoulos, N., Papalexandris, S., Papalada, A., Papacostas, E. The role of stretching in rehabilitation of hamstring injuries: 80 athletes follow-up. *Medicine & Science in Sports & Exercise* 36(2004):756–9.

McClure, S. M., Laibson, D. I., Loewen-stein, G., Cohen, J. D. Separate neural systems value immediate and delayed monetary rewards. *Science* 306(2004): 503–7.

McEwen, B. *The End of Stress As We Know It.* Washington, DC: The Dana Press, 2004.

Means, K. M., Rodell, D. E., O'Sullivan, P. S. Balance, mobility, and falls among community-dwelling elderly persons: Effects of a rehabilitation exercise program. *American Journal of Physical Medicine & Rehabilitation* 84(2005):238–50.

Menec, V. H. The relation between everyday activities and successful aging: A 6-year longitudinal study. *Journal of Gerontology Series B: Psychological Sciences and Social Sciences* 58(2003):S74–S82.

Miller, E. R., Pastor-Barriuso, R., Dalal, D., et al. Meta-analysis: High-dosage vitamin E supplementation may increase all-cause mortality. *Annals of Internal Medicine* 142(2005):37–46.

Moore, A. A., Gould, R., Reuben, D. B., et al. Longitudinal patterns and predictors of alcohol consumption in the United States. *American Journal of Public Health* 95(2005):458–65.

Morris, M. C., Evans, D. A., Bienias, J. L., et al. Dietary niacin and the risk of incident Alzheimer's disease and of cognitive decline. *Journal of Neurology, Neurosurgery and Psychiatry* 75(2004):1093–99.

Mukamal, K. J., Kuller, L. H., Fitzpatrick, A. L., et al. Prospective study of alcohol consumption and risk of dementia in older adults. *Journal of the American Medical Association* 289(2003):1405–13.

Murtaugh, M. A., Jacobs, D. R. Jr., Jacob, B., Steffen, L. M., Marquart, L. Epidemiological support for the protection of whole grains against diabetes. *The Proceedings of the Nutrition Society* 62(2003):143–9.

Newberg, A., Alavi, A., Baime, M., Pourdehnad, M., Santanna, J., d'Aquili, E. The measurement of regional cerebral blood flow during the complex cognitive task of meditation: A preliminary SPECT study. *Psychiatry Research* 106(2001):113–22.

Nissen, S. E., Tuzcu, E. M., Libby, P., et al. Effect of antihypertensive agents on cardiovascular events in patients with coronary disease and normal blood pressure: The CAMELOT study: A randomized controlled trial. *Journal of the American Medical Association* 292(2004):2217–25.

North American Menopause Society. Recommendations for estrogen and progestogen use in peri- and postmenopausal women: October 2004 position statement of The North American Menopause Society. *Menopause* 11(2004):589–600.

Olshansky, J., Passaro, D. J., Hershow, R. C., et al. A potential decline in life expectancy in the United States in the 21st century. *New England Journal of Medicine* 352(2005):1138–45.

Paffenbarger, R. S. Jr., Hyde, R. T., Wing, A. L., Hsieh, C. C. Physical activity, all-cause mortality, and longevity of college alumni. *New England Journal of Medicine* 314(1986):605–13.

Palmore, E. Predictors of the longevity difference: A 25-year follow-up. *Gerontologist* 22(1982):513–18.

Pargament, K. I., Koenig, H. G., Tarakeshwar, N., Hahn, J. Religious struggle as a predictor of mortality among medically ill elderly patients: a 2-year longitudinal study. *Archives of Internal Medicine* 161(2001):1881–5.

Pate, R. R., Pratt, M., Blair, S. N., et al. Physical activity and public health. A recommendation from the Centers for Disease Control and Prevention and the American College of Sports Medicine.

Journal of the American Medical Association 273(1995):402–7.

Persson, G. Five-year mortality in a 70-year-old urban population in relation to psychiatric diagnosis, personality, sexuality and early parental death. *Journal of Psychosomatic Research* 24(1980):244–53.

Peters, A., von Klot, S., Heier, M., et al. Exposure to traffic and the onset of myocardial infarction. *New England Journal of Medicine* 351(2004): 1721–30.

Petersen, R. C., Thomas, R. G., Grundman, M., et al. Vitamin E and donepezil for the treatment of mild cognitive impairment. *New England Journal of Medicine* 352(2005):2379–88.

Pew Internet & American Life Project. *The Internet and Daily Life.* 2004. http://www.pewinternet.org/

Poynter, J. N., Gruber, S. B., Higgins, P. D., et al. Statins and the risk of colorectal cancer. *New England Journal of Medicine* 352(2005):2184–92.

Prigerson, H. G., Maciejewski, P. K., Rosenheck, R. A. The effects of marital dissolution and marital quality on health and health service use among women. *Medical Care* 37(1999):858–73.

Rami, T., Shih, H. T. Update of implantable cardioverter/defibrillator and cardiac resynchronization therapy in heart failure. *Current Opinions in Cardiology* 19(2004):264–9.

Raskind, M. A., Peskind, E. R., Wessel, T., and the Galantamine USA-1 Study Group. Galantamine in AD. A 6-month randomized, placebo-controlled trial with a 6-month extension. *Neurology* 54(2000):2269–2276.

Rea, T. D., Breitner, J. C., Psaty, B. M., et al. Statin use and the risk of incident dementia: The Cardiovascular Health Study. *Archives of Neurology* 62(2005): 1047–51.

Reisberg, B., Doody, R., Stoffler, A., et al. Memantine in moderate-to-severe Alzheimer's disease. *New England Journal of Medicine* 348(2003):1333–41.

Rennie, M. J. Claims for the anabolic effects of growth hormone: A case of the Emperor's new clothes? *British Journal of Sports Medicine* 37(2003):100–5.

Rimm, E. B., Ascherio, A., Giovannucci, E., et al. Vegetable, fruit, and cereal fiber intake and risk of coronary heart disease among men. *Journal of the American Medical Association* 275(1996): 447–51.

Rimm, E. B., Stampfer, M. J. Diet, lifestyle, and longevity — The next steps? *Journal of the American Medical Association* 292(2004):1490–2.

Rozmus-Wrzesinska, M., Pawlowski, B. Men's ratings of female attractiveness are influenced more by changes in female waist size compared with changes in hip size. *Biological Psychology* 68(2005):299–308.

Ruitenberg, A., van Swieten, J. C., Witteman, J. C., et al. Alcohol consumption and risk of dementia: The Rotterdam Study. *Lancet* 359(2002):281–6.

Sano, M., Ernesto, C., Thomas, R. G., et al. A controlled trial of selegiline, alpha-tocopherol, or both as treatment for Alzheimer's disease. *New England Journal of Medicine* 336(1997):1216–22.

Schneider, R. H., Alexander, C. N., Staggers, F., et al. A randomized controlled trial of stress reduction in African Americans treated for hypertension for over one year. *American Journal of Hypertension* 18(2005):88–98.

Schneider, R. H., Alexander, C. N., Staggers, F., et al. Long-term effects of stress reduction on mortality in persons > or = 55 years of age with systemic hypertension. *American Journal of Cardiology* 95(2005):1060–4.

Sesso, H. D., Chen, R. S., L'Italien, G. J.,

et al. Blood pressure lowering and life expectancy based on a Markov model of cardiovascular events. *Hypertension* 42(2003):885–90.

Shenk, D. *Data Smog: Surviving the Information Glut.* New York: HarperCollins, 1997.

Sherman, S. E., D'Agostino, R. B., Cobb, J. L., Kannel, W. B. Physical activity and mortality in women in the Framingham Heart Study. *American Heart Journal* 128(1994):879–84.

Shoghi-Jadid, K., Small, G. W., Agdeppa, E. D., et al. Localization of neurofibrillary tangles and beta-amyloid plaques in the brains of living patients with Alzheimer disease. *American Journal of Geriatric Psychiatry* 10(2002): 24–35.

Shumaker, S. A., Legault, C., Rapp, S. R., et al. Estrogen plus progestin and the incidence of dementia and mild cognitive impairment in postmenopausal women. The Women's Health Initiative Memory Study: A randomized controlled trial. *Journal of the American Medical Association* 289(2003):2651–62.

Simon, S. R., Chan, K. A., Soumerai, S. B., et al. Potentially inappropriate medication use by elderly persons in

U.S. Health Maintenance Organizations, 2000–2001. *Journal of the American Geriatric Society* 53 (2005):227–32.

Singer, T., Seymour, B., O'Doherty, J., Kaube, H., Dolan, R. J., Frith, C. D. Empathy for pain involves the affective but not sensory components of pain. *Science* 303(2004):1157–62.

Small, G., Vorgan G. *The Memory Prescription: Dr. Gary Small's 14-Day Plan to Keep Your Brain and Body Young.* New York: Hyperion, 2004.

Small, G. *The Memory Bible: An Innovative Strategy for Keeping Your Brain Young.* New York: Hyperion, 2002.

Small, G. W., Silverman, D. H., Siddarth, P., et al. Brain function and physical effects of a 14-day healthy lifestyle program. *9th International Conference on Alzheimer's Disease and Related Disorders*, 2004.

Small, G. W. What we need to know about age related memory loss. *British Medical Journal* 324(2002):1502–5.

Smith, G. D., Frankel, S., Yarnell, J. Sex and death, are they related? Findings from the Caerphilly cohort study. *British Medical Journal* 315(1997): 164–5.

Soeken, K. L., Lee, W. L., Bausell, R. B., Agelli, M., Berman, B. M. Safety and efficacy of S-adenosylmethionine (SAMe) for osteoarthritis. *Journal of Family Practice* 51(2002):425–30.

Spiro, H. What is empathy and can it be taught? *Annals of Internal Medicine* 116(1992):843–6.

Springer, M. V., McIntosh, A. R., Winocur, G., Grady, C. L. The relation between brain activity during memory tasks and years of education in young and older adults. *Neuropsychology* 19(2005):181–92.

Stanton, R., Reaburn, P. R., Humphries, B. The effect of short-term Swiss ball training on core stability and running economy. *Journal of Strength and Conditioning Research* 18(2004):522–8.

Stevens, C., Tiggemann, M. Women's body figure preferences across the life span. *Journal of Genetic Psychology* 159(1998):94–102.

Takahashi, M., Nakata, A., Haratani, T., Ogawa, Y., Arito, H. Post-lunch nap as a worksite intervention to promote alertness on the job. *Ergonomics* 47 (2004):1003–13.

Takano, T., Nakamura, K., Watanabe, M. Urban residential environments and senior citizens' longevity in megacity areas: The importance of walkable green spaces. *Journal of Epidemiology and Community Health* 56(2002):913–18.

Thomsen, D. K., Mehlsen, M. Y., Hokland, M., et al. Negative thoughts and health: Associations among rumination, immunity, and health care utilization in a young and elderly sample. *Psychosomatic Medicine* 66(2004): 363–71.

Travis, F., Arenander, A., DuBois, D. Psychological and physiological characteristics of a proposed object-referral/self-referral continuum of self-awareness. *Consciousness Cognition* 13(2004): 401–20.

Turner, R. B., Bauer, R., Woelkart, K., Hulsey, T. C., Gangemi, J. D. An evaluation of *Echinacea angustifolia* in experimental rhinovirus infections. *New England Journal of Medicine* 353(2005): 341–8.

USC Annenberg School Center for the Digital Future. *The Digital Future Report.* 2004. http://www.digitalcenter.org/

van der Valk, R., Webers, C. A., Schouten, J. S., et al. Intraocular pressure-lowering effects of all commonly used glaucoma drugs: A meta-analysis of randomized clinical trials. *Ophthalmology* 112(2005): 1177–85.

Van Gaal, L. F., Rissanen, A. M., Scheen, A. J., et al. Effects of the cannabinoid-1 receptor blocker rimonabant on weight reduction and cardiovascular risk factors in overweight patients: 1-year experience from the RIO-Europe study. *Lancet* 365(2005):1389–97.

Verghese, J., Lipton, R. B., Katz, M. J., et al. Leisure activities and the risk of dementia in the elderly. *New England Journal of Medicine* 348(2003): 2508–16.

Verhagen, E., van der Beek, A., Twisk, J., Bouter, L., Bahr, R., van Mechelen, W. The effect of a proprioceptive balance board training program for the prevention of ankle sprains: A prospective controlled trial. *American Journal of Sports Medicine* 32(2004):1385–93.

Vermeire, K., Brokx, J. P., Wuyts, F. L., et al. Quality-of-life benefit from cochlear implantation in the elderly. *Otology & Neurotology* 26(2005):188–95.

Vijan, S., Hayward, R. A.; American College of Physicians. Pharmacologic lipid-lowering therapy in type 2 diabetes mellitus: Background paper for the American College of Physicians. *Annals of Internal Medicine* 140(2004):650–8.

Villareal, D. T., Holloszy, J. O. Effect of

DHEA on abdominal fat and insulin action in elderly women and men: A randomized controlled trial. *Journal of the American Medical Association* 292(2004):2243–8.

Wager, N., Fieldman, G., Hussey, T. The effect on ambulatory blood pressure of working under favourably and unfavourably perceived supervisors. *Journal of Occupational and Environmental Medicine* 60(2003):468–74.

Wang Y., Wang, Q. J. The prevalence of prehypertension and hypertension among U.S. adults according to the new joint national committee guidelines: New challenges of the old problem. *Archives of Internal Medicine* 164(2004): 2126–34.

Wannamethee, S. G., Camargo, C. A. Jr., Manson, J. E., Willett, W. C., Rimm, E. B. Alcohol drinking patterns and risk of type 2 diabetes mellitus among younger women. *Archives of Internal Medicine* 163(2003):1329–36.

Wansink B., Lee, K. Cooking habits provide a key to 5 a day success. *Journal of the American Dietetic Association* 104(2004):1648–50.

Wansink, B., Linder, L. R. Interactions between forms of fat consumption and restaurant bread consumption. *International Journal of Obesity* 27(2003): 866–8.

Weuve, J., Kang, J. H., Manson, J. E., et al. Physical activity, including walking, and cognitive function in older women. *Journal of the American Medical Association* 292(2004):1454–61.

Williams, F. M., Cherkas, L. F., Spector, T. D., MacGregor, A. J. The effect of moderate alcohol consumption on bone mineral density: A study of female twins. *Annals of the Rheumatic Diseases* 64(2005):309–10.

Wilson, R. S., Evans, D. A., Bienias, J. L., et al. Proneness to psychological distress is associated with risk of Alzheimer's disease. *Neurology* 61(2003):1479–85.

Zelinski, E. M., Gilewski, M. J., Anthony-Bergstone, C. R. Memory Functioning Questionnaire: Concurrent validity with memory performance and self-reported memory failures. *Psychology and Aging* 5(1990):388–99.

Index

allergies (*continued*)
  bedding and, 202–3
alternating overhead stretch, 271
Alzheimer's disease, 21, 30, 37, 38, 49, 58
  coenzyme Q_{10} and, 373
  dancing and, 257
  diet and, 308–9, 312–13
  free radicals and, 308
  ginkgo biloba and, 375–76
  gum disease and, 399
  medications and, 313
  omega-3 fats and, 312–13, 375
  physical activity and, 243
  prevention and treatment of, 58–59,
    355, 357–61, 372–76
  stress and, 108, 154
  vitamins and, 371, 373–74
amino acids, 300, 309, 311, 324, 382
amitriptyline, 363
anger, 172–74
  letting go of, 101–2, 136, 175
angioplasty, 339–40
Antell, Darrick, 227
antihistamines, 347
antioxidants, 298, 300, 308–9, 310–11,
  325, 364, 371–74
apartments, toxins in, 225
appetite, 155, 338
  sleep and, 201–2
apple crumble à la mode, 425

brain (*continued*)
    meditation and, 160
    multitasking and, 164–65
    prefrontal cortex of, 164, 183
    right and left sides of, 43
    see also mental sharpness
breast lifts, 388
Brondolo, Elizabeth, 107
Buber, Martin, 26
buttermilk dressing, lowfat, 426
bypass surgery, 339

caffeine, 179, 188
cake, 299, 303
calcitonin, 352
calcium, 312, 351, 358
calf strengthener, 279–80
calories, 134, 252, 259, 264, 304–5, 314
cancer, 24, 85, 339, 340–41
    curcumin and, 374
    diet and, 298, 300, 312, 314, 318
    free radicals and, 308
    hormone therapies and, 380–81
    meditation and, 161
    physical activity and, 243-44
    smoking and, 227
    stress and, 154–55
    sun exposure and, 229
    treatments for, 341, 355
    vitamins and, 371–72
    wine and, 303

carbohydrates, 299, 300, 302, 303, 321–22, 323
    glycemic index and, 317–18, 318–320, 323–24
    whole grains, 300, 316–22, 324, 325
cardiovascular conditioning, 23, 251, 252–59, 265, 270
cardiovascular disease, *see* heart disease
cataracts, 308, 365
cat stretch, 288–89
Celebrex, 356
Celexa, 363
cell phones, 164, 210, 217
cellulite, 393–94
chair squat, 278–79
cheat eats, 303–4, 325
cheese
    pesto with pasta, 427–28
    Roquefort dressing, 432
chemical peels, 396–97
chest stretch, 287–88
chi, 180
chi gong, 192, 261
cholesterol, 30, 313
    pets and, 146
    treatments for, 25, 340, 354–55, 378
    yoga and, 191
cholinesterases, 358–59
chondroitin, 376–77
chores, 258–59

diabetes (*continued*)
  stress and, 155
  vitamin C and, 372
diet, 20, 21, 23, 24–25, 27, 298–99, 416
  setting goals for improving, 420–21
  stress and, 155
  weight and, 298–99, 302, 304, 309,
    312, 316, 324, 325, 331–32
  see also Longevity Diet
dip, caramelized onion, 426–27
disease and illness, 22, 23, 26
  diet and, 298
  free radicals and, 308
  spirituality and, 85–87
  stress and, 107–8, 153, 205
  see also specific conditions
donepezil (Aricept), 58, 59, 358–59
dopamine, 246–47
driving
  air pollution and, 223–24
  safety and, 230–31
  sleep and, 177–78
dust, 224, 226
dust mites, 203

eating, *see* diet; Longevity Diet
echinacea, 377
education, 38, 44
Eight Essential Strategies, 20
  mindful awareness in, 26–27
  see also environment; Longevity Diet;

environment (*continued*)
   safety and, 231, 235–36
   setting goals for improving, 420–21
   smoking and, 227–28
   sun exposure in, 229–30, 383
   technology in, 209–17
   television in, 178, 179, 204, 217–20
   workspace, 189, 220–22
ergonomics, 189, 220–21
estrogen replacement therapy, 351,
   367–68, 378–80
Exelon, 358, 359
exercise, *see* fitness and exercise
eye diseases, 364–66
   cataracts, 308, 365
   macular degeneration, 365, 373–74, 376
eye surgery
   cosmetic, 389
   Lasik, 389–90

face lifts, 387–88
faces and names, remembering, 54–56,
   165
fat injections, 393
fats, 298, 300, 303, 309, 312–16, 324
   omega-3, 300, 312–13, 314, 325, 375
   unhealthy, 313
feelings
   anger, 101–2, 136, 172–74, 175
   depression, *see* depression
   negative, 90–103, 113, 136

happiness (*continued*)
    of spouse, 140
    see also positive outlook
hearing problems, 222, 366
heart attack, 305, 338, 340, 350, 355
    air pollution and, 223
    physical activity and, 243–44
    sexual activity and, 133–34
    smoking and, 228
    vitamin E and, 371–72
    workplace stress and, 187–88
heart disease (cardiovascular disease),
    24, 26, 354
    air pollution and, 223
    alcoholic beverages and, 303
    anger and, 173
    diet and, 298, 300, 312–13, 316, 318
    exercise and, 252
    free radicals and, 308
    gum disease and, 399
    laughter and, 175
    meditation and, 161, 191
    omega-3 fats and, 300, 312–13, 314, 375
    pets and, 145
    physical activity and, 243, 244
    smoking and, 227
    stress and, 108, 155
    treatments for, 339–40
    vitamin E and, 371
heart failure, 349
heart rate, 86, 87

heart rate (*continued*)
  anger and, 173
  exercise and, 253–54
  laughter and, 175
  meditation and, 161
  stress and, 154, 155
  target, 253–54
Hedge, Alan, 222
HEPA filters, 226
high blood pressure (hypertension), 22,
  30, 305, 349–50, 407
  air pollution and, 223
  anger and, 173
  diet and, 316
  drugs for, 25
  exercise and, 244–45, 252
  eye disease and, 364
  laughter and, 175
  medications for, 340, 345, 346, 347, 350
  meditation and, 86, 87, 161
  music and, 200
  pets and, 146
  relationships and, 108
  stress and, 154–55, 186
  workplace and, 186
  yoga and, 191
hip abduction, 277
hip extension, 277–78
hip stretch, 273
hip twist, 294

Koenig, Harold, 86
Krause, Neal, 101
Kubey, Robert, 218

Lancet, 353
Langevin, Hélène, 181
Lao-Tzu, 26
laser resurfacing, 394
　Fraxel, 394–95
Lasik eye surgery, 389–90
latanoprost (Xalatan), 365
lateral lift, 283
lateral thinking, 59
laughter, 175–76
learning, 39–40, 42
leg lifts
　back, 293
　forward, 276
legumes, 300, 321–22
　soybeans, 311–12, 316
leisure activities
　mentally stimulating, 37–38, 44–45
　qualities of, 41
Leisure World Cohort Study, 31
leptin, 155
Levitra, 368
Levy, Becca, 81
Lewis, C. S., 104
libido, 22, 367–69
Librium, 347

memory (*continued*)
    training of, 46–48, 51–54
    working, 46–47
    see also Alzheimer's disease; mental
        sharpness
Memory Prescription, The (Small), 19–20
menopause, 379, 380
mental sharpness, 20–21, 35–76, 407
    brain mass and, 45–48
    checklist for improving, 408–9
    lateral thinking and, 59
    mental aerobics and puzzles for, 21,
        27, 35–37, 38, 43, 44–45, 46, 48,
        59–74, 164, 435–42
    mindful awareness and, 26
    perseverance in, 40–41
    presence and focus in, 40, 41, 51–52,
        165, 191, 192
    quality of information and, 41
    questioning and curiosity in, 41
    setting goals for improving, 420–21
    see also Alzheimer's disease; memory
mesotherapy, 393–94
metformin, 353
Miacalcin, 352
microdermabrasion, 394
milk, 311, 312, 313, 315–16
mindful awareness (mindfulness), 26–27, 86
    Longevity Diet and, 299, 305–07
    sex and, 136

mindful awareness (*continued*)
    stress and, 26, 160–61
minoxidil, 398
mold, 224–25, 226
money
    family issues and, 148–49
    saving for the future, 182–85
moral behavior, 90
Motrin, 313, 356
muffins, raisin-bran, 431–32
multitasking, 142, 164–66
muscle relaxation exercise, 176–77
music, 84, 200
    listening before bedtime, 179

Namenda, 358–59
names and faces, remembering, 54–56, 165
nanotechnology, 337–38
naproxen sodium, 313, 356
naps, 179, 189–90
Nature, 45, 313
negative thoughts and feelings, 92–102,
    136
    anger, 101–2, 136, 172–74, 175
    unhealthy relationships and, 112–13
    see also depression
New England Journal of Medicine, 37,
    341, 377
9/11 disaster, 83
"no," saying, 167–72

noise, 200
  in bedroom, 200, 203–4
  hearing problems from, 222, 366
  in workplace, 222
NSAIDs (nonsteroidal anti-inflammatory drugs), 356
nursing homes, 234
nutrition, *see* diet; Longevity Diet
nuts, 300, 315, 325

olive oil, 298, 313, 314, 325
omega-3 fats, 300, 313, 314, 325
  supplements of, 375
onion
  caramelized, dip, 426–27
  fennel, and orange salad, 429
optimism, *see* positive outlook
orange, fennel, and red onion salad, 429
organization, 187, 217
  clutter and, 23–24, 193, 205–8, 209–10, 216, 232, 235, 238, 407
  multitasking and, 164–66
organizations, 443–60
osteoarthritis, 355–57
  see also arthritis
osteoporosis, 263–64, 350–52
overhead press, 285
overhead stretch exercise, 271

pain, 21, 362

pain (*continued*)
  acupuncture and, 180–81
  back, 135, 192, 203, 267–69
  exercise and, 267–69
  mindful awareness and, 26
  pets and, 145–46
  positive outlook and, 79
  relationships and, 108
  self-hypnosis and, 192
  sound and, 200
parents and adult children, 124, 147–49,
  233–34
Pargament, Kenneth, 85
paroxetine, 363
pasta
  cheesy pesto with, 427–28
  mixed seafood and linguini, 430–31
Pavlov, Ivan, 218
Paxil, 363
pea soup, lowfat split, 433
pelvic tilt, 292–93
perseverance, in mental sharpness, 40–41
pesto with pasta, cheesy, 427–28
pets, 145–46
photofacial, 396
physical activity, 242–45
  housework and gardening, 258–59
  sleep and, 179–80
  stress and, 193
  see also fitness and exercise
Pilates, 249, 251, 262, 268

Roman Room Method, 57
rosiglitazone, 353

safety
   driving and, 230–32
   in the home, 235–36
salad dressings
   buttermilk, lowfat, 426
   Roquefort, 432
salads
   fennel, orange, and red onion, 429
   white bean, 434
salt, 305
SAMe (S-adenosylmethionine), 377–78
Schulz, Charles M., 297
seafood, 314–15
   mixed, and linguini, 430–31
self-confidence and self-esteem, 22, 42,
      82, 87–89
   attractiveness and, 146, 383
   building, 89–91
   Inner Critic and Rebuttal exercise,
      90–91
   moral behavior and, 90
   relationships and, 88, 108–9
   sexual activity and, 135, 136
self-hypnosis, 160, 192
Seligman, Martin, 98
Senior Scholars Program, 44
serotonin, 155, 181

stretching (*continued*)
  at work, 188–89
stroke, 305, 340, 349, 354
  anger and, 173
  diet and, 312–13, 316
  exercise and, 244–45
  gum disease and, 399
  omega-3 fats and, 312–13, 375
  smoking and, 227
  stress and, 155, 186
  workplace and, 186
sulfonylurea drugs, 353
sun exposure, 228–230, 383
supplements, 347, 369–78
  curcumin, 374–75
  echinacea, 377
  ginkgo biloba, 344, 346, 375–76
  glucosamine and chondroitin, 376–77
  omega-3, 375
  policosanol, 378
  SAMe, 377–78
  vitamin, 309, 344, 346, 351, 364, 371–74
surgery, cosmetic, 385–91
  breast lifts, 388
  eyelid surgery, 389
  face lifts, 387–88
  hair enhancement, 390–91
  Lasik eye surgery, 389–90
  liposuction, 388–89
swimming, 256
Swiss balls, 262–63

Taczanoski, Eva, 227
tai chi, 191–92, 261
technology management, 209–17
teeth, 399–400
television, 217–20
  watching before bedtime, 179, 204
temperature
  in bedroom, 204
  in workplace, 222
tennis, 257
testosterone, 134, 367, 368, 380–81
therapy
  cognitive, 97–98
  marital, 140–42
Thermage, 395
timolol (Timoptic), 365
Tofranil, 363
Tomlin, Lily, 151
travel, 42–43
travoprost (Travatan), 365
triceps extension, 284
Tucker, Sophie, 405
Tylenol, 356

upper arm stretch, 287
upper-body floor stretch, 294–95
upright rows, 282

Valium, 347
vegan diets, 312

weight (*continued*)

    exercise and, 244–45, 251, 252, 254, 264, 304

    ideal, 246

    Longevity Diet and, 325, 331–32

    mindful awareness and, 26, 159

    sleep and, 178, 201–2

    stress and, 155

    television and, 219

weight lifting, 263–67, 352

    equipment for, 265–67, 270

whole grains, 300, 316–22, 324, 325

wine, 302–3

work

    air pollution and, 223–24

    contaminants at, 226

    environment at, 189, 220–22

    ergonomics and, 189, 220–21

    retirement plans at, 182–85

    stress at, 107–8, 186–89

wrinkles, *see* skin; youthfulness and attractiveness

Xalatan, 365

Xanax, 347

yoga, 160, 191, 251, 262

youthfulness and attractiveness, 89, 245–47, 382–83

    makeup and, 383, 384–85

    smoking and, 227

The employees of Thorndike Press hope you have enjoyed this Large Print book. All our Thorndike and Wheeler Large Print titles are designed for easy reading, and all our books are made to last. Other Thorndike Press Large Print books are available at your library, through selected bookstores, or directly from us.

For information about titles, please call:

(800) 223-1244

or visit our Web site at:

www.gale.com/thorndike
www.gale.com/wheeler

To share your comments, please write:

Publisher
Thorndike Press
295 Kennedy Memorial Drive
Waterville, ME   04901

The Sister Jane series

Outfoxed

Hotspur

Full Cry

The Hunt Ball

The Hounds and the Fury

The Tell-Tale Horse

Hounded to Death

Fox Tracks

Let Sleeping Dogs Lie

Books by Rita Mae Brown with Sneaky Pie Brown

Wish You Were Here

Rest in Pieces

Murder at Monticello

Pay Dirt

Murder, She Meowed

Murder on the Prowl

Cat on the Scent

Sneaky Pie's Cookbook for Mystery Lovers

Pawing Through the Past

Claws and Effect

Catch as Cat Can

The Tail of the Tip-Off

Whisker of Evil

Cat's Eyewitness

Sour Puss

Puss 'n Cahoots

The Purrfect Murder

Santa Clawed

Cat of the Century

Hiss of Death

The Big Cat Nap

Sneaky Pie for President

The Litter of the Law

Nine Lives to Die

The Nevada series

A Nose for Justice

Murder Unleashed

Books by Rita Mae Brown

Animal Magnetism: My Life with Creatures Great and Small

The Hand That Cradles the Rock

Songs to a Handsome Woman

The Plain Brown Rapper

Rubyfruit Jungle

In Her Day

Six of One

Southern Discomfort

Sudden Death

High Hearts

Started from Scratch: A Different Kind of Writer's Manual

Bingo

Venus Envy

Dolley: A Novel of Dolley Madison in Love and War

Riding Shotgun

Rita Will: Memoir of a Literary Rabble-Rouser

Loose Lips

Alma Mater

The Sand Castle

LET SLEEPING DOGS LIE

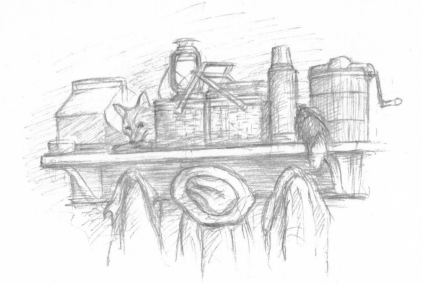

LET SLEEPING DOGS LIE

A NOVEL

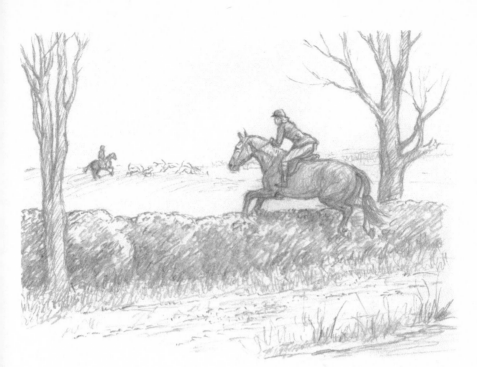

RITA MAE BROWN

ILLUSTRATED BY LEE GILDEA, JR.

BALLANTINE BOOKS

NEW YORK

Copyright © 2014 by American Artist, Inc.

Illustrations copyright © 2014 by Lee Gildea, Jr.

Published in the United States by Ballantine Books, an imprint of Random House, a division of Random House LLC, a Penguin Random House Company, New York.

BALLANTINE and the HOUSE colophon are registered trademarks of Random House LLC.

Library of Congress Cataloging-in-Publication Data
Brown, Rita Mae.
Let sleeping dogs lie : a novel / Rita Mae Brown ;
illustrated by Lee Gildea, Jr.—First edition.
pages ; cm
ISBN 978-0-553-39262-3 (hardcover : acid-free paper—ISBN 978-0-553-39263-0 (ebook)
1. Arnold, Jane (Fictitious character)—Fiction. 2. Murder—Investigation—Fiction.
3. Fox hunting—Fiction. 4. Virginia—Fiction. I. Gildea, Lee, Jr., illustrator. II. Title.
PS3552.R698L48 2014
813'.54—dc23   2014030600

Printed in the United States of America on acid-free paper

Image on page xxiii copyright: © iStock.com / © Lindybug

www.ballantinebooks.com

2 4 6 8 9 7 5 3 1

First Edition

Dedicated in Loving Memory
to
Idler, American Foxhound, Bywaters blood
Who patiently taught me to carry the horn

CAST OF CHARACTERS

Jane Arnold, "Sister" is Master of Foxhounds, MFH, of The Jefferson Hunt in central Virginia. In her early seventies, she's strong, bold, loves her life, the people and animals in it. Like many people who live a deep life, she endured a terrible loss, her son, which ultimately taught her to cherish life, especially the simple things.

Shaker Crown, the hunt's long-serving huntsman, is loyal, reliable, mostly quiet. He and Sister are two peas in a pod when it comes to hunting philosophy.

Gray Lorillard, retired from a powerful accounting firm in Washington, D.C. He grew up in central Virginia and even when working in D.C., would come to the old home place on weekends for hunting. He's smart, handsome, judicious. As an African American man in his late sixties he has a broad overview of how things really work. He's in love with Sister and she with him.

Sam Lorillard is Gray's younger brother. A wonderful horseman, a Harvard graduate who threw it all away thanks to a long tango with the bottle. Dried out, he works for Crawford Howard. He and his brother share the old Lorillard house with its lovely graveyard embracing two hundred years of Lorillards and Laprades.

Mercer Laprade is the cousin of Gray and Sam. He's a successful bloodstock agent. His family has closely worked with an important family of Thoroughbred breeders, the Chetwynds. He, too, has hunted with The Jefferson Hunt since childhood. (Children and grooms ride in the rear, a hunting tradition that allowed latitude where social customs at the time did not.)

Daniella Laprade at 94 can run her son crazy. Proud, imperious, so proud that when she married in 1940 she kept her maiden name as her husband lacked social cachet. Her sister, Gray and Sam's mother, took her husband's name, Lorillard, being less enchanted with social standing. Graziella Lorillard has passed on. Daniella is triumphantly alive.

Walter Lungrun, M.D., Joint Master of foxhounds, is a relatively new Master often amazed at what one must learn and do. His medical reputation is skyrocketing, his riding is much improved, and he loves Sister, has since a child. Walter is the outside son of Sister's late husband. Mr. Lungrun never knew or never let on if he did. Sister didn't know until shortly before tapping Walter to be her Joint Master. Made her love him more somehow.

Phil Chetwynd owns and runs Broad Creek Stables, a Thoroughbred breeding operation that has ridden the ups and downs of that most daring of employments since the 1870s. He grew up with Mercer and his cousins. Loves Mercer, teases him incessantly, and vice versa. They've made good money together, too.

Betty Franklin, as Sister's best friend and a good twenty-five years younger, is also a whipper-in, honorary, which means she isn't paid. She is a kind woman and a good one.

Anne Harris, "Tootie" lives with Sister, taking night classes at UVA. She left Princeton to be with The Jefferson Hunt. Her dream is to become an equine vet and to be a whipper-in. She is sweet, determined, and shockingly beautiful. She is also African American, born to one of the richest men in Chicago who can't fathom why anyone would want to work outside or with animals.

Crawford Howard is probably as rich as Tootie's father and equally as stubborn and egotistical. When Sister did not choose him to be her Joint Master he flew off in a huff and started an outlaw pack that seems to be spectacularly unsuccessful. With all the faults of a self-made man and many of the virtues, he is a force to be reckoned with. He cares a great deal about young people and their education and gives generously.

Ben Sidell has been sheriff of the county for three years. Since he was hired from Ohio, he sometimes needs help in the labyrinthine ways of the South. He relies on Sister's knowledge and discretion.

Kasmir Barbhaiya, widowed and in his midforties, moved to central Virginia to be close to his college roommate after his wife died. He is impossibly rich, having made his fortune in pharmaceuticals in India. He is generous, loving, helpful, and finally able to think about truly living again. He's also a very good rider.

Ed and **Tedi Bancroft** are in their early eighties, ride to three hunts a week, and are dear friends of Sister's. The Bancrofts and Sister have seen one another through desperate sorrows as well as many joys.

Sybil Fawkes is the Bancrofts' daughter and the other Jefferson Hunt whipper-in. Always impeccably turned out and beautifully mounted, there's nothing she can't do on a horse. She's divorced and her two sons are close to grown.

Penny Hinson, DVM, takes Tootie with her on Mondays. She likes the young woman, loves her patients.

Alida Dalzell, from North Carolina, comes to central Virginia on a foxhunting vacation and to rethink her career. Perhaps tipping over into her forties, she is flat-out gorgeous, and better, she can ride and adores hounds.

Jane Winegardner, MFH of Woodford Hounds in Lexington, Kentucky, is a dear friend of Jane Arnold, so this Jane is known as O.J., the Other Jane. An inspired Master, a natural leader, she gets things done and makes riding Thoroughbreds look easy.

Ginny Howard is O.J.'s hunting buddy; married to a man who knows horses as well as his wife, she hunts with his support. She has insight into people that she usually keeps to herself except for O.J.

Justin Sautter, new JT-MFH of Woodford, is young, good with people, and has the wonderful fortune of having a wife, Libby, who can ride right up there with him.

Meg Jewett is Justin's aunt. She loves all animals, being the proprietress of glorious Walnut Hall in Kentucky. She has an incredible eye for structure, beauty, harmony.

Alan Leavitt, married to Meg, presides over Walnut Hall and still breeds Standardbreds for which this lovely place is famous. It is in Lexington, Kentucky, and the Kentucky Horse Park is on former Walnut Hall land. Like his wife, Alan is public-spirited, farsighted, and generous.

THE AMERICAN FOXHOUNDS

Sister and Shaker have carefully bred a balanced pack. The American foxhound blends English, French, and Irish blood, the first identifiable pack being brought here in 1650 by Robert de la Brooke of Maryland. Individual hounds had been shipped over earlier, but Brooke brought an entire pack. In 1785, General Lafayette sent his mentor and hero, George Washington, a pack of French hounds whose voices were said to sound like the bells of Moscow.

Whatever the strain, the American foxhound is highly intelligent and beautifully built, with strong sloping shoulders, powerful hips and thighs, and a nice tight foot. The whole aspect of the hound in motion is one of grace and power in the effortless covering of ground. The American hound is racier than the English hound and stands perhaps two feet at the shoulder, although size is not nearly as important as nose, drive, cry, and biddability. It is sensitive and extremely loving and has eyes that range from softest brown to gold to sky-blue. While one doesn't often see the sky-blue eye, there is a line that contains it. The hound lives to please its master and to chase foxes.

Cora is the strike hound, which means she often finds the scent first. She's the dominant female in the pack and is in her sixth season.

Asa is in his seventh season and is invaluable in teaching the younger hounds.

Diana is the anchor hound, and she's in her fourth season. All the other hounds trust her, and if they need direction she'll give it.

Dragon is her littermate. He possesses tremendous drive and a fabulous nose, but he's arrogant. He wants to be the strike hound. Cora hates him.

Dasher is also Diana and Dragon's littermate. He lacks his brother's brilliance, but he's steady and smart. A hound's name usually begins with the first letter of his mother's name, so the D hounds are out of **Delia.**

Giorgio is a young entry and just about the perfect example of what a male American foxhound should be.

Other hounds

Trinity, Tinsel, Trident, Thimble, Twist, Tootsie, Trooper, Taz, Tattoo, Pookah, Pansy, Dreamboat, Ardent, Parker, Pickens, Zane, Zorro, Zandy

THE HORSES

Sister's horses are **Keepsake,** a Thoroughbred/Quarter Horse cross (written TB/QH by horsemen), an intelligent gelding of twelve years; **Lafayette,** a gray TB, fourteen now, fabulously athletic and talented, who wants to go; **Rickyroo,** an eleven-year-old TB gelding who shows great promise; **Aztec,** a ten-year-old gelding TB, also very athletic, with great stamina and a good mind; and **Matador,** a gray TB, also ten years old, sixteen hands, a former steeplechaser.

Shaker's horses come from the steeplechase circuit, so all are TBs. **Showboat, Hojo, Gunpowder,** and **Kilowatt** can all jump the moon, as you might expect. Betty's two horses are **Outlaw,** a tough QH who has seen it all and can do it all, and **Magellan,** a TB given to her by Sorrel Buruss, a bigger and rangier horse than Betty was accustomed to riding, but she's now used to him. Kilowatt is a superb jumper, bought for the huntsman by Kasmir Barbhaiya.

Nonni, tried and true, takes care of the sheriff.

Matchplay and **Midshipman** are TBs from Roughneck Farm.

THE FOXES

The reds can reach a height of sixteen inches and a length of forty-one inches, and they can weigh up to fifteen pounds. Obviously, since these are wild animals who do not willingly come forth to be measured and weighed, there's more variation than the standard just cited. **Target;** his spouse, **Charlene;** and his **Aunt Netty** and **Uncle Yancy,** and **Earl** at Old Paradise are the reds. They can be haughty. A red fox has a white tip on its luxurious brush, except for Aunt Netty, who has a wisp of a white tip, for her brush is tatty.

The grays may reach fifteen inches in height and forty-four inches in length and may weigh up to fourteen pounds. The common wisdom is that grays are smaller than reds, but there are some big ones out there. Sometimes people call them slab-sided grays, because they can be reddish. They do not have a white tip on their tail but they may have a black one, as well as a black-tipped mane. Some grays are so dark as to be black.

The grays are **Comet, Inky, Georgia, Tollbooth,** and **Grenville.**

Their dens are a bit more modest than those of the red foxes, who like to announce their abodes with a prominent pile of dirt and bones outside. Perhaps not all grays are modest nor all reds full of themselves, but as a rule of thumb it's so.

THE BIRDS

Athena is a great horned owl. This type of owl can stand two feet and a half in height with a wingspread of four feet and can weigh up to five pounds.

    Bitsy is a screech owl. She is eight and a half inches high with a twenty-inch wingspread. She weighs a whopping six ounces and she's reddish brown. Her considerable lungs make up for her small stature.

    St. Just, a crow, is a foot and a half in height, his wingspread is a surprising three feet, and he weighs one pound.

THE HOUSE PETS

Raleigh is a Doberman who likes to be with Sister.

    Rooster is a harrier, willed to Sister by an old lover, Peter Wheeler.

    Golliwog, or **Golly,** is a large calico cat and would hate being included with the dogs as a pet. She is the Queen of All She Surveys.

SOME USEFUL TERMS

Away. A fox has gone away when he has left the covert. Hounds are away when they have left the covert on the line of the fox.

Brush. The fox's tail.

Burning scent. Scent so strong or hot that hounds pursue the line without hesitation.

Bye day. A day not regularly on the fixture card.

Cap. The fee nonmembers pay to hunt for that day's sport.

Carry a good head. When hounds run well together to a good scent, a scent spread wide enough for the whole pack to feel it.

Carry a line. When hounds follow the scent. This is also called working a line.

Cast. Hounds spread out in search of scent. They may cast themselves or be cast by the huntsman.

Charlie. A term for a fox. A fox may also be called **Reynard.**

Check. When hounds lose the scent and stop. The field must wait quietly while the hounds search for the scent.

Colors. A distinguishing color, usually worn on the collar but sometimes on the facings of a coat, that identifies a hunt. Colors can be awarded only by the Master and can be worn only in the field.

Coop. A jump resembling a chicken coop.

Couple straps. Two-strap hound collars connected by a swivel link. Some members of staff will carry these on the right rear of the saddle. Since the days of the pharaohs in ancient Egypt, hounds have been brought to the meets coupled. Hounds are always spoken of and counted in couples. Today, hounds walk or are driven to the meets. Rarely, if ever, are they coupled, but a whipper-in still carries couple straps should a hound need assistance.

Covert. A patch of woods or bushes where a fox might hide. Pronounced "cover."

Cry. How one hound tells another what is happening. The sound will differ according to the various stages of the chase. It's also called giving tongue and should occur when a hound is working a line.

Cub hunting. The informal hunting of young foxes in the late summer and early fall, before formal hunting. The main purpose is to enter young hounds into the pack. Until recently only the most knowledgeable members were invited to cub hunt, since they would not interfere with young hounds.

Dog fox. The male fox.

Dog hound. The male hound.

Double. A series of short sharp notes blown on the horn to alert all that a fox is afoot. The gone away series of notes is a form of doubling the horn.

Draft. To acquire hounds from another hunt is to accept a draft.

Draw. The plan by which a fox is hunted or searched for in a certain area, such as a covert.

Draw over the fox. Hounds go through a covert where the fox is but cannot pick up his scent. The only creature who understands how this is possible is the fox.

Drive. The desire to push the fox, to get up with the line. It's a very desirable trait in hounds, so long as they remain obedient.

Dually. A one-ton pickup truck with double wheels in back.

Dwell. To hunt without getting forward. A hound who dwells is a bit of a putterer.

Enter. Hounds are entered into the pack when they first hunt, usually during cubbing season.

Field. The group of people riding to hounds, exclusive of the Master and hunt staff.

Field master. The person appointed by the Master to control the field. Often it is the Master him- or herself.

Fixture. A card sent to all dues-paying members, stating when and where the hounds will meet. A fixture card properly received is an invitation to hunt. This means the card would be mailed or handed to a member by the Master.

Flea-bitten. A gray horse with spots or ticking that can be black or chestnut.

Gone away. The call on the horn when the fox leaves the covert.

Gone to ground. A fox who has ducked into his den or some other refuge has gone to ground.

Good night. The traditional farewell to the Master after the hunt, regardless of the time of day.

Gyp. The female hound.

Hilltopper. A rider who follows the hunt but does not jump. Hilltoppers are also called the Second Flight. The jumpers are called the First Flight.

Hoick. The huntsman's cheer to the hounds. It is derived from the Latin *hic haec hoc,* which means "here."

Hold hard. To stop immediately.

Huntsman. The person in charge of the hounds, in the field and in the kennel.

Kennelman. A hunt staff member who feeds the hounds and cleans the kennels. In wealthy hunts there may be a number of kennelmen. In hunts with a modest budget, the huntsman or even the Master cleans the kennels and feeds the hounds.

Lark. To jump fences unnecessarily when hounds aren't running. Masters frown on this, since it is often an invitation to an accident.

Lieu in. Norman term for go in.

Lift. To take the hounds from a lost scent in the hopes of finding a better scent farther on.

Line. The scent trail of the fox.

Livery. The uniform worn by the professional members of the hunt staff. Usually it is scarlet, but blue, yellow, brown, and gray are also used. The recent dominance of scarlet has to do with people buying coats off the rack as opposed to having tailors cut them. (When anything is mass-produced, the choices usually dwindle, and such is the case with livery.)

Mask. The fox's head.

Meet. The site where the day's hunting begins.

MFH. The Master of Foxhounds; the individual in charge of the hunt: hiring, firing, landowner relations, opening territory (in large hunts this is the job of the hunt secretary), developing the pack of hounds, and determining the first cast of each meet. As in any leadership position, the Master is also the lightning rod for criticism. The Master may hunt the hounds, although this is usually done by a professional huntsman, who is also responsible for the hounds in the field and at the kennels. A long relationship between a Master and a huntsman allows the hunt to develop and grow.

Nose. The scenting ability of a hound.

Override. To press hounds too closely.

Overrun. When hounds shoot past the line of a scent. Often the scent has been diverted or foiled by a clever fox.

Ratcatcher. Informal dress worn during cubbing season and bye days.

Stern. A hound's tail.

Stiff-necked fox. One who runs in a straight line.

Strike hounds. Those hounds who through keenness, nose, and often higher intelligence find the scent first and press it.

Tail hounds. Those hounds running at the rear of the pack. This is not necessarily because they aren't keen; they may be older hounds.

Tallyho. The cheer when the fox is viewed. Derived from the Norman *ty a hillaut,* thus coming into the English language in 1066.

Tongue. To vocally pursue a fox.

View halloo (halloa). The cry given by a staff member who sees a fox. Staff may also say tallyho or, should the fox turn back, tally-back. One reason a different cry may be used by staff, especially in territory where the huntsman can't see the staff, is that the field in their enthusiasm may cheer something other than a fox.

Vixen. The female fox.

Walk. Puppies are walked out in the summer and fall of their first year. It's part of their education and a delight for both puppies and staff.

Whippers-in. Also called whips, these are the staff members who assist the huntsman, who make sure the hounds "do right."

THE JEFFERSON HUNT CLUB

EST. 1887

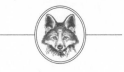

LATE WINTER 2014
FEBRUARY

Sat., Feb. 1	Jt. Meet Woodford Hounds in their Territory	10:00 A.M.
Tues., Feb. 4	Oakside	10:00 A.M.
Thurs., Feb. 6	Tattenhall Station	10:00 A.M.
Sat., Feb. 8	Mill Ruins	10:00 A.M.
Tues., Feb. 11	After All	10:00 A.M.
Thurs., Feb. 13	TBA	10:00 A.M.
Tues., Feb. 18	Prior's Woods	10:00 A.M.
Thurs., Feb. 20	Skidby	10:00 A.M.
Sat., Feb. 22	Orchard Hill	10:00 A.M.
Tues., Feb. 25	Close Share	10:00 A.M.
Thurs., Feb. 27	Punchbowl	10:00 A.M.

MARCH

Sat., Mar. 1	Foxglove	10:00 A.M.
Tues., Mar. 4	Litany Brook	10:00 A.M.
Thurs., Mar. 6	Oakside Jt. Meet Woodford Hounds	10:00 A.M.
Sat., Mar. 8	After All	10:00 A.M.
Tues., Mar. 11	Beveridge Hundred	10:00 A.M.
Thurs., Mar. 13	Tattenhall Station	10:00 A.M.
Sat., Mar. 15	Roughneck Farm Closing Meet	10:00 A.M.

Hounds Always Have Right of Way

Hunting 540-111-1111

Mrs. Raymond Arnold, MFH
Dr. Walter Lungrun, Jt-MFH
Mr. Shaker Crown, Huntsman

. . . . .

1. Hunting license and State Forest permit required by law.
2. Negative Coggins and signed liability waiver required.
3. Formal Dress, Saturdays and Holidays. Proper ratcatcher for Tuesdays, Thursdays.
4. Damage to fences, crops, lawns must be reported to the Field Master immediately.
5. No smoking in the hunt field.
6. Obey the Field Master and give staff precedence in the field.
7. Give every consideration to landowners, through whose kindness hunting is possible.

. . . . .

CAP FEES

For adults on Saturdays and holidays	$100.00
For adults on Tuesdays and Thursdays	$75.00
Juniors (17 and under) & grooms	$15.00

. . . . .

www.facebook.com/sisterjanearnold

Kennels: 540-111-1122

LET SLEEPING DOGS LIE

C H A P T E R   1

Two women, both named Jane, heads down, horses' heads down, rode into driving sleet. Even their horses had sleety, icy bits stuck to their long eyelashes.

O.J., Jane Winegardner's nickname, standing for the Other Jane, shouted to the tall older woman riding next to her. "It's an ill wind that blows no good."

"So much for the weather report," said Jane Arnold, generally known as "Sister." Chin tucked into her white stock tie, collar of her heavy frock coat turned up, she blinked to keep the sleet out of her eyes.

A stone fence appeared up ahead, then disappeared. The two walked their mounts in that direction.

Sister turned toward O.J. "Can't hear a thing. You think we'd hear the horn."

"I hope Glen has the hounds up by now," said O.J., Master of Woodford Hounds, mentioning her huntsman.

When the joint meet started out on Saturday, February 1, low clouds blanketed the Kentucky sky, the temperature at ten in the morning hung at 34°F. The first cast started off hopefully: the Woodford Hounds, named for Woodford County, found a coyote line right off. The Jefferson Hunt, central Virginia, rode right up with the Woodford people, a courtesy extended to them by their host. Eighty people charged up over a hill from the main barn at Shaker Village in Mercer County.

Upon well-groomed horses, the riders in their best hunt gear had little trouble negotiating the hill as the ground remained frozen. So far the two degrees above freezing had no effect. The slipping and sliding would start in perhaps an hour. The cold air felt invigorating, the cry of the hounds exciting.

Like The Jefferson Hunt, Woodford Hounds did not hunt to kill but rather to chase. The Virginia hunt chased more fox than the Kentucky group, who flew across fields on coyotes running straight and fast. Usually the quarry would speed out of the hunt's territory. Riders would pull up, waiting for huntsman and staff to bring hounds back, often grateful for a breather.

That's how both Janes thought the day would go: hard runs, retrieving hounds and then casting them again for another fast go. O.J., MFH, along with Robert Lyons and new Joint Master, Justin Sautter, asked Sister Jane to ride with O.J. The two ladies would whip in, which means riding at the edge of the hounds where the huntsman assigned them. This was a bit like playing first base or third. The Masters didn't expect Sister Jane to really whip in but all knew if she trotted out with O.J., she'd be rewarded with great views of the excellent hound work.

"The girls" were flying along when, within five minutes, a low howl came from the west: an unnerving noise. Neither woman paid much attention, the pace was too good. Sister Jane knew the sound of approaching wind well, as much as her huntable land nestled east, at the foot of the sensuous Blue Ridge Mountains. Sometimes the wind would howl overhead, not touching those below. Other times it cut you to the bone.

A few moments passed after the ominous sound, then trees bowed before the onslaught. The two Masters were hit full in the face. Clouds lowered, bringing an impenetrable freezing fog, what the tribes called a pogonip. The colonists kept the word. Sleet slammed the riders like the palm of a giant open hand. They could neither see nor hear.

O.J. knew this place intimately. She pulled up. She knew where she was when the sleet and fog hit but now had to feel her way, hoping a landmark would appear through the fog.

Turning her wonderful mare around, O.J. had the good sense to head back to the barn. The mare had a better sense of direction than she did.

The two women rode right up on the stone fence.

O.J. hollered, "Sister, if we back up to jump it, we won't see it until we're right on it. Let's walk around to the right. We should come up on a creek. There's a small hand gate there."

Slipping, sliding now as the ground sloped down, their horses carefully walked along, keeping their heads low. Finally, they reached the creek and O.J. saw the small gate nearby when a swirl cleared her vision for a moment.

Sister Jane dismounted before O.J. could protest. Once both horses passed through, the older woman closed the gate.

"I'll hold your horse," O.J. yelled.

Seeing that her saddle seat was already covered with sleet, Sister thought the better of plopping in the middle of it. Her hands throbbed. She couldn't feel her feet. "I'll be warmer walking." She ran up her stirrup irons, lifted Rickyroo's reins over his head to walk on his left between both horses. That would shield her a bit from the fierce winds.

She opened her mouth to add something, but in a second it was full of ice bits. Sister Jane loved foxhunting. She loved being a Master but at this exact moment she questioned her sanity. She questioned O.J.'s, too.

. . .

Shaker Village in Mercer County, Kentucky, flourished between 1806 and 1923 when Mary Settles, the last Shaker, passed away. Like all Shaker settlements, this one died out due to the fact that Shakers did not believe in sexual congress and therefore no children were born in the villages. People joined the sect with children in tow. Eventually those children became seventy, eighty, a few even ninety years old. Without new recruits, these visually beautiful communities died out. Time passed them by.

Americans lost interest in the spiritual, quiet development fostered by the Shakers. While the lack of sex surely deterred many, another cause for the demise of such an unusual sect was the Industrial Revolution. This force grew and grew, devouring much in its path, most especially the desire to live simply.

Sister patted Rickyroo on the neck. A ten-year-old Thoroughbred, nearing eleven, he'd learned his job, carrying it out with energy, but even this kind fellow had found the going difficult.

"Couldn't they smell it coming?" O.J.'s mare asked.

"No," Rickyroo replied. *"You have to think for them."*

Another seven miserable minutes and the two lone humans finally made it to the barn. They could just see the outline of the roof. Inside was a much-needed welcoming party, Betty Franklin, Anne "Tootie" Harris, and Ginny Howard.

Although one is not supposed to dismount inside a barn, O.J. couldn't stand one minute more of that lashing wind outside. Her friend Ginny Howard helped her down, putting O.J.'s hands between her own. Ginny took off her gloves, then rubbed the Master's hands. The mare stood by patiently, grateful to be inside.

Betty Franklin, Sister's best friend, quickly untacked Rickyroo, for Sister couldn't uncurl her fingers.

Tootie, a beautiful young woman, who had left Princeton in her freshman year to the horror of her socially conscious Chicago family to work with Sister, came up with a heavy blanket for Ricky-roo.

"Honey, before you put that blanket on, rub some Absorbine on his back and down his legs," said Sister, teeth chattering. "Wet a chamois cloth, make it warm, good and warm. Put that on his back just for a couple of minutes. Then wipe him down and toss the blanket on."

Tootie spoke to both human and horse: "You must be frozen."

"Hateful," came the human's one-word reply.

"Hateful," Rickyroo echoed.

Betty took off Sister's gloves, blew on her hands to rub them as Ginny was doing. "Your hands are cherry red."

"They throb. The thought of taking my boots off fills me with dread."

"Gray went back to your room to get things ready for you," Tootie said.

"That's a happy thought." Sister loved her boyfriend for his thoughtfulness. That he was handsome didn't hurt. She called him her gentleman friend—ever proper Sister.

"Ginny, what happened?" O.J. asked. "It was like a curtain of fog, sleet, and wind dropped."

"That's what happened. There was no hope so we turned back, everyone turned back."

"Did Glen get the hounds up?"

"You bet he did." Ginny smiled. "They didn't want to be out either."

"Good." O.J. breathed relief.

Both Sister and O.J. loved their hounds. Being Masters, they were, in effect, the chief executive officers of their respective hunts. An overwhelming number of chores dropped into their lap but Sister sometimes thought her most important function was to patiently listen.

"Everybody ready?" O.J. asked.

"I haven't cleaned my tack yet." Sister wondered if her hands could do it.

Betty, saddle over her forearm, bridle over her shoulder, announced, "I'll do it in my room. You rest. Don't forget you need to be at your best at the dinner."

Sister smiled. "We all need to be at our best. Woodford never does things halfway."

Both Sister and Tootie, along with many other Jefferson Hunt members, stayed in the Long House at Shaker Village. Each of the original rooms remained as they had been built, though were now guest rooms with a shower and sink. No TV. No radio. Scrubbed wooden floors, chairs hung up on pegs to create more space, a nice bed with blankets, all bore testimony to the pure design of Shakers.

Standing outside the door to their room, Sister knocked, wincing as she did so.

Gray opened the door. "Honey, I've been so worried about you."

Stepping inside, she allowed him to peel her out of her heavy frock soaked at the shoulders. She then wriggled her arms out of her vest. "The storms knocked out my cell phone, plus in that freezing torrent I couldn't use it anyway." She inhaled deeply.

"Here, sit in the chair." He pulled a second one down off the wall for her. "I'll undo your tie."

"You're an angel. There's no way I could unfasten the pin."

Gray expertly freed the long titanium pin, a gift from a friend, Garvey Stokes, owner of Aluminum Manufacturers, and also unfastened the two safety pins to hold down the ends of the tie.

She began to fill him in on the adventure. "A pogonip."

Gray, African American and well versed in the old stories, murmured. "A bad sign."

"Well, that's what the Virginia tribes always said."

"My grandmother, too." Their eyes met. "Okay, beautiful. Be

brave. You have got to get your boots off." He pulled the big boot-jack over for her. They always took a big bootjack when they traveled, just as she always took a heavy down comforter, a real necessity in these rooms without insulation. A few of the Shaker lodgings had horsehair in the walls but the wind rattled the hand-blown glass, finding every crack in the walls.

"Come on. I'll hold the handle along with you but you need to get your boots off before the warmth makes your legs swell."

"What warmth?" She felt a wedge of cold air from the window reach her as she stood with one foot on the bootjack the other in the slot where the heel would rest.

He laughed. "Come on. Better a short, sharp pain than a long, drawn-out one."

"Dear God." She gasped as she freed one foot.

"One more." He encouraged her and she did pull her foot out of the boot, pressing her lips together so she wouldn't scream.

"Will I ever walk again?"

He put his arms around her. "I don't know, but I know you'll ride again. You get the rest of those cold, wet things off. I'll start the shower. All you have to do is step inside. I'll have your Constant Comment ready when you step out."

"Weren't we smart to bring the electric teapot?" She gingerly stepped to the bathroom as he preceded her.

Feeling had returned to her frozen feet and they hurt like hell.

Once cleaned up, wrapped in her heavy robe, she sat on a ladderback chair across from him.

Gray scanned the room. "I admire Shaker design, don't you?"

"I do. It reminds me that I have too much stuff. Whenever we come here, I feel cleansed."

Holding the heavy mug in her hands felt restorative as did a sip. Tea always lifted Sister's spirits as did the sight of a horse, hound, or Gray.

"Funny, how we remember the old tales, isn't it? I mean the stories about freezing fogs."

"I wouldn't disbelieve them and you were lucky to get through that pogonip, those damn winds. What in the hell were you doing out there?"

"I told you. We whipped in on the left side and within five minutes, *whammo*."

"Actually, it was pretty much that way in the field, too. I don't remember anything quite like it." He took a sip of his own tea. "I'm looking forward to the dinner at Walnut Hall. I've never been inside."

"It's fabulous. But then everything that Meg and Alan Leavitt do is pretty fabulous," she said, referring to the owners of Walnut Hall.

Meg Jewitt was the aunt of the new, young Joint Master, Justin Sautter, about whom O.J. was thrilled. Well, she should be. Young people bring with them energy, new ideas, and physical strength.

"I remember a pogonip when I was in grade school," said Gray. "The teacher wouldn't let us walk home. Took forever for our parents to fetch us and, of course, my mother had to go on about unhappy spirits being released during a pogonip." He paused. "And you know, it was February first like today."

Sister sipped again. "Do you believe that stuff about unhappy spirits?"

He shrugged. "I don't know."

In a sense, they were about to encounter one.

C H A P T E R   2

Nestled in Gray's big-ass Land Cruiser, Sister felt warm at last. The SUV's heater was a godsend. He exited the drive from Shaker Village, turning right.

"It's more scenic if you turn left," Sister offered.

"Takes longer, too." His iron-gray military mustache curved up at one end as he teased her, "You know, I could install a steering wheel on your side."

She turned to face him, as always admiring his handsome profile. "You say."

He laughed. "So, I do. The sun won't set until five-thirty. I love the light. I mean, winter has its beauty but sometimes the darkness gets me. We now have an hour's more light than on December twenty-first. Never seems to bother you."

"Doesn't. How do people live without the seasons? That would get me. I'd go stark raving mad. I measure time, even emotion, by those shifts."

"Mmm." He paused for a moment, then turned another right

onto one of Kentucky's highways. "Boy, this state has done a lot of work on the roads."

"Yes, it has. They have a good governor in Beshears and they have had some good ones before. Some real stinkers, too."

"It's the legislature that's the problem." Gray, a retired accountant from a high-powered firm in D.C., kept up with financial incentives and disincentives in government. Although he'd made a career as a tax lawyer of impeccable repute, he knew only too well how the system could be gamed from either end.

"Right now we Virginians can't really hold our heads up either. Hopefully, McAuliffe will prove more rigorously honest than the governor before him, who I thought was pretty good until the stories came out about accepting money, a watch, etc., for favors. So very foolish." She noticed a huge sycamore in the middle of a field that meant water was nearby. "What is it about old trees that call to one?"

"Old spirits."

"That's one of the things I liked about the Harry Potter movies; the trees talked and moved. Well, all that started long before that, remember the story about Apollo chasing Daphne? Just as Apollo grabbed her, Daphne called to her Mother Earth, who snatched her out of Apollo's arms, putting a laurel tree in Daphne's place. Apollo created a laurel wreath to console himself. Somehow the laurel wreath was used ever after to crown victors in the real Olympics. It was used for artistic contests, too. I'd love to see that now. You know, current Olympians crowned with laurel leaves, the Wimbledon winner, the winner of the golf U.S. Open, that sort of thing. There's something beautiful about it."

"You think about things that would never occur to me." He loved that about Sister most times.

On a few occasions, it became tedious.

"I'll take that as a compliment. Gray, we've got the Chetwynds and the Bancrofts coming to this. Those families once raced against

Meg's grandfather, when everyone raced harness horses. There were a few Thoroughbreds at the farm, too."

"I thought L.V. Harkness was a Standardbred man through and through," Gray remarked.

"He was, and Meg and Alan still are. Every now and then I think Mr. Harkness slipped in a Thoroughbred but in those days, the turn of the last century and before, sulky racing was the thing. Think of Dan Patch," she continued. "As big a star as later Secretariat was." She wrapped her arms around herself, beaming. "How it pleases me to be driving through Kentucky knowing the last winner of the Triple Crown, one of the greatest Thoroughbreds ever, was bred in Virginia."

"I'd keep that to myself tonight."

"I will." She frowned for a moment. "Harness racing ought to prove to all of us not to take anything for granted. You and I could live to see the fraying of flat racing."

"Don't you think it already is?"

"Yes, but there's hope for it being reversed. It comes down to three things, honey: visionary leadership, unimpeachable training practices, and slots."

"Well, that's another subject we'd best not get on tonight. Too close to home. Don't get Mercer on it." He mentioned his cousin, who did business in Kentucky and elsewhere as a bloodline/breeding consultant. Gray's mother and Mercer's mother were sisters.

It was a sore subject since the Kentucky legislature repeatedly voted down, always with a terrific fight, not to allow other forms of gambling at the racetracks. As to good treatment of horses by trainers, the issue was made more difficult as each state had different drug rules. Barn practices, cleanliness, proper food, and so forth proved far less difficult to monitor than drugs.

Many members of Woodford Hounds made their living through breeding, selling, and racing Thoroughbreds. Phil Chetwynd, one of The Jefferson Hunt's members, had kept up his family tradition and stayed in the Thoroughbred business, which was small in Virginia compared to Kentucky. The Chetwynds, four generations' worth, were kept afloat financially through their stallions. People still vanned mares from New York, Pennsylvania, Maryland, West Virginia, and even Kentucky to breed to Broad Creek Stables stallions, each of whom carried impeccable blood.

"For Kentuckians, the frustration has to be wild. All anyone needs to do is cross the Ohio River into Indiana and walk onto a riverboat." Sister shook her head.

"As an accountant, I have mixed feelings about gambling."

"Gray, I don't. No one puts a gun to someone's head and says you will wager away your salaries. And face it, there is a thrill."

"There is no thrill to bankruptcy."

"You've got me there, but really, do you think we can protect people from themselves?"

"No. On the other hand, we don't have to enshrine foolishness."

"You are so right. That's why we elect it."

He laughed. "Now I know you're warmed up."

"Slow down. No, I'm not backseat driving but we're only twenty minutes from Walnut Hall and we don't want to be the first ones at the do." She thought for a moment and reconsidered. "Oh, don't slow down. Having a few moments with Meg and Alan, Justin and Libby, too, surely they'll be there early, that's a treat. They are so literate. I love being around people who read."

"It's always an elite, you know. Throughout history. One can know how to read but not exercise the ability. Now people look at their phones, their iPads, their computers."

"Useful stuff but makes you passive." She announced this with conviction, absentmindedly fingering the pearls at her throat. God forbid a Southern lady be without her pearls.

"I understand how film and TV makes one passive but I'm not so sure about the other stuff."

"Okay. When you read a book, it's just you, a white piece of paper with black marks on it. You know what the black marks mean but they explode in images in your head. So you and I can read the same passage from *Moby-Dick* but your whale looks different from mine. We use our imaginations. When the image is preselected as it is in electronic media, you are looking at someone else's whale. I mean, some of the electronic books even have moving images."

"Ah." A few moments passed. "You're certainly philosophical."

"The near-death experience in the pogonip. Crystallized my mind."

He burst out laughing as he turned down Newtown Pike. Kentucky Horse Park was at one time part of Walnut Hall. Now Walnut Hall as well as the Sautter house were behind it. Originally the giant property was granted to William Christian in 1777. Christian moved his family near Louisville in 1785 but was soon killed by Indians that same year. The western territories seethed with danger. Over time, as those dangers abated and Christian's daughter Elizabeth Dickerson persevered, more settlers moved to the lands.

Dickerson sold a section of her land. Down through the nineteenth century it was passed along, being subdivided over time. L.V. Harkness bought the land in 1895 from the estate of Captain Sam Brown who had won the Kentucky Derby in 1884 with his horse, Buchanan. Harkness renamed the place Walnut Hall, owning 2,000 acres.

A late sun drenched the large still-bare trees in pale light, for the skies had cleared and the winds stood still. Just another demonstration of the variability of Kentucky weather.

The manicured grounds exuded a subdued grace.

"What's going on over there? No one dead, I hope." Gray knew no person was, for they slowly drove by the oldest horse cemetery in

America, where rested fifty-eight of the greatest of the early Standardbreds. A statue of the horse Gus Axworthy, 1902–1933, announced the lovely final finish line of their lives.

At the edge of this hallowed ground, Sister observed two men working to dislodge a huge shard of engraved slate. The slab had broken over the only Thoroughbred there, Benny Glitters, 1892–1921. A large tree limb could be seen upturned at the side of the large flat tomb marker that covered the entire equine grave. So great was the force of the earlier wind that the branch must have fallen onto the slate with such ferociousness that it drove the broken sharp edge into the grave itself. The odd rise of the temperature after the storm was turning the hard frozen ground into mud.

Arriving at the door to Walnut Hall, Gray handed the keys to the gentleman there to park the cars.

"We aren't the first." He took Sister's arm as he escorted her to the door.

"And it's six o'clock. If people are that eager to get here you know it will be some party."

Standing by the door to greet his guests, Alan Leavitt kissed Sister on the cheek, shook hands with Gray. "How good to see you. Sister, you light up every room you enter." Alan meant that, but as he was a gentleman he wisely knew to flatter the ladies.

People were pushing in behind them. Alan continued greeting guests. Meg was easy to find, you followed the laughter.

The party, in full swing at 6:30 P.M., was the typical foxhunters' gathering. There were people there of great wealth like Kasmir Barbhaiya, a portly Indian gentleman who had moved to Virginia to be part of The Jefferson Hunt. He'd made a billion dollars plus in pharmaceuticals in his native India. A widower, he was beset by many women who liked his money and therefore liked him. No fool, he trusted that when he did find a person to whom he could give his heart, his late wife would tell him. This he firmly believed and, having told Sister, she believed it, too.

The deepest things in life are not logical.

The elegant rooms filled with Woodford people and Jefferson people. Old silver trophies, continually polished over generations, reflected light, adding their own silver glow. Old and new gossip was rapidly dispensed with so folks could get to the real conversation: horses and hounds.

Walnut Hall represented both accumulated wealth and excellent taste. In a sense, it was like an old European home where generations refined the art of living and in the case of Meg, of giving. Kasmir was another giver.

Mingling among those who had financial great fortune in their lives were those who barely had two nickels to rub together. Apart from those two poles, the bulk of the group watched their pennies, got along, and enjoyed life with what they were able to earn.

Exuberance, love of nature, physical energy counted for more than money. And of course, character counted most of all. Foxhunters, like any group of humans anywhere in the world, provided a rich assortment of the good, the bad, and the plain old rotten to choose from.

O.J. found Sister in the scrum. "Took me two hours to thaw out."

"I'd still be blue if it weren't for Gray," said Sister. "He helped me take my boots off, got me in the shower, then handed me a cup of tea. I think that's the coldest I have ever been. Then he picked out tonight's clothing, insisting I wear this cashmere sweater with a wraparound skirt. He said I needed to stay warm."

Eyes twinkling, O.J. laughed, then said low into Sister's ear, "Remind me of the connection between the Chetwynds and the Laprades? Didn't the Laprades work for them since World War One?"

"Before and after. The Laprades had and still have a great eye for a horse. The Chetwynds were smart enough to use it."

"As long as they stand Guns and Roses and Loopy Lou, people will haul mares to Virginia. They've also got St. Boniface, young, his first year crop looks good."

"O.J., you remember your horses."

"So do you. So much of what's good in Virginia goes back to Mr. Mellon's stud, the Chenerys, of course. But tell me about the Laprades." O.J. leaned in closer.

"Related to Gray. Gray's mother, Graziella Lorillard, and Daniella Laprade were sisters. I add, they weren't close but they more or less got along. The Laprades made a lot of money with the Chetwynds. Not so much in salary but in betting at the track, or so I'm told. Mercer"—she indicated a well-dressed man in his fifties—"still advises Phil Chetwynd as well as others. Gray says he makes money at the track as well."

"Well, he doesn't look poor," said O.J. "Anyone riding in a Hermès saddle isn't poor."

"Drives Gray nuts." Sister shook her head. "Gray does not believe in flash."

"You might remind Gray that a Hermès saddle will last at least three generations and if it fits you and your horse, it's worth the price." O.J. grinned. "The Chetwynd money isn't all from horses, right? I thought their fortune started with coal in West Virginia."

"Did. They still own the mines. Phil"—she nodded at the Chetwynd standing nearby next to Gray, towering over him actually—"doesn't run the mines. His brother does. Phil is in charge of the breeding and racing operation, Broad Creek Stables. Phil works closely with Mercer. There's always been the thought that they are related back through Phil's grandfather and Mercer's grandmother. No one says this outright but Gray told me and he wondered if it ended there. He's good about so-called sexual sins but prior generations lied through their teeth. Phil comes to Kentucky regularly for the big races but he does most of his business in the mid-Atlantic."

"Dear Lord, Sister, the way things are going, racing might shift to the mid-Atlantic."

"Kentucky will always be first in Thoroughbreds," Sister predicted.

"Sister, each year over five hundred million dollars shoots out of this state into Indiana casinos. And we can't get slots in the racetracks. It's crazy."

"It's kind of like killing the goose that laid the golden egg." Sister had no idea how immense was the financial drain Kentucky was experiencing.

Both their heads turned when they noticed their host Alan Leavitt opening the front door to the two men, Fred and Arnie, who had been at the graveyard. After a quick conversation, Alan hastily threw on his overcoat and left with them, shutting the door behind him.

He returned within fifteen minutes, said something to Meg.

Meg's expression changed from calm to disbelief. "Alan, that can't be," Sister heard her say.

"Well, come see."

As others overheard this exchange, curiosity rose.

Alan looked over his shoulder as he stepped outside the door. "Come on. Might as well see this, but put on a coat. Sun has set and it's getting cold again."

Sister, Gray, O.J., Betty, Phil Chetwynd, Mercer Laprade, who was in the front hall, Tootie, Kasmir, and a group of the Woodford members dutifully put on their overcoats and went outside to trod upon the sodden ground squishing beneath their feet.

For the ladies in heels, this was not a good idea.

At the Walnut Farms burial grave site, Fred and Arnie pointed down. Fred held a strong flashlight while Arnie knelt down, slinging away mud.

"Who was Benny Glitters?" Tootie asked, then quickly shut up.

"What's that?" Meg exclaimed, for a smashed gold pocket watch and chain caught the gleam from Fred's flashlight.

Arnie scraped around a bit more and a dog skull appeared, possibly that of a small terrier, then a thumb and human forefinger also appeared not far from the watch. The forefinger was bent toward the unseen palm.

Sister inhaled sharply, then whispered. "Death beckons."

CHAPTER 3

Tuesday, February 4, some clouds and some sun hinted that the weather might turn in the foxhunter's favor. Sister Jane knew better than to be too hopeful. She'd lived through whopping snowstorms as late as mid-April in central Virginia. As a rule of thumb, though, the last frost was around April 15 and she fervently hoped this year would run true to form. However, it was now February, a notoriously difficult month.

Tuesdays, Thursdays, and Saturdays were The Jefferson Hunt days. Back from Kentucky, Sister, her hounds, her huntsmen, and two whippers-in prepared for what they hoped would be a good day. As so many people worked, Tuesdays and Thursdays drew smaller numbers. When the season passed New Year's Day, the die-hards slipped away from work as they knew the last half of hunt season always flew by faster than the first half.

As Field Master, the seventy-three-year-old Sister led the riders in First Flight, those who took the jumps. Bobby Franklin, Betty's husband, a man of prudent judgment, led Second Flight. Mostly they didn't jump, although they might pop over a log.

The pasture—dull brown, patches of old snow here and there—lay below them. Within two months it would shine bright green.

Another reason people came out on this particular Tuesday was that they were hunting a new fixture, Oakside. It takes a season to learn a fixture, sometimes more, both for hounds and staff.

Led by Cora, an older, wiser hound, the pack fanned out over the lower pasture. They'd lost the line, easy to do in even the best of conditions, for the fox is every bit as smart as the old myths and stories tell us.

Noses down, concentration intense, the Jefferson pack made Sister proud. Shaker Crown, her huntsman of many years, knew when to urge them on and when to sit tight and shut up. This was a sit-tight-and-shut-up situation.

Pookah, young, a trifle silly, was momentarily distracted by the pungent odor of a bobcat. *"Hey, this smells kind of interesting."*

Diana, an outstanding hound in her prime, walked over, checked it out. *"Pook, that's a bobcat. You know that's a bobcat. Why waste your time?"*

"Well, if we can't pick up the fox again this could be fun. I want to have fun."

"Shut up. Forget it and go to work." Cora growled convincingly.

Pookah immediately did as she was told. You didn't cross Cora.

Most members of the field want to gallop along. The more they gallop, the better they think the hunting. Granted, moving along at pace is always a thrill, but for Sister, staff, and those fox-hunters who loved hounds, they marveled at the work below. This pack performed beautifully.

Dreamboat was one of the D line, for foxhounds take the first initial of their name from their mother's name. He stopped, sniffed, sniffed more, his tail started to flip like a windshield wiper. Now Dreamboat was not a particularly brilliant hound. He was the good foot-soldier type. He had always been overshadowed by his litter-mates, Diana, Dragon, and Dasher. He did his job, was always in the middle of the pack but today was his day.

"Here he is!" he sang out in his resonant voice.

As Dreamboat was a reliable fellow none of the lead hounds bothered to check the line. Within seconds, Dreamboat up front, the pack spoke in unison.

Shaker, on Hojo, the perfect huntsman's horse, bold, fast, and handy, fell in behind the pack. Way out on the right of the pack rode Betty Franklin, whipping in. On the left, just now dipping down into a swale, rode Sybil Fawkes, also whipping in.

Sister waited for a moment before trotting down the hill, riding behind Shaker by about thirty yards. Just behind her rode Maria and Nate Johnson, owners of Oakside. Out of the corners of their eyes they caught sight of their daughter, Sonia, behind Sybil by about a football field in length, riding tail. Sister wanted to train young people for staff positions and as Sonia was in her early twenties and could ride, this was working out.

The Johnsons rode up to direct Sister, who did not yet know the territory that well. Good thing, too, because the fox crossed a shallow creek, headed into a woods, and burst out again. Of course he didn't run in a straight line, so everyone looped in the woods a bit. When they emerged, an old fence line dividing the Johnsons' property from their neighbors' appeared and so did the fox. The crafty fellow paused for one moment, looked back at the approaching hounds, then scooted under the fence and put on the after-burners to create havoc.

Knowing that the neighboring farm wasn't available for hunting, Shaker had to halt his pack. Taking hounds off a hotline is miserable work because, in a sense, you are punishing them for doing their job. Hounds have little sense of human boundaries and if they did, they wouldn't care.

To make matters worse, the entire field could view this beautiful red while watching the whippers-in jump the three-board fence to bring back the hounds.

Shaker pulled up to blow them in. Had he gone on, the hounds would have taken that as a signal they could continue. If the huntsman was right behind them, they were right. Like any huntsman, Shaker, frustrated, blew his horn three long notes in succession, and prayed his whippers-in could do their job. Not an easy one.

Betty rode right up on the pack's shoulder, looking down at Thimble and Twist. "Leave it."

"It's red-hot!" Thimble protested.

On a blindingly fast Thoroughbred, Sybil called out the same order on the left side where Giorgio, a hound of stunning beauty, obeyed.

Sonia, without being told, rode past Sybil, got in front of the pack, slightly turned toward them and cracked her whip. That sounded like rifle fire and scared the hounds. They slowed down.

Then Betty and Sybil, who had worked with the pack for decades, knew everyone and vice versa, called again. *"Leave it!"*

Diana stopped so the others did, too, as Diana and Cora had the respect of all the hounds. Hounds, like humans, are pack animals. Some have natural authority and often they build on this, earning trust by their work.

"Not fair! Not fair!" Trident howled.

"How could they do this to us?" Dasher cried.

"Good hounds. Good hounds." Betty praised them, which offered some salve.

"Come on. Come along," Sybil pleasantly ordered, turning her horse back toward the fence.

"Why do they do this? Why?" Trident, who had been right behind Dreamboat, spoke in misery.

"Humans are perverse," Trooper replied.

"True, but you have to admit, they rarely break us off a line," Cora counseled.

Back at the fence, the hounds wiggled back under it while Betty, not under pressure, looked for a place with a top board off to jump. Yes, she could and just did jump a three-board fence, but it wasn't her preference. She rode Outlaw, her tough Quarter Horse, who had that odd little engine push when he jumped.

Thoroughbreds' jumps were usually smooth, often seemingly effortless; they spoiled their riders. Quarter Horses could jump without a doubt, but they always felt—to Betty, at least—as if there was a little extra wiggle there in the rear.

Sybil didn't think anything about the fence being three boards. She leapt back over, as did Sonia.

The hounds gathered around Shaker, who lavishly praised them.

The medium-built, muscular huntsman leaned over, citing Dreamboat directly for all to hear; hounds, horses, and humans.

"Dreamboat, you were a star."

"Me?" The good fellow gazed up, then realized *"Me!"*

Dreamboat stood on his hind legs as Shaker leaned over, reaching down, and took the offered paw.

The happy hound rejoined the pack. Shaker paused for a moment, looking to his master.

Sister asked Maria, "If we follow the creek south then turn back toward your farm, think we'll be okay?"

"Sure."

"If we find another fox that runs out of the fixture, we'll just deal with it," the elegant Master said.

A narrow path followed the creek. Resuming the search, hounds headed south, a few floated into the woods.

As Sister rode along, she memorized suitable crossings on the new fixture's creek. As the waters were clear she could see the bottom, a big help. Nothing like getting into water only to sink in nasty silt.

Fifteen minutes passed, then twenty. Betty, on the other side of the water, picked her way through, as there wasn't a path on that side. The problem was always those tendrils hanging from trees, Virginia creepers, and little bushes with loathsome thorns. It was a good horse that willingly plunged into the stuff, which Outlaw did. Not that he didn't complain about it.

Twenty minutes. Twenty-five. The temperature, midforties, felt warm, especially if one had put on extra layers, since it was below freezing at ten o'clock when hounds were first cast.

Thirty minutes.

"Hey, gray," Dreamboat called out, having picked up a scent. *"Fading,"* he cautioned.

He moved along a bit faster, hooked into the woods on the path side, then opened in earnest, his resonant hound baritone sounding beautiful.

Another run, maybe ten minutes followed, but it seemed longer as there were many obstacles to dodge. Finally the scent pooped out.

By now it was twelve-thirty. Two and a half hours seemed sufficient, given conditions and the newness of the fixture. Sister didn't want to risk heading into forbidden territory should they get another line.

So many times a decision a Master must make isn't good for hunting but necessary for landowner relations. She hoped, in time, the neighbor would learn that the club did no harm and was happy to do some good if you needed a gate fixed or perhaps useful information. She would call upon the neighboring farm after this first season down here and hope for the best.

Oakside's neighbors, new people, were not country people. Like most new people, especially those moving from cities or suburbs, their property lines seemed inviolate to them. This is deeply unrealistic but it was best folks learn this lesson in a gentle manner. That didn't necessarily mean Sister would someday be able to hunt that land but it did mean that hounds can't read. You can post all the NO TRESPASSING signs you want, won't do a bit of good to four-legged hounds with a snoutful of scent.

Walking back, the group came up to the old, now unused Saddlebred barn. The Johnsons had their hunting barn up by the house. The five-stall Saddlebred barn, built decades ago by an owner of these lovely horses, rested farther away and had been let go by an interim owner. The abandonment gave it a sorrowful air.

As she rode by, Sister noticed glowing skulls with red eyes pushing up from the ground, red paint on the sides of the barn reading, Murder, Help, I'm Being Held a Prisoner, plus a mannequin hanging from the rafters.

Maria and Sonia, with Nate's help, had created a haunted barn as a fund-raiser for the pony club last year. A haunted barn it remained.

"Those darn skulls get me. It's the damned red eyes," Sister remarked to Maria.

"Scared the devil out of the kids." Maria laughed.

Walking behind Sister, Phil Chetwynd teased Maria, "If you ever have a big fight with Nate, we'll know where to look."

Mercer, next to Phil, chirped, "I don't know, Phil, I'd worry *more* about you. Taking all those road trips."

Phil grinned. "Truthfully, I think sometimes my wife is glad to get rid of me."

"Hear! Hear!" Sister called out and people laughed, most especially Phil.

Once back at Roughneck Farm, a forty-five-minute drive from Oakside, hounds were carefully checked for barbed-wire cuts, sore pads, anything unusual.

Betty and Tootie untacked horses to clean them as Sister and Shaker checked, then fed hounds.

The Master and huntsman watched the boys eat. The boys ate first, then the girls. Shaker figured if any of the girls were going into heat early the scent would linger and might cause a ruckus among the boys. And the boys always knew before humans had a sign. Of course, given that all had just hunted together without a hint of someone coming into season early, hounds were safe but Shaker stuck to his program. Sister rarely interfered. Her philosophy was if you have a good huntsman who doesn't drink, run women, or is cruel to horses, leave him or her alone.

Shaker hadn't gone to Kentucky. Sometimes he'd go along to away meets but mostly he didn't want to be far from his hounds. He did enjoy riding with other huntsmen and had struck up a friendship with Glen Westmoreland at Woodford as well as Danny Kerr, huntsman at Camargo Hunt, another rousing Kentucky hunt. Shaker enjoyed talking shop. Most huntsmen did, especially as they were few in number, 162 in North America, give or take one or two depending on circumstances.

"Dreamboat, this was your day. It was the best day you ever had," Sister called to the racy-looking hound as he enjoyed his food, drizzled with corn oil for the taste and also the shine it put on the coats.

"Funny, isn't it?" Shaker smiled, for he liked the hound so much. "He really did me proud."

"I love this pack. It's taken a lifetime of breeding and work and I've always loved my hounds, but Shaker, I think this is the steadiest, hardest-working pack I've ever had and of course, much of the credit belongs to you and our whippers-in."

"No shortcuts." Shaker appreciated the compliment and she knew it.

The two of them had spent many an hour poring over bloodlines and performance. They also attended other hunts, singling out the special hounds there. The research never ended, the study, the planning, and they never wanted it to.

Sister's cell phone beeped. She fished it out of her barn jacket, as she'd already taken off her good hunt coat. Peering down, she read a text:

"Call me. O.J."

"Excuse me a minute." She walked back into the tidy office and called Kentucky.

"Hey."

"Sister, Alan and Meg notified the authorities as you would think they would. So Benny Glitters's tomb has been opened with, oh, I don't know what you call them, forensic people, I guess were there. Anyway, they found an entire human skeleton. Found the watch chain, no other jewelry. Bones and a watch."

"What about the dog?"

"Buried with the human skeleton. No one can say for sure but it looks like the skeleton of a little terrier, you know, like a Norwich. The snout wasn't long enough to be a Jack Russell. Oh, the human skeleton is male."

"I'll be damned. Did they find anything else?"

"Well, Benny Glitters."

"Yes. Remind me again about Benny Glitters."

"The owner, Captain Brown, of Walnut Hall before L.V." Like most people, O.J. called Mr. Harkness by his first initials, as though he were still alive. "Brown was a very successful Thoroughbred horseman."

"Right."

"Before he died, he'd bred Benny Glitters. Everyone thought this would be the next great one. It surely looked like it. Well, Captain Brown died in 1894. The year Benny was eligible to race, he was sold along with the farm to L.V. L.V. was a harness-racing man but he wouldn't have minded winning the Derby. Anyway, Benny started out brilliantly, winning everything and then just fizzled. No one knows why. He was sound. L.V. retired him, hoping he might prove useful as a stud. But then Lela, L.V.'s one daughter, he had two, fell in love with Benny, who was sweet. He became her favorite horse. She foxhunted him and when he died in 1921, she created a memorial. Benny is the only Thoroughbred buried in that graveyard, placed a little off to the side, under the trees."

"She must have loved him very much."

"It's a wonderful story. The Chetwynds, your Chetwynds, did a lot of business in Kentucky, as you said. Old Thomas Chetwynd and L.V. were pals, according to Meg. Kindred spirits perhaps. Thomas had the big slate covering the tomb made, cut, engraved, and brought it out from Virginia to here. I guess there are a lot of slate quarries in central Virginia."

"Yes. We hunt a fixture with an abandoned quarry on it. A seam of land running under a few counties, kind of like your limestone, I guess."

"Anyway, that's how Benny came to rest. The first Standardbred buried in what we all now know as the cemetery was Notelet, who died in 1917, and of course by then L.V. was gone. He died in 1915."

"I don't suppose anyone has an idea who it was down there with Benny," said Sister, her interest piqued, inflamed really.

"No. It surely seems to be murder. You don't just reopen a grave and stick someone and their dog in it."

"True enough and it couldn't have been a robbery. No one would leave a gold watch."

"Meg said police took the watch with them after looking it over carefully at the site. No initials on it but a horsehead is engraved on the back. So I suspect whoever was down there was in the business."

"Or an inveterate gambler," speculated Sister.

"Didn't think of that."

"No good will come of this. I don't care how long someone has been entombed, when you disturb them, troubles follow." Sister shivered for a second as she felt the old evil of the deed.

"I wonder if troubles will follow finding and moving Richard the Third." O.J., an avid reader and history buff, had followed that recent news story with great interest. The bones of the former English king—killed in 1485 in the Battle of Bosworth Field—were found under a parking lot.

"In one way or another it will, but I'm sure the British are equal to it. My worry is this is our problem. Well, I certainly hope it doesn't bring trouble to Meg and Alan, or others that we know."

"Sister, isn't it creepy to think someone has been down there for one hundred and thirteen years and no one knew?"

"That's just it. Someone did know."

CHAPTER 4

Clutching a bottle of hyaluronic acid, Crawford Howard leaned over the counter of the Westlake Equine Clinic. Barbara Engles, the receptionist, printed out the receipt just as one of the partners in the clinic emerged from the rear of the facility.

"Crawford, how are you and how is Czpaka?" asked the veterinarian, Penny Hinson.

"Good. This stuff works. I take it myself. Physicians warn us not to use vet products but hyaluronic acid is hyaluronic acid and it's a lot cheaper here."

Wise in the ways of bumping up any human pharmaceutical cost, Penny nonetheless didn't want to counter a human doctor's caution. She smiled. "So both you and your horse have good working joints."

"Marty's horse, too," he said, mentioning his wife and her horse.

Kasmir Barbhaiya came through the door. "A convocation!" he exclaimed.

Crawford Howard, a self-made man originating along with his fortune from Indiana, respected Kasmir. Crawford felt that anyone who made wagonfuls of money was smarter than someone who didn't. "How's Nighthawk?"

A large smile wreathed the kind fellow's face, for Kasmir, like most foxhunters, dearly loved his equine partner. "A bad boy. Oh my, yes, a very bad boy."

Penny unzipped her coveralls, smears of mud and some blood on them. "What did he do now?"

"Stole my Borsalino. Oh, a lovely navy hat it was, and he snatched it right off my head."

"Did he put it on his?" Penny smiled at Kasmir.

"No, he ran all the way to the end of his paddock, all the way back, then dropped it in his water trough."

Crawford chuckled. "Give him credit for good taste. You never wear anything shabby."

"You are too kind," Kasmir demurred. "I wish you would rejoin the hunt club, Crawford. Yes, I do." Kasmir held up both hands palm outward as this was a vexing subject. "You must hear what happened in Lexington, Kentucky. A most remarkable thing."

He told the three about the sudden pogonip, the sleet, the long ride back to the barns and then the discovery at the Walnut Hall dinner.

"A gold watch?" Crawford stroked his chin.

"Oh, that poor little dog." Barbara couldn't care less about the watch.

"Did they find a body?" Penny got down to business.

"I read *The Lexington Herald* online," Kasmir informed them. "They did, but whose body they don't know. A stray skeleton, ah, too many deaths, I think."

"How do they go about notifying the next of kin if they can't identify the remains?" Crawford remarked.

"Who would know?" Kasmir replied.

"Exactly," Penny sensibly said as Mercer Laprade came through the door.

"Ah, Mercer," said Kasmir. "I was just telling the ladies and Crawford about the branch cracking the slate covering the horse's tomb."

Mercer was careful around Crawford, as he hoped one day the rich man would breed Thoroughbreds to Mercer's profit. "It was a joint meet with one excitement after another."

"You two should come hunt with me." Crawford then added with vigor, "The hell with the MFHA and who would know? My Dumfriesshires are good hounds."

He mentioned the Master of Foxhounds Association of America and a type of hound that originated in Scotland, hence the name. As Crawford ran or tried to run an outlaw pack, members of recognized hunts could not hunt with him without jeopardizing their status with other recognized hunts. The rub was how does one enforce this and Crawford well knew it. He had no intention of submitting to MFHA rules, hence the term outlaw pack.

Kasmir inclined his head in a small bow. "You are most hospitable." Then he quickly changed the subject, turning to Mercer. "You would remember, what was the name of the horse whose memorial covering was smashed?"

"Benny Glitters," Mercer quickly answered as he, too, wanted to slide away from the outlaw pack discussion.

"Yes, yes, that's it."

Mercer was eager to share his knowledge, hoping Crawford would be a bit impressed. "Benny Glitters was a son of the great Domino. Captain Brown, who owned him and the farm then called Senorita, thought he would equal his sire on the track. A beautiful fellow, Benny. Alas, he went up like a rocket and came down like a stick, which was unusual since Domino usually passed on talent. His son, Commando, for example, another great horse."

Crawford placed the bottle back on the counter. "Benny washed out?"

"The farm was bought by L.V. Harkness, who changed the name to Walnut Hall," said Mercer. "One of his daughters fell in love with Benny, who more or less went with the farm. He lived to a ripe old age, twenty-nine. He was so loved he was buried at the farm, the only Thoroughbred in the graveyard. So that's how Benny wound up where he did. His father, by the way, is buried at Hira-Villa, Kentucky. Domino died in 1897. A great, great horse. You can never trace pedigree back far enough."

"It's worked for you." Crawford nodded, acknowledging Mercer's success. For Crawford, success meant money, which led to prestige.

"A bit of care and most people can see some profit in Thoroughbreds." Mercer was shrewd and knew not to push it. He also did not expand on his views concerning the upsetting graveyard incident.

"Um." Crawford picked up the bottle again. "Well, I'm on my way to Old Paradise."

Both Kasmir and Mercer held their breath for an instant, and Penny's eyebrows rose.

"A place steeped in history." Kasmir always felt the romance of Old Paradise. His holding, Tattenhall Station, lay across the road from Old Paradise. Both places encompassed thousands of acres.

"Steeped in history and stupidity," said Crawford. "The Du-Charme brothers, thanks to their ridiculous feud, never realized the profits the place could bring. The last smart DuCharme was the one who created the place and that was after the War of 1812. The rest drifted along." Obviously, he disdained the distinguished old family.

"Perhaps," Kasmir said noncommittally. Although a recent resident of this beautiful area, he took pains to learn the history of the farms as well as the people.

"Perhaps? The brothers are idiots and all over a woman. This was back in the 1960s." He laughed. "And it's not like Binky's wife is Helen of Troy."

No one said a word.

Then Penny remarked diplomatically, "Your efforts are bringing the place back. The sad Corinthian columns, all that's left from the great fire—the sight of them always gives me chills."

"Marty says that, too." Crawford had often heard this from his wife.

"Crawford, you like history." Mercer fed him a compliment. "The boars on top of the pillars to your entrance were the symbol of Warwick the Kingmaker, the man who put Edward the Fourth on the throne."

Crawford lapped it up. "A man who knew how the world truly works. I have always admired him and when I first went to England I visited where he is buried."

"Back to dead bodies again." Penny giggled.

"The truth will all come out sooner or later," Mercer replied.

"Did the dog carry the gold pocket watch?" Barbara couldn't resist.

They all smiled.

"Well, I'd better get over there to see Arthur and Margaret." Crawford named Arthur DuCharme's daughter, a sports physician. Arthur was Binky's brother.

"I do hope you will allow us to continue on to Old Paradise if the hunted fox leaves Tattenhall and crosses the road." Kasmir smiled.

As Kasmir had more money than Crawford, the late-middle-aged man softened his words. "Of course. I respect the traditions, but it goes in reverse, Kasmir. You won't throw me off of Tattenhall if my hunted fox heads east."

"Never." Kasmir smiled broadly.

"Good to see you all." Crawford left.

Mercer breathed out through his nose, then said, "He lives to make us miserable."

"Not us," Kasmir corrected him. "Sister Jane."

Penny knew the story. "And all because she didn't choose him to become Joint Master."

"How could she?" said Mercer. "He's like a bull in a china shop. Every week she'd have to put out brush fires started by his ego. She's a good Master and yes, his money would have been terrific and he would have spent freely but my God, we would have paid for it."

Penny nodded. "Subtlety isn't his strong suit."

"The first time he met me, he looked into my eyes and said, 'You must have a lot of white in you.'" Mercer's light hazel eyes flashed.

"I hope you said, 'Sure, my bad half.'" Penny looked at the wall clock.

"You know, I didn't say anything. I figured why bother on someone that dense? You know, it is possible to be rich and stupid."

Kasmir burst out laughing. "I know."

"Kasmir, I never meant you," Mercer quickly apologized.

"A man can be smart about one thing and dumb about another, or as my late wife used to say, 'A man can be smart during the day but dumb at night.'"

CHAPTER 5

Wednesday, February 5 was fair, in the midthirties, and began with a glorious welcome sunrise. Sister, Shaker, Betty, and Tootie walked the hounds from the kennels along the farm road. On their right was a large pasture with stone ruins in the middle of it, a huge tree beside the ruins. The old fence line had three stout logs as a jump not too far from the ruins, all that was left of the first tiny dwelling from the mid 1780s. Horses took this log jump seriously, whereas an airy jump, some spindly sticks, often set them off.

The group walked on foot. To their left reposed a lovely apple orchard, its trees gnarled. Inky, a black fox, kept a cozy clean den here, from which she would sally forth at night for hunting as well as to visit the kennels. She enjoyed chatting with hounds as long as they were on the other side of their heavy chain-link fencing.

A huge old walnut growing at the edge of the ruins provided a spacious accommodation for Comet, a gray fox. While not as good a housekeeper as Inky, he wasn't a total slob like Uncle Yancy, a red fox who threw everything out of his den. Even a human not well acquainted with wildlife would know whoever lived in Uncle Yancy's den was messy.

Foxes, like people, evidenced distinct personalities and habits.

Asa, an old hound beloved by all, walked up front. He could only hunt one day a week now but he still hunted well. Then, like many an old gentleman, he needed some extra rest, the canine version of Motrin, and a bit of extra love.

"Inky, I know you're in there," Asa good-naturedly called as the pack walked by.

A voice from within the den hollered, *"And I'm staying in."*

"Saucy devil." Sister laughed as she heard the little yip.

On the right side of the pack, Shaker grinned. "The only thing better than being a fox on this farm would be being a hound or a horse. Then again, being a human isn't so bad." He looked over toward the ruins, where Comet did not stick his head aboveground. "Give any thought to breeding Giorgio?" The huntsman greatly admired this hound.

"I have. I'm not sure yet to whom or if we should take him to another club. You know, Princess Anne has some wonderful girls, old Bywaters blood." She mentioned an exciting hunt located on the mighty Lower James River.

Sister, like any Master who breeds, studied bloodlines. Since childhood, she had favored Bywaters blood, a hound bred for Virginia's demanding conditions. She also strongly liked Orange County blood, another Virginia hound bought from William Skinker, the Virginian who bred them, by a rich northerner, Harriman, over one hundred years ago. That old, fine blood coursed through Orange County's kennels.

They walked on, the dirt road firm.

Tootie glanced up toward the top of Hangman's Ridge. "Looks like it's blowing up there."

Betty also looked up. "Hard."

"That's what's so odd," said Sister. "Sometimes the wind will barrel right down the edge to us and other times it literally skims over our heads. You'd think after living here all these decades I'd have figured it out."

Walking out hounds, always a high spot in the day for the staff of The Jefferson Hunt, seemed to put things in perspective. Each time Sister would walk along with her friends and hounds, she knew how lucky she was to be strong and healthy and, best of all, to live out in the country where she could open her door to a beautiful world unfolding before her. She often thought of the millions of people all over the world whose primary view was a set of red taillights in front of them only to be followed by a computer screen. And then there were how many millions of women in Africa who walked miles to a well for a bucket of water? Were taillights an improvement over such hardship? Sister feared urbanization and had no answers to counter the destruction of so many unique environments. But she did know she'd fight like the devil to protect Virginia.

"Did you read in the paper about the next bypass meeting?" Betty inquired. "This western bypass has been in contention for, what, forty years?"

"Actually, I didn't read it," said Sister. "I did find out from O.J. that there was an entire man's body in the horse's grave. I told you that, though, didn't I?"

"You left a brief message. Well, whoever he was, God rest his soul," Betty intoned. "Seems to me all they have to do is go through the papers from 1921 to see who went missing."

"I don't know but I do know we'll be hunting from Tattenhall Station tomorrow and I will bet any of you one hundred dollars that Crawford will hunt from Old Paradise."

"He did that last season and at the beginning of this one, and made a fool out of himself both times," said Shaker. "He can't be that stupid." He laughed because Crawford would lose his pack or more accurately, whoever was hunting his hounds would lose the pack. Now on his fourth huntsman in three years, Crawford couldn't stop from meddling, from thinking he knew more than the person he hired to hunt his hounds.

"No one's going to bet me one hundred dollars?" Sister wheedled.

"I will." Tootie took her up on it.

"And if you lose the bet, where are you going to find the money?" Sister smiled at her.

"Betty will lend it to me," the beautiful young woman teased.

"Ha." Betty loved Tootie, as did they all.

"I'll bet one hundred dollars," Trident offered, the young hound listening in.

"You don't have anything worth that much," Dragon, a few years older, taunted him. *"You aren't even worth a hundred dollars."*

At that, the pack laughed that funny dog laugh where they puff out a little air, their eyes brighten.

"Just wait," said Trident. *"I'll show you all tomorrow that I'm worth more than one hundred dollars."*

And so he would.

Tattenhall Station, a clapboard train station with lovely Victorian flourishes, rested on the west side of the Norfolk and Southern rail line. The Western County Volunteer Fire Department sat across from this on the eastern side of the tracks. It was the westernmost fire station in the county.

Tattenhall, once busy thanks to passenger trains, had fallen into disuse, and was finally abandoned by the railway in the early 1960s. Kasmir Barbhaiya bought the station, all the land abutting it on the south side, and had added bits and pieces of more property over the last two years. His holdings, now two thousand acres, give or take, bordered such historic properties as Old Paradise to the west, Little Dalby and Beveridge Hundred to the south.

Across from this charming station, restored by Kasmir, sat the picturesque Chapel Cross on the northeast quadrant of the crossroads that bore its name. Apple orchards abounded along with pastures. Across from the church, shielded by pines, Binky and Milly DuCharme's Gulf Station still sported the old blue and orange Gulf sign. His son, Art—in his midthirties, often called Doofus behind his back—sometimes acted as a go-between for the brothers, as did Margaret, Arthur's daughter. The two cousins got along just fine, despite feuding fathers.

Horse trailers parked in the paved lot at the station. Sister knew the fixtures around here as well as her own farm. She'd hunted them for over forty years, thinking of her landowners as a large family, filled with old stories, resentments, loves, dreams.

Across from the fire station, Mud Fence was yet another fixture, so Sister had thousands of acres at her disposal, barring Old Paradise now controlled by Crawford. Recently, she'd also picked up some new fixtures.

The DuCharmes were desperate for money; what choice did they have but to turn out their old friend Sister when Crawford offered to pay big bucks to hunt there? This was also a violation of MFHA strictures. Land had to be offered, not paid for. Knowing this, Sister bore no grudge but she sorely missed Old Paradise. Crawford rented it, improved it, but did not own it . . . yet.

Phil Chetwynd, Mercer Laprade, Ronnie Haslip, Gray, the Bancrofts, were a few of the people whose trailers Sister had noticed as she drove in earlier. People were out in full force, for the day looked promising and February could wind up with snowstorms canceling hunt days. Why miss a good day?

Once everyone was mounted, Sister quietly said to Shaker, "Hounds, please," the traditional request from Master to huntsman meaning, "Let's go."

Looking down at all those upturned faces, Shaker smiled, and replied, "Hup-hup."

He trotted up the slight hill behind the station, calling out,

"Lieu in," then blew the note followed by four short ones. Hounds moved out in a semicircle going forward, noses down.

Trident spoke loudly. Never one to be outshone by any other hound, Dragon checked the line. Trident was right. Dragon, fussy because he didn't go out Tuesday, tried to push ahead of the well-built tricolor but Trident was a touch younger and fast. All of Sister's younger hounds had speed. She had deliberately picked up the pace in these last three hound litters.

The pack ran so close together one could have thrown a blanket over them, as the old foxhunting saying goes. The horses followed. Shaker rode Kilowatt, purchased for him by Kasmir, and felt as though he'd gone from 0 to 60 in three seconds. A few in the field parted company from their mounts, as the acceleration caught them off guard.

Bobby Franklin always assigned someone to ride tail to pick up the pieces. Fortunately, no one was hurt, but there's always that delay for a person on the ground to mount, which is why someone stays back. The field must move on, and move on they did.

Happy for a fast start, Sister felt Aztec stretch out underneath her. Like so many Thoroughbreds, Aztec had a long stride, so compared to other horses in the field it looked as though he wasn't laboring or trying very hard. And like all Thoroughbreds, he was born to run. The hounds charged into the thick woods a half mile from where they picked up the fox. Narrow trails necessitated slowing and taking some care, lest you leave your kneecap on a tree trunk.

Even with leaves off the deciduous trees, Sister couldn't see well. Behind her, Bobby's voice, loud and clear, stopped her short.

"Tallyho," came his booming, deep voice.

This was followed by a chorus of the same.

Sister couldn't easily turn around. She heard hoofbeats coming toward her. Aztec didn't want to back into the woods with its low bushes, but a hard squeeze did the trick.

"Huntsman!" Sister shouted.

With difficulty, people got their horses into the woods, heads pointing outward. In this way, the huntsman and Kilowatt didn't risk a kick. A hard kick could break a leg.

Flying as fast as he could given conditions, Shaker, mindful of the members, touched his crop to his cap. As he burst out into the open he saw Bobby, horse turned toward the north, cap off in his right hand, arm extended fully. This told the huntsman the line of the fox.

Sister was still in the woods and not liking it. She shot out of the underbrush to Aztec's delight, then thundered past the people in the woods. Following by placement, one by one, they emerged. Phil Chetwynd, who had ridden right behind Sister, was the next out. Ronnie Haslip, the club's treasurer, was next, and so they went. This is a sensible arrangement because usually horses in the rear are slower than horses in front, so if the people in the back came out first they would slow everyone down.

As she reached the pasture, Sister saw nothing. Bobby, as he should, followed the huntsman. She hit the rise, looked down and saw hounds, huntsman, Betty on the right, Sybil on the left, and Bobby leading Second Flight behind. As Sister rode down, hard, Bobby veered off to the side so she could slip behind Shaker, leaving a good forty yards between huntsman and herself. The faster you rode, the more space you left, just in case.

Once the entire First Flight emerged, Bobby fell in behind them. The fox, which no one saw, crossed the railroad tracks and cut north into Mud Fence farm.

The riders had to cross above the railroad tracks, then carefully cross the tertiary road, climb a small bank, take three steps, and pop over a coop that, having sunk with age, couldn't have been more than two and a half feet high. Sister was over in a flash, as were those close behind her, including the Bancrofts who, nearing eighty, were always perfectly mounted for their abilities, high, and their ages, also high.

Bobby knew where a hand gate was. This cost him a good ten minutes even though the last person with a companion closed it so he could get forward. You never leave anyone alone at a gate when horses are moving off. So it's always two people.

Bobby heard the horn blowing "Gone Away" again. Standing in his stirrups to see over the rise, he beheld all in front of him and pushed on.

Sister, flying, just flying, reveled, in her element. The fact that this was a fox they didn't know also excited her. Given the hard winter, breeding season had been interrupted by heavy snows, so she was sure this was a visiting dog fox.

She passed a collapsed shed, then the entire pack, Trident still in front, turned west, headed for Chapel Cross. A narrow ditch divided the church land from Mud Fence and it was full of running water from melting snows higher up. Aztec leapt it. Sister didn't look down. Never a good idea to look down.

They clattered by the graveyard, right past the small lovely church and had to cross the north/south road, which meant Sister was right at the Gulf station. Apron on, Milly stood in the picture window with DuCharme Garage written in the top. She waved to the people, which made a few horses shy.

Sister waved back but kept moving. The fox crossed the east/west road almost at the crossroads, shot into the edge of Old Paradise, and ran along the snake fencing. A roar above them announced Crawford Howard's Dumfriesshire hounds, who joined them.

To Sister's relief, the two packs ran together. The music was incredible. The cry of these hounds must have reverberated over the mountain all the way to Stuarts Draft.

The new, larger pack soared over the snake fencing, crossed the road again, this time a good mile from the crossroads. Trident was still in the lead and to Sister's surprise, Dreamboat was pushing his way forward.

Sister was so proud of him. His great day at Oakside had emboldened him. He now believed he could lead and he was right up there.

She easily jumped over the snake fence, hit the road, slowed for a moment, then rode along the three-board fence marking Kasmir's land. A new coop beckoned; it was stout. Again, as it was close to the road, she had only a few strides to hit it right and sail over, which she did; but like any rider, a little wiggle room was always desirable.

Within seconds she was right back in the woods and hounds just tore through those woods, finally losing their fox at a small meadow with large fallen trees on it bordered by a tributary feeding into a larger creek.

How did the fox lose them? Scent vanished.

Hounds cast about, Shaker patiently waited, moving a bit here, a bit there, but that boy was gone.

Everyone pulled up. Some slumped over, trying to catch a deep breath.

The two packs kept trying to pick up a lead. Shaker called them over and Crawford's hounds followed, as though part of the Jefferson pack. He headed the group south, and try as he might for the next hour, their efforts were fruitless.

They'd been out for three hours, so Shaker turned back toward Tattenhall Station. Once again, hounds opened.

This brief run took them down to the larger creek. After fifteen blazing minutes, that was over.

Although she had hunted since childhood, Sister never deluded herself into thinking she understood scent. Only the fox understood scent. Hounds could smell it but they didn't understand it either.

Oh, she knew the basics. She knew a fox could jump into the creek and run in the water to destroy scent, which this fox may well have done. A clever fox with some den openings into a creek bed could get in and out without leaving much of a trace, or so Sister thought. He could roll in running cedar or cow dung, which threw hounds off for a time. He could also, if he knew where one was, go straight to a carcass. That never failed to confuse hounds.

But those thoughts were the thoughts of reason. The fox didn't care what she thought.

The group of humans chatted excitedly on the way back to Tattenhall Station. If hounds had spoken, the people would have quieted. Sister had them well trained. Crawford's hounds merrily tagged along. A gabby field drove her bats. Her people respected tradition. The human voice can bring a hound's head up, the last thing you want to do. They need their full powers of concentration. The only thing worse than bringing a hound's head up was kicking one. Turning a fox back into the hound pack ranked right up there with these cardinal sins as it meant certain death for the fox. Sister didn't want to kill foxes nor did most other Masters.

Fortunately The Jefferson Hunt people, most all of them, rode to hunt as opposed to hunting to ride. Observing hounds when they could was a goal for many of them.

Sister motioned for Tootie to catch up to her.

"See anything?" she asked.

The younger woman shook her head, then added, "Well, I did see Lila Repton take that coop on the road. Her horse didn't."

"She all right?"

"Yes. I stayed back to get her up."

"Could she make the jump then?"

"She was a little put off so I jumped her horse over. She climbed on the coop and mounted up while I untied Lafayette from the fence line. He's so good, that horse."

"Well, that was good of you."

"Lila is desperate to ride First Flight. I figured maybe this would help."

"Mmm. Good run." Sister beheld both packs walking quietly up ahead. "How long before he tears down here with his hound trailer and raises holy hell?"

Turns out, Crawford didn't show up.

Sister, Shaker, and the whippers-in put up the Jefferson Hounds and Phil Chetwynd kindly allowed Crawford's hounds to rest in his horse trailer. His horse and Mercer's horse, Dixie Do—tied outside, happily munching away at feed bags—didn't mind.

The station had a long kitchen at one side. Kasmir had outfitted the place so the club could enjoy hot breakfasts. Old railway benches pushed up to long tables provided seating. Once people selected what they wanted from the food tables outside the kitchen, they were glad to sit and not stand holding plates. There was also a cook in the old kitchen to scramble eggs, flip pancakes, fry bacon. This was pure luxury.

The old station exuded an ambience of time gone by. To Kasmir's credit, he did not dispense with the sign over a door that said Ladies Waiting Room nor the old one that spelled out Colored. He talked to many hunt club people about it but Gray settled the issue for him. Gray simply said, "It's our history. Let's not hide it."

History infused the place. As people excitedly replayed the hunt, some could imagine ladies in long dresses, bonnets, repairing to their waiting room where their delicate sensibilities would not be offended by the unwanted attentions of men.

The Southern concept is that every man surely wants to be in the company of a lady.

Sister figured there was some truth to that and she swept her eyes down the long tables to see the women, flushed from the exercise, exuberant. Even those not especially favored by nature became attractive. And then there were the ones like Tootie, so beautiful, so young and sweet, that she took a man's breath away. Tootie had no idea of this. That made her even more beautiful.

Unfortunately, not enough young men hunted but when one did show up in the hunt field he gravitated toward her.

Tootie's dream was to hunt hounds one day after becoming an equine vet, a dream that infuriated her ever-so-rich Chicago father and didn't much please her socially-conscious mother either. Why would their beautiful, brilliant daughter want to operate on horses as well as be an unpaid amateur huntsman?

On and on the assemblage chattered. Sister, coat hanging on the rack at the door along with everyone else's, pulled her grandfather's gold pocket watch from her vest. Snapping it shut with a click, she laughed, for Phil, Mercer, Gray, and Betty had imitated her with their pocket watches.

"Grandfather's." Phil smiled. "I know that's our grandfather's."

Betty chimed in. "Dad's."

"What about you, Mercer?" Sister asked.

"Bought it at Horse Country. You know the case of antique jewelry? Couldn't resist." Mercer smiled.

"The workmanship on those old pieces is, well, I don't know if people can make jewelry like that anymore." Sister again pulled out her grandfather's pocket watch, admiring the filigree and his initials in script, JOF for Jack Orion Fitzrobin. Sister was a Fitzrobin on her mother's side and an Overton on her father's. She'd had a wonderful childhood of hunting with both grandfathers and grandmothers.

Betty, Phil, and Mercer again pulled out their pocket watches, opened them, and then all four clicked watches together, which gave them a good laugh.

After the breakfast, Sister kissed her Thoroughbred Aztec, then along with Betty and Sybil, rendezvoused at the hound trailer, also known as the party wagon.

Betty asked the obvious, "What do we do about Crawford's hounds?"

"Take them to him. I think they'll load into our trailer." Sister put her hands on her hips. She had no desire to see Crawford. However, she would always help hounds.

As his trailer was near the hound trailer, Phil overheard. He and Mercer usually hauled their horses together using a top-of-the-line four-horse conveyance.

"Sister, I'll take them to Crawford. I pass his farm on the way to mine and our guys will be fine with hounds all around them, plus we have the dividers. As long as they have their hay bags they don't care."

Dividers, a padded type of guard hung on a hinge, could be used to separate horses.

"That's kind of you."

"I don't mind a bit." Phil smiled broadly.

When Phil rumbled down Crawford's long drive, at the turnoff, Sam Lorillard met him with a truck and led him back to the kennels, on which—like everything else—Crawford Howard had spared no expense.

Phil had called ahead to Sam, Gray's brother, who worked for Crawford. No one else would give the former alcoholic a job, including his brother. Crawford took a chance on him, paid him handsomely, and was well rewarded by Sam's loyalty and labor.

Sam unloaded the hounds. "How was the hunt?" he asked.

"Good," Phil replied. "Where's Crawford?"

"Up at the house. He drove in about an hour ago."

"Well, his hounds hunted nicely under Shaker, if that matters to him," Mercer piped up.

Sam nodded. "He fired the huntsman in the middle of today's hunt. We will now be looking for number five."

"Man would have to be a fool to take that job." Mercer didn't monitor his opinion.

Grateful as Sam was to Crawford, he knew Mercer was right.

"He'd do better with a woman," Phil declared.

"Why's that?" Sam watched the last hound walk into the well-lit kennel.

Phil folded his long arms over his chest. "I think women are better at dealing with difficult people."

Mercer pulled out his pocket watch and as he did so he told Sam about the four people closing their watches at the same moment. "You know we'd better shoot out of here before he sees us and we hear the lamentations of Crawford Howard," Mercer advised.

"Something elegant about a pocket watch," said Sam.

Mercer said, "One of our relations had a gold pocket watch and he walked into a whorehouse and never walked out—remember that old story?"

Phil tilted his head. "Must have been a hell of a transaction."

Eye on the big house, Mercer recalled, "Great-Aunt Jessamy would shake her head and say they never found anything of Grandpa Harlan's. They found an empty wallet and his clothes were neatly folded in the laundry room of the establishment. Of course, the authorities couldn't tell Jessamy that, but they told enough others. Word got around." He looked at his cousin. "Funny what one remembers."

Moving toward the driver's door, Phil said, "Maybe some things are better forgotten."

CHAPTER 6

The long polished table gleamed under the soft lights which, though subdued, were bright enough to take notes by. The board of trustees for Custis Hall met regularly once a month, more if the occasion demanded. The paneled room was in the original building.

Founded in 1812 as a school for young women, it remained true to its originating principles, now being one of the best prep schools in Virginia. The original funding came from the owner of Old Paradise, a grand lady who had made a great fortune running supplies through the British lines during the War of 1812. Had this indomitable woman been able to return she would have been satisfied, thrilled even, at how the school had flourished over the years. She would have been much less impressed had she visited Old Paradise.

These days, Crawford Howard, a board member, was slowly putting the holding's owners, the DuCharmes, in his back pocket with money and improvements calculated to help Arthur again keep cattle. Crawford's long-term goal was to buy Old Paradise. The

DuCharmes would first fight among themselves but he could play a waiting game.

On moving to central Virginia, Crawford committed the mistake of building a garish new home designed to look old. He garnered attention. Not a penny was spared. Over time he learned that showing off his riches like this put a mark by his name as a vulgarian, even though he tried to make the place look historic. Far better to buy an historic estate. Even if one lived in one that was falling down, that still trumped the look of new money. Every place has its ways and Virginia remained steadfast in her habits, for both good and ill.

To Crawford's credit, he cared about young people. One of his passions was education and he gave generously—as in six figures per annum—to Custis Hall. Young and attractive, Headmistress Charlotte Norton proved adept at managing him, a quality Sister Jane admired since she had failed to pacify Crawford when he was a hunt club member. Crawford's business acumen also proved vital to Custis Hall.

Sister was now in her fortieth year on the board of trustees, for she kept getting re-elected. She valued Crawford's contribution even as she disdained him personally. While lacking his degree of business sense, she had a bit. Moreover, she was one hundred percent committed to a strong humanities curriculum, which meant foreign languages, structured classes, knowing your country's history along with world history. As a former professor of geology at Mary Baldwin College, the huntmaster was passionate about the natural sciences.

The board had wisely corralled a bank president, head of one of the best local law firms, and one music star—who worked very hard, to everyone's surprise, as they thought she'd more or less show up for one meeting a year. Turned out that Mary Sewell Wainwright was as enthusiastic about all the arts as Sister was about the natural sciences.

The two women clicked, despite a thirty-year age gap.

Elected just last year and still finding their way were Phil Chetwynd and Mercer Laprade. The Chetwynds served on many boards but this was Phil's first turn at Custis Hall, where his oldest daughter was a sophomore. Mercer was determined to create scholarships for young women of color, a much cherished goal.

Nancy Hightower, also African American, addressed the gathering. "My fear is that this interference will create a backlash."

She referred to the S.O.L.'s, the Standard of Learning rules laid down by the federal government and then enforced by the state government.

"Not for us." Phil put his pencil down. "Custis Hall exceeds all the criteria."

"Let me be more clear, the backlash I fear is accusations about elitism. We outperform most every state school and we are right up there against St. Catherine's and St. Christopher's, Collegiate, St. Gertrude's, Foxcroft, Madeira. We hold our own and better."

"Private schools can't be compared to state schools," said Phil. "We can be far more demanding than the state."

"Yes, we can and we should be," Mercer agreed, his light voice clear, pleasant. "But the bulk of our students come from homes that are stable, value education, and strongly support same. We need more scholarship students."

"Mercer, forty percent of our students receive some form of student aid," said Isadore Rosen, head of personnel.

Now in his midfifties, Isadore had taken his job decades ago, thinking it would be temporary. But he had found his calling and stayed, to the benefit of all.

The six o'clock news anchor at a network station in Richmond and a Custis Hall alumna, Frances Newcombe agreed. "Mercer has a point. Private schools are seen as elitist and there is resentment about children not getting in because they can't afford it. We all at this table know it takes more than money, what it really takes is aptitude, a willingness to work hard and frankly, there's not enough of that as I would wish. This is a generation that expects to have everything given to them."

Sister weighed in. "With all due respect, Frances, there are plenty of young people out there who would make good use of an education here if they could swing it. Custis Hall is expensive as are all the prep schools. It's not just the expansion of scholarship funding, it's also the housing, the food. You all see our budget statements. Lord, just keeping the physical plant and the grounds up to form costs us thousands upon thousands. And then if we could increase enrollment of scholarship students, could we raise the money to pay for it? Where would we build a new dorm without risking the historical character of this place? Custis Hall is one of the most beautiful secondary schools in the United States."

In his commanding voice, Crawford said, "There is another way."

The eleven other trustees stared at him as did the headmistress, Isadore, and the two other school administrators present.

"How?" Charlotte asked.

Never averse to being the center of attention, Crawford paused for a moment, then launched in. "We can't create scholarships without creating more infrastructures as has been noted." He couldn't bring himself to credit Sister but she enjoyed that he had to acknowledge her concerns. "Custis Hall can create outreach programs. There's no reason why we can't rent space for early evening classes, weekend classes in Charlottesville, Waynesboro. Bringing in students who don't live on campus is cheaper than construction. Yes, it takes planning and we would need to augment salaries for those on the faculty willing to do this. But even if we had to hire some new people, it's more cost-effective than housing twenty or thirty new students on campus."

A long silence followed this, then everyone talked at once, sparked by Crawford's vision.

Sister, who always made a point of sitting next to him on the principle that you keep your enemies close, touched his forearm. "Brilliant, Crawford. Thank you."

He nodded, then looked up as Phil called over the chatter, "Crawford, the old Chetwynd offices are serviceable in downtown Charlottesville. They need a bit of rehab but I could do that as a gift to Custis Hall if the board pursues this."

Charlotte pounced but softly. "Phil, that is extraordinarily generous. Well, Crawford, you've given us all something exciting to consider. I don't want this to slip away, frittered away in committees, so may I ask the following to be done for our next meeting? Crawford, would you examine our curriculum and determine what you think would be suitable for satellite locations or even e-courses? Most all students have access to a computer now."

Apart from the reception to his idea this flattered Crawford, who assumed she'd always limit his input to financial matters. "Of course."

"Phil, given your family's long association with the area, might you explore other potential locations?"

"Are you willing to decentralize enough so that we could offer classes in Waynesboro and over by Zion Crossroads?" Phil inquired. "In that way, we could bring in students from western and eastern counties. Zion Crossroads could serve Louisa, Fluvanna, possibly even Orange. There are a lot of bright kids out there."

"Hear. Hear," Mercer said.

"Mercer, are you willing to secure, or even procure, the numbers of students in area schools who score in the top ten percent at their school, the ones with good grades?"

"Of course, but Charlotte, there are kids who aren't doing well scholastically who would if we could just reach them." Mercer truly cared.

The headmistress smiled for she, too, wanted to find those diamonds in the rough. "You're right, but we may have to work up to that or find an efficient way to identify them. I know test scores aren't always the answer; the answer is and always will be educators who take an interest in their students, which brings me to you, Lucas." She addressed Lucas Diamond, who had worked in the State Education Department. "Find those teachers."

He looked up at the ceiling, then around the table. "Well, if you all can do what you're going to do, I will do my part." Then he laughed.

"What about me?" Mary Wainwright asked plaintively.

"Mary, this board and me in particular are going to shamelessly abuse you." That got everyone's attention. "Once we have a plan, you are going to give a concert to raise money."

All eyes were on Mary as she dramatically breathed in, then said saucily, "I will raise so much money you'll be able to build a satellite campus."

The room cheered. Sister thought it was the best board meeting she'd ever attended.

As it broke up, knots of people conferred and she found herself with Phil and Mercer by the long polished sideboard against the wall.

"Hey, to switch the subject, Sister, I know Lafayette is getting on. That fellow has to be fourteen or so, right?" asked Phil.

"We're both getting up there." She smiled at the thought of her aging horse.

"Keepsake and Rickyroo must be close to their early teens, too, if I recall," Phil continued.

Mercer teased, "I feel a horse deal coming on."

"I have a two-year-old and a three-year-old. One is by Guns and Roses and the other by St. Boniface, out of solid mares but they don't have the speed for the track. They have good minds. Why don't you come have a look?"

Crawford joined the group. "Phil, thank you for bringing my hounds back the other day."

Knowing the history between Crawford and The Jefferson Hunt, Phil said, "It was Sister's idea."

As this transpired, Mercer glanced at his iPad, which showed he had a new e-mail. He checked on the message. "Sister, thank you," Crawford said, doing the right thing.

"Crawford, they hunted wonderfully well under Shaker and they are in good flesh. Very handsome hounds." Sister smiled.

Clearing his throat he responded, "Thank you."

"What the hell?" Mercer exclaimed, then looked up. "Sorry."

"Well, what the hell?" Sister teased him.

"Justin Sautter, with the help of Meg and Alan, have gone through the family papers and found a note about the delivery of Benny Glitters's slate memorial. Roger Chetwynd"—Roger was old Tom Chetwynd's son—"Lucius Censa, the Chetwynd's stable manager, and a Negro worker accompanied the memorial. The Kentucky forensic people said the skeleton is that of an African American male, early forties, old break in the left leg. Anyway, they think the skeleton might be of the man who accompanied the slate memorial from here in Virginia to there. They also found a note in Lela's hand about the slate and the man escorting it, whom she described as a 'fine dark man with an adorable little dog.' I'll bet that was my grandfather!" Mercer said with excitement.

"I thought your grandfather walked into a whorehouse and never walked out," Phil remembered.

"Am I missing a good story?" Sister leaned toward Mercer.

"Grandpa Harlan did," said Mercer, "but I didn't mention that the whorehouse was in Lexington, Kentucky."

Phil calmly replied, "Mercer, even if it is your grandfather, why would he end up in a grave with a horse and a dog? It makes no sense."

"It makes sense to someone," Mercer's voice rose.

"I'm sure they are all dead," Phil replied.

"Well, they may be but that doesn't mean someone who is alive doesn't know," Sister stated as Crawford, Mercer, and Phil looked at her.

"If you all will excuse me, I'm going to concentrate on the living." Crawford withdrew.

"Me, too." Phil smiled.

Mercer drew close to Sister. "You're right. Someone might know. Wait until I tell Mother. I want to know who killed my grandfather and why. Mother's become very intrigued, too."

"I can understand that, Mercer, but you don't know for sure that this body was your grandfather's. As it was 1921, he must have had late children."

"He did and my father, his son, had me in his middle years. In my family, we stay, um, virile and healthy a long time."

"I hope so." She winked at him.

CHAPTER 7

Cold seeped into Uncle Yancy's bones. At ten, for a red fox he was old. Quick thinking and cleverness kept him alive when other foxes fell by the wayside. He wondered when his spouse would leave her earth, a spacious den. A nag, Aunt Netty had plucked his last nerve and he had moved out. She said she threw him out. Over the last three years Netty's expulsions became an annual event based, she said, on his messy ways. She prided herself on a clean den. His version was she didn't know what she wanted and had turned into an old crank.

Then spring would come, Aunt Netty would need help with one project or another, something usually involving killing rabbits, and she'd woo him back.

This night, twenty-two degrees outside but cozy in the mudroom at the Lorillard home place, Uncle Yancy swore he wouldn't fall for it this spring . . . if spring ever arrived.

Yancy had chewed a hole through the floorboards from underneath the mudroom to crawl up next to the tack trunk. A few of the floorboards were rotten, which made it easier. Sam Lorillard had thrown a pile of washed red rags in the corner, then forgot them. The fox, smelling crumbs and other tidbits would push the rags aside, enter through, then push them back. Once in the mudroom he had many places to hide, including jumping from shelf to shelf until he was on the highest one. To him, the mudroom was a little bit of heaven. The temperature inside hovered in the low fifties. The grasses and old towels in his den in the graveyard, another under the front porch, were all right if he curled up, but this was true luxury.

Uncle Yancy recognized the Lorillard brothers, Gray and Sam. The two kept the home place, having bought out their snotty sister, Nadine, who was now a leading light in Atlanta, wanting nothing to do with country life. She certainly wanted nothing to do with Sam.

Gray would stay home maybe two nights a week, less if he was called in for a consulting job in Washington where he retained a convenient small apartment. The rest of the time he stayed at Sister's.

Uncle Yancy knew many of the humans in his territory. The Bancrofts' farm touched the Lorillard farm on the Lorillards' western edge. He also knew Sister, Shaker, Betty, and Sybil and he even recognized some people in the hunt field. From time to time the hounds, all of whom he also knew, would pick up his scent and he'd lead them a merry chase until he tired of it. Usually he'd dump them at Hangman's Ridge, an eerie place. Too many ghosts and too many minks—those nasty little devils with their sharp teeth. He hated them. It was mutual, but their strong odor almost always threw off the hounds, and many's the time when Uncle Yancy walked down the backside of Hangman's Ridge. Just in case, he marked every gopher hole and abandoned fox den along the way. You never knew when you'd need it.

On the top shelf, he rested his head on his outstretched right arm.

The kitchen was next door, a wood-burning stove heating most of the wooden house with a little help from a newly installed heat pump. There Sam sat on a chair, bucket between his feet, bridle in his hands. Uncle Yancy could smell the special saddle conditioner, a type of saddle butter, that the wiry man always ordered from Grangeville, Idaho.

The men's voices carried into the mudroom and the fox found their deep timbre oddly soothing. He liked Sam, who he saw more than Gray. Something sad and lonely about the man affected the creature. Most all of the higher vertebrates can sense emotions in others. Humans deny this ability in animals, but then they also deny their own emotions. Uncle Yancy had nothing to hide, therefore he was open to all information.

"That stuff really is the best." Gray leaned back in the wooden chair. "But it takes so long. First you have to strip down the leather, wash it good, use some saddle soap, then let it dry. Half the time I don't have the time."

"Brother, when do you clean your own tack? You pay Tootie to do it for you."

Sheepishly, Gray agreed. "Most times I do but, you know, those spring days, you smell the apple blossoms, then it's a joy to sit outside and clean tack or clean anything, really. The rest of the time, not so much."

"I never knew how beautiful this place was until I left for college. Harvard, well, it's in the city, grand as the place is, but I thought I would perish of homesickness."

"Me, too, not so much at college but all those years in D.C." Sam rose to start heating water on the stove. "I feel like hot chocolate. What about you?"

"Sounds good. I've been thinking about what you told me. What Sister told you after the Custis Hall meeting last night. Mercer's one brick shy of a load."

Gray smiled. "He's always been excitable."

"Excitable, hell, he's all over the map. Lorillard men aren't supposed to be, well, you know. Anyway, he treats me like a slug, a sea slug."

"Because you don't have any money. Sam, he's not that bad."

"Hell, he's not. The only reason he's nice to me is when he nudges me a little to try to get business out of Crawford. Oh, how Mercer loves to make money and be around money."

"His side of the family has had money for a long time. While he's not exactly Crawford or Phil's equal, he's not poor by a long shot. And give him credit, he knows his business."

"He can recite bloodlines and sales figures. I told him once, forget blabbing about bloodlines. People don't care. Just talk about how much the sire won or the dam and what their progeny is doing on the track. But he keeps blabbing on, showing off."

Gray mixed the hot chocolate powder, the hot water releasing the enticing smell. "Here."

"Thanks. You taking a break from female companionship?"

"Sam, I usually spend Monday and Friday nights here if I can. Sometimes it is good to have one's little space."

"*A Room of One's Own.*" Sam cited the Virginia Woolf book, as he was well educated.

"Something like that."

"I don't know if I will ever enjoy female companionship. Been a long dry spell." Sam started rubbing in the saddle butter using the warmth of his hands to help the waxes penetrate the leather. "Mostly I really do enjoy women but sometimes the way they think drives me over the cliff. Too emotional."

Gray shrugged. "That's painting with a broad brush."

"Yeah, but my experience is women notice the damnedest things. I mean stuff that just makes no sense. Kind of like Mercer." He burst out laughing.

Gray laughed, too. "The Laprade side of the family is given to emotional drama."

"They live for it. I'll bet you twenty Georges that if that body is our grandfather or great-grandfather or whoever the hell he is, some family relation, Mercer will be beside himself."

Gray touched his mustache, smoothing it outward. "Nero Wolfe. He'll have to solve the crime."

This set them both to laughing.

"I'm surprised Mercer hasn't driven to Lexington to offer up his saliva for a DNA test." Sam could hardly finish the sentence, he was laughing so hard.

"I don't get the science behind that but it must work." Gray finished his drink. "I wonder if we want to know too much. Maybe it's better not to know. Someday, someone will find Amelia Earhart or pieces of something that will solve her disappearance. What good does it do? She's gone. Same with the princes in the tower. Remember that, when the two little bodies were found under a stairwell in the Tower of London? Anyway, that was before DNA testing, but so many people are convinced these are the murdered sons of Edward the Fourth."

"Gives academics and novelists a field day. You know, did Richard the Third kill them, or did Henry Tudor once he became king after killing Richard at Bosworth Field? I'm curious I guess. Yeah, I am."

"You always liked history," said Gray. "I read some and I know we need to know what came before but Sam, I can't say as I care much. I care about now. I care about the future."

"But that's just it, the past is prologue."

"Teach you that at Harvard?" Gray smiled.

"Did. The guilt of throwing away that education haunts me. Christ, what a mess I made of my life, your life, anyone around me."

Gray had paid for two drying-out clinics. The second one took. As Sam had remained sober for nine years now, Gray began to relax, yet in the back of his mind was always the fear that somehow for some reason, Sam would relapse.

"It's all over, done. I don't know what was worse, not capitalizing on Harvard or losing your chance as a steeplechase jockey. You could have set up business after the competitive days were over but you're still in horses, you can still set up a sideline." He leaned down and picked up the saddle butter jar. "Build a better mousetrap."

"That saddle stuff really is the better mousetrap." Gray wiped his hands on a cloth, then rose to wash them.

Gray took his cup over to the sink, looked out the window. "Black as the ace of spades. Low cloud cover."

"Half moon tonight. The good thing about a low cloud cover is it keeps a little heat on the earth. Those cold clear nights make it hurt when you breathe."

"Tonight's cold even with the cloud cover," Gray remarked.

Sam opened the door to the mudroom, flinging two used towels toward the back door. "I swear I smell fox."

Uncle Yancy, flattened low on the shelf, watching with his glittering deep yellow eyes.

Gray joined Sam at the door. "Does. Probably the graveyard fox."

"Well, he has one hell of a signature if it's this strong in the mudroom." Sam closed the door.

Had the brothers walked into the mudroom, turned around and glanced upward, they would have seen the tip of a magnificent brush just falling over the shelf. Uncle Yancy was hiding in plain sight.

It would have been a good lesson for all to learn before it was too late.

CHAPTER 8

That same Friday night Sister's fountain pen glided over perfectly lovely cream stationery, the hunt club crest centered at the top. She sat at the graceful desk in her library, its smooth writing surface highly polished. This regal piece of furniture commanded the room. While Sister considered this her main desk she was one of those people who scribbled wherever she could. At the end of the day, after her shower, she would often troll through the house's rooms, picking up and reading through her notepads, finding much that could prove useful.

Golliwog, her insufferable long-haired cat, sprawled on the back of the leather sofa, her tail slightly swaying to and fro. Plopped on the sofa cushions the two house dogs snored; Raleigh, a beautiful male Doberman and Rooster, a harrier bequeathed to Sister at the death of an old lover, Peter Wheeler. He also willed her his estate, Mill Ruins, on which an enormous waterwheel, ever turning, could have been restored to grind grain should anyone be so inclined. Mill Ruins was rented for ninety-nine years by Sister's Joint Master, Walter Lungrun, M.D., a fellow in his prime, early forties.

Peter had always sworn to Sister that he would leave her everything, but she'd thought he was joking. He wasn't and she found herself with two sizable farms to run, combined with the great good luck of owning desirable property.

Conscious of her wonderful luck, Sister realized there are people who resent anyone with resources. She accepted that blind hatred, and she had no real answer as to why the Wheel of Fortune had placed her on the upswing. She herself was not an envious person. She did, however, like very much that her position allowed her to be useful to others—specifically young people and animals. She cared little about anyone else's status or bank account. She either liked you or she didn't, and being Southern, if she knew you needed some financial help she often found a way to do that without embarrassing you. Many Virginians had a lot of pride and would not take what they considered a handout. She worried about so many people out of work, she worried about people sliding out of the middle classes into poverty, and she also was angered at those few who abused public trust whether on Wall Street, Silicon Valley, or Washington, D.C.—people who profited secretly or openly from the distress of others.

She was just one person. All she could do was to shoulder the load with people she knew. Sister was not one to write checks to organizations. She had to know to whom money was going and she had to respect them. If nothing else, she was consistent.

She'd written a check this Friday to Custis Hall for a scholarship for a fourteen-year-old whom Mercer sponsored. He wrote the other half of the check for the girl's first year.

Sister did not think of herself as a particularly loving or good person. She thought of herself as a clear-eyed responsible one. What others thought of her mattered precious little if at all. This quality above all others drove her enemies wild. Over the years, Crawford had dug, parried, and derided her, yet she never bothered to respond. Worse, she sought him out at the board meetings and remained friendly with his wife—or as friendly as she could under the circumstances.

Some of this impressive lady's supreme self-confidence was rubbing off on Tootie, who walked into the library.

"Bills?" asked the lovely young woman.

"You know, just when you think you're in the clear, the mailbox is filled with some more." Sister capped the pen, turning to view Tootie, who had recently turned twenty-one.

"Did you hear that Felicity got promoted?" Tootie mentioned a brilliant schoolmate of hers who had gotten pregnant. Unable to go off to college, Felicity took night courses toward a degree.

"Garvy Stokes knows talent when he sees it. I'm behind on seeing Felicity. I haven't visited my godson in two weeks."

"He doesn't stop talking." Tootie smiled. "Not at all like his mother," she quipped.

"And how is your mother, speaking of mothers?"

Tootie shrugged. "Same as always."

"You haven't visited Chicago in over a year. Why don't you go once hunt season is over?"

Tootie sat on the couch next to Raleigh. The Doberman raised his head only to drop it in Tootie's lap, give her a loving gaze, then close his eyes.

Golly, on the other hand, opened her lustrous eyes. Far be it for the cat to miss anything.

"I don't want to," said Tootie. "It's always the same old thing. They make me miserable, angry, and finally bored."

"That's a harsh judgment on your mother and father."

"Sister, you've met them."

"I have, and I know your father doesn't much like me but he's still your father and he loves you the only way he knows how. And as for your mother, she does what most good wives do, she props him up, tries to get him to see reason or at least have some emotional understanding. She loves you, too."

"You know what, Sister? I don't care." A flash of defiance flared from that beautiful face.

Picking up the fountain pen, Sister twirled it. "You've been with me one and a half years now and you've taken courses at UVA. You've kept your word about that. Things come so easily to you—riding, college courses. I don't know if that's good or bad."

"Not everything. I signed up for organic chem. That might not be easy."

"We'll see. You know Dr. Hinson will help." Sister named the veterinarian, a woman who liked Tootie.

"I'm trying to be like you." Tootie smiled. "I'm writing letters."

Sister beamed. "It's the only proper way to communicate, or at least to communicate some things. I was just writing O.J. to invite the Woodford group here in March. We've talked about it but a formal invitation is needed. Wouldn't it just be silly if they all get here and we have a storm?"

"What was it you called the storm in Lexington?"

"A pogonip, a freezing fog. The superstition is that it brings bad luck."

"Well, it did, didn't it?"

"I suppose it did."

"I found some old pictures of Benny Glitters."

"You did?" Sister asked, surprised and curious.

"Sure. I'll show you." Tootie rose, walked to a simple desk tucked in a corner, upon which was Sister's computer. The young woman sat down and quickly pulled up images from Google. "Look."

Sister stood behind her. "I keep promising to move the computer out of here to a better place, a bigger place, and move that little desk. Well, that's irrelevant, I fear. I'll never be able to use it like you do."

"You don't have to. You have me." Tootie clicked and sure enough there appeared an old sepia photograph of a petite woman in hacking attire, presumably Lela Harkness, astride a well-built bay.

"How about that? Don't you love that Lela looks like a magazine model? People dressed for the occasion in those days." Sister leaned forward, squinting a bit. "Benny Glitters looks like a handsome bay horse. Well, Thoroughbreds are usually some form of bay or chestnut with the occasional gray. Look how sturdy his forelegs are."

"I found other pictures, too." Tootie flipped through old photographs, some from the turn of the last century going up through the 1920s. "Here's one of Phil Chetwynd's grandfather, I guess."

"Roger was the grandfather. Old Tom, Phil's great-grandfather, started Broad Creek Stables. Both Phil and his brother—the one who lives in Charleston, West Virginia—resemble their father, also named Tom in honor of the original patriarch. I vaguely remember Roger. What I recall is that he was so competitive. When people had money in those days, they really had it."

"Look at this." Tootie filled the screen with photographs of L.V. Harkness's daughters, and others of Walnut Hall through the years.

"Go back to Benny," said Sister.

"Sure."

"Okay, now can you find me a picture of Domino?"

"That's easy. He was so famous. There's lots of photographs." Tootie proved her point.

"Hmm. It's hard to tell how much Benny looks like his sire. Pull up one of Domino's most famous son, Commando."

Tootie did. "He looks a little more like Domino. I mean, it's hard to tell bays apart."

"'Tis. I'll tell you a secret. Always start at the hoof. Then go up the legs starting from the rear. Pause at the gaskin, the large muscle at the top of the hind legs often called the second thigh. Now look at the hip angle. Okay, go to the forelegs. Same trajectory. Right? Now look from the withers to the hindquarters. Okay, set that in your mind. Look at the shoulder angle, look at the angle of the neck from that shoulder, look at the chest. Finally, go to the head."

"I did that."

"Now pull up a photograph of Man o' War. He ought to be easy to find."

He was.

Tootie looked at the great horse as Sister had instructed her. "Well, they don't look alike but they are both really handsome horses."

"Yes, they are. A sharp eye can help you a lot, save mistakes." Sister paused lest she rattle on, although Tootie was a ravenous listener. "And after all the conformation talk, I tell you the most important thing about horses, hounds, and people: You can't put in what God left out."

Tootie quietly registered all this. "You mean the mind, the mind first."

"Indeed I do, especially for a hunting horse. You can get killed out there, Tootie. Sometimes I think people who foolishly ride a beautiful horse with a bad mind are just asking for it. I don't have but so much sympathy."

The two studied Man o' War, a delight for any horseman. Tootie clicked back to Domino, and they examined him again.

"Look at these photographs of Broad Creek Stables. This one is from 1902!" said Tootie.

"Old Tom Chetwynd. He had to be incredibly smart to found that coal business and then the stables, too. I often wonder why Phil doesn't leave for Lexington, but he's big beans in the Mid-Atlantic."

Tootie remarked, "Some people like my father have to be the big shot, you know?"

"I know, but Phil covers it up well." Sister watched as Tootie scrolled through more photographs.

"Stop." Sister pointed to a photograph of Roger Chetwynd and Lucius, the stable manager. Behind them stood some stable hands and a well-dressed African American. Farther back were horses in paddocks. "I'll be damned," said Sister.

Tootie studied the photograph. "I see it."

The natty African American had Mercer's chin and his high cheekbones. There was a resemblance but then again many people could have those features. Catching both their attention too was the adorable, bright-eyed Norwich terrier at his feet.

Tootie looked up at Sister. "Should we tell Mercer?"

Sister took a long time, leaned on the back of the sofa.

"I was here first," Golly complained.

Rooster opened one eye and regarded the cat. *"Shut up, Golly."*

"Methuselah's dog. Worthless old fart." Golly swished her tail.

Without rising, Rooster lifted his head, growling.

"That's enough," Sister commanded.

Golly eyed the harrier with malicious glee.

"No, we shouldn't tell Mercer about the resemblance," Sister finally declared.

"Why?"

"Mercer can be like a helium balloon. *Pfft.*" She moved her forefinger up in the air like a helicopter blade.

"I have a terrible feeling about those old bones. Mercer, well, I just think he could stir up a hornet's nest."

"But that could really be his grandfather." Tootie was confused.

"It was so long ago," Sister said. "The reverberations from violent crimes never quite stop. That's easy to see in the cases of"—she thought about earlier conversations with O.J.—"Lincoln's assassination, stuff like that. That's a significant political event but any murder is an event that touches others and can continue to do so. We should be careful."

"But we don't have anything to do with it."

"Tootie, if we are too interested or find some useful information, we *will* have something to do with it. That man was killed over money, a lot of money. You don't kill someone for a few bucks. Don't get me wrong. I want to find out what I can. Seeing that fore-finger, the watch, and little dog skull really got me. But something tells me to be careful. That had to be murder."

"A woman. Men kill over women."

"He wouldn't be buried with a horse and his dog. He would have been shot in passion or stabbed. This is deliberate. You know how I told you to look at a horse from the hoof up, well, look at this from the ground up, so to speak."

"Didn't Mercer say his grandfather's clothes were found at a whorehouse?" Tootie was realizing that Sister was extremely practical when it came to emotions.

Mercer, on the other hand, was volatile and emotional. Strangely enough, at the same time, he was shrewd and patient concerning business.

"Apparently, that was a ruse," said Sister. "Whoever murdered Harlan Laprade thought it through. People would be more than willing to believe a man would go to a house of ill repute, an expensive one, and fall into trouble. Especially if he's away from home. Men visit such places every day all over the world."

Young and idealistic, Tootie said, "That's horrible. Disgusting."

"Honey, most men, no matter where they are, high or low, Asia, Africa, the Americas, you name it, most men feel they are entitled to sex."

"Gross!"

"I can't judge. I can only tell you that if a fellow doesn't have a girl in every port, so to speak, he's happy to pay for a night of pleasure. In fact, it's easier. No strings. A straight cash transaction. Whoever left those clothes folded in the laundry room at the whorehouse was very, very clever and probably knew the victim would be there— or visit, then leave. How easy to kill him in an alley, take his clothes back to the whorehouse. Pretty easy, I think. First of all, no one would tell a wife her husband's clothes were found in an exclusive whorehouse. So there's one line of inquiry shut down."

"They would now." Tootie was incredulous.

"But not then. Remember the time. 1921. Secondly, the murder victim probably had a reputation for chasing skirts. Those who knew him would be surprised at his disappearance but not really shocked. I mean it, Tootie, if a Laprade really is the victim, we need to be careful. Whoever killed him is long gone but the effects of that murder might not be, especially if it was over a boatload of money and it was done or conceived by someone highly intelligent." Sister put her hand on Tootie's shoulder. "Let's walk softly."

"Maybe we should hope Mercer doesn't find any photos," Tootie remarked. But he had.

CHAPTER 9

"Don't you have a brighter lamp?" Mercer fussed as he peered at old photographs.

"Use this little flashlight." Phil pulled open the narrow desk drawer, retrieved a small promotional LED light, and handed it to him.

Looking at the light, Mercer remembered. "This thing has to be four years old."

"It is. Gave them out at Keeneland back at the stables." Phil sat shoulder to shoulder with Mercer at his office desk in the old main barn.

"Last really good sale anyone had. This economy has to get better," Mercer grumbled.

"It will. Always does. The secret is to pare down and hang on. I forgot that Daddy saved all this stuff. Fortunately, he kept it in a metal box up at the house. Glad you made me look for old family photos."

"We don't have any that go that far back. That's my granddad Harlan," Mercer said, squinting at the sepia photograph. "Can't be anyone else." He flipped it over, and along with the filly's name, Topsail, was Harlan Laprade.

Shirtsleeves rolled up, bowtie, what looked like summer flannel pants and a snappy boater, Harlan stood next to the filly. Both stared straight at the camera.

"Knew how to show a horse," Phil said admiringly.

Mercer carefully sifted through more photographs in the pile from the metal box. A few were of back barns and run-in sheds being built, the main barns in front. Others cataloged mares, colts, fillies, and four standing stallions.

"Navigator. 1923. Bone." Mercer appreciated the bay stallion. "He had some age on him in this photo but he looks incredible. Just incredible." Mercer remarked on the heavier denser bone the horse displayed compared to so many of today's horses, who are more fragile.

"Had to have bone then. Still should. But so many races were a mile, a mile and a quarter. Few seven furlong runs then, I think." Phil tidied up the photographs. "Dad said that was the biggest change he'd seen in his lifetime, the jigging of race conditions to favor weaker horses."

A furlong is one-eighth of a mile.

"Mmm," Mercer half listened, his eye again drawn to his grandfather. "Good clothes run in the family."

"Seems so. Funny, I didn't know Dad kept so many photos."

"Mother advised me to ransack the old barn for photographs, files. I think my dear mama lost some things like photographs between moves and husbands back in the day."

Phil took the photograph of Navigator from Mercer's hand. "Would you like me to make a copy of this?"

"Mother would like that," said Mercer. He was a bachelor and lived just next door to Daniella Laprade, which most folks would think was too close by.

"Looking at these photos, I wonder if they were happier then. Was life really simpler?"

"No. Nothing changes, Phil. I'm convinced of that. Technology changes how fast we can travel, communicate. Medicine changes, but people, no. People don't change."

"Yeah, I guess. You know, maybe I'll make two copies of this and send one to the Lexington Police Department."

"What can they tell from a photograph? All they have are bones, but now I'm sure they are my grandfather's. Did anyone at the farm keep records? Not breeding records and accounts but, you know, a diary?"

"Not that I know about but, Mercer, even if my great-grandfather Old Tom did or his son, my grandfather, did, no one would record the clothing being found in a house of ill repute, then send it on to the family. One didn't talk about stuff like that, especially if a woman might find the records and Dad always said that Grandpa and Great-grandpa were circumspect, especially where women were concerned. A trait I'm trying to pass on to my boys, but maybe they're too young."

"Ten and twelve, that's not too young."

"If whoever was in that grave had his throat slit, any kind of flesh wound, there won't be a trace. The only way to know how he was killed is if a bone was shattered or lead pressed into it." Phil switched back to the unidentified bones in the equine grave.

"Maybe our dentist has records. Worth a try. We've gone to the same family dentist since Christ went to Chicago," Mercer replied.

The old Southern expression made Phil chuckle. "A long time and I don't know as the Good Lord was able to reach the Chicago heathen."

"O ye of little faith," Mercer chided him. "Thanks for finding this stuff. It's not like you don't have other things to do."

"We all do," said Phil. "Overcommittment is the great American vice." He smiled. "Anyway, I enjoyed looking at the photographs. I think both our grandfathers were driven men—had to be, to be successful. People like that usually accomplish a lot but they miss a lot, too. Dad said he hardly ever saw his dad and when he did, the old man paid little attention to him. Maybe that's why he was such a good father to me."

"Different times." Mercer shook his head. "Look, I know in *my* bones that was my grandfather, Harlan, in that grave. He didn't return to Virginia, obviously, from delivering the slate memorial. Has to be him that was under it."

"It's a good guess but don't jump the gun, Mercer. All that does is create confusion."

"It's Mother that worries me. She wants to know. She's looking for dental records. She wants to know now."

"Mercer, no one can handle your mother and you aren't going to learn now. If you find Harlan's dental records and if they match the corpse's, what then? There's only so much you can do."

"If they match, Mother will not rest until the story is told. Who murdered him and why."

"Even if it leads to the whorehouse?"

"Even so. This is a different day. That won't embarrass her. I think it probably offends me more."

Phil closed the metal box, looked at his old friend with surprise. "Why?"

"I really believe prostitution harms women."

Phil turned his chair to face Mercer more directly as they'd been sitting side by side at the big desk. "Not if a woman chooses the profession."

"If they had equal opportunity, would any woman?"

"Hell, yes." Phil slightly raised his voice. "It's fast money and you know the Sims sisters from central Virginia? They opened and ran the most elite whorehouse in Chicago, The Everleigh Club, at the turn of the last century. Those two girls made millions, millions."

That gave Mercer pause. "Millions?"

"Millions before income tax!"

"Well, maybe the Sims sisters chose running a house but what about the women who worked for them?"

"Mercer, I don't know. People make choices in life and some are made for you. If I were a young, poor woman, had beauty, I'd rather do that than flip burgers. It's one way to work your way through college, as well."

"Maybe," Mercer said, unconvinced. "How did we get on prostitution?"

"Harlan's clothes being found in a house of prostitution."

"Oh, right."

"Mercer, are you all right?"

"I am. I am." He breathed deeply. "It's Mother."

"Sorry." Phil, having grown up with the Laprades around him, knew how demanding and imperious Daniella could be on her good days. The bad days were hell.

Daniella's sister, Graziella—Gray and Sam's mother—exhibited a totally different personality. Diplomatic, polite, reserved, you never knew what the older sister was thinking. With Daniella, the world knew. Both women had been smashingly beautiful as had their mother, Andrea. Suspicion lingered that Phil's father, Roger Chetwynd, flourished in Andrea's company. Knowing winks, nods, whispers behind hands, fueled the suspicions. The boys, when boys, had no idea and both their parents shielded them from loose talk. As they grew to manhood, of course, they heard. Neither one discussed it with the other. Nor did Gray or Sam ever bring it up with their cousin.

Many were the beautiful women, nowhere near prostitution, who made the most of their beauty. Then and now. Mercer's mother and grandmother were no exception, as Phil now pointed out.

"Andrea and Daniella received a monthly stipend from my grandfather as long as he lived. Mother said when Roger would visit she'd be sent to Graziella's. I learned early to not ask questions about that." Mercer rose, rolled his chair back to the wall. "You know, I want to know and I don't. Part of me wants to know if my mother is your grandfather's daughter. Part of me doesn't. Part of me feels if those bones are Harlan's, I should give him a respectable funeral." He shrugged. "I really won't have a choice." Then he returned to Phil's desk, snatched the little LED flashlight off the top. "I need one of these. 'Broad Creek Stables' green and gold. Easy to find. Anything black is hard to find."

"Chiseler." Phil smiled at him.

Mercer pocketed the flashlight, made in China. "I'm just recognizing your marketing skills."

"Get out of here." Phil laughed at him. "See you in the morning."

CHAPTER 10

A light shone in Daniella Laprade's living room window at six-thirty that same evening. Mercer pulled into his mother's driveway, stepped out of his Lexus SUV, glad for the lamppost at the walkway to the front door, for darkness enveloped everything. A stream of cold breath gave evidence to the plunging mercury. Hurrying to the red front door, he knocked, then opened it.

"Mother."

Daniella looked up from *By the Light of Other Suns*, which she was reading with intense interest. "Where's your coat, son?"

"Left it in the car."

"Well, it won't do you any good there. Are you trying to die before I do?" She closed the heavy book, carefully marking her place with a satin ribbon.

"You'll outlive us all, Mother." He leaned over, kissed the 94-year-old on her rouged cheek, then sat opposite her in a chintz-covered comfortable chair. "Good book?"

"Remarkable. It's about the diaspora of our people after 1865. Of course, we never left."

Mercer smiled. "Better the devil you know than the devil you don't."

"Indeed. Laprades and Lorillards live by that." Her diamond earrings, bracelet to match, long wool navy skirt, and cowl-necked sweater marked Daniella as a proper woman of a former generation.

Smartly turned out even at home, Daniella was always presentable, should an unannounced caller arrive. A lady can never be too careful about her appearance, age be damned.

Tapping her finger on the volume, she ordered, "Fetch me a drink. Make one for yourself. We could both use a lift."

Mercer repaired to the well-stocked bar tucked into a corner of an equally well-stocked pantry with wooden folding doors to hide the cans. He quickly returned, a stiff bourbon in one hand and a cut crystal glass filled with ice cubes and locally made ginger ale in the other. Then he returned, poured himself a thimble of scotch with his own ginger ale chaser. The ginger ale sometimes seemed to pack more punch than the liquor. That stuff could pucker your lips. The Laprades regarded clear spirits as inferior. If you were going to drink, it had better be bourbon, whiskey, scotch, or rye.

Sinking in the chair as his mother drank half her bourbon with one smooth draw, he held up his scotch, stuck his tongue in first, then took a tiny sip. A wonderful warm sensation traveled down his throat.

Daniella raised her glass, "God bless the state of Kentucky."

He nodded, holding up his shot glass. Then he said, "Mother, how are you feeling?"

"Now? Good." She placed her glass on the coaster. "Good, all things considered. I haven't been idle today. I called Dr. Zazakos about my father's dental records. As you know our family has used the Zazakos family since the earth was cooling and they keep records. Well, they keep everything, don't they?" She referred to each generation's habit of collecting something. "I swear they never see a piece of paper they don't want to save. Naturally, the wives throughout the years are far more intelligent. They collect diamonds." She half smiled.

"Well, Mother, you didn't do so bad yourself."

"I had many admirers. In my day, men showed their appreciation in useful fashion. Don't you want to know what I found out?"

"I expect you'll tell me."

"They have Harlan's records and Peter Zazakos promised to e-mail them to the Lexington authorities. This should hasten the identification of those bones which I know, I know in my own bones, are my father's."

"Indeed, you haven't been idle," Mercer said admiringly.

"Did you and Phil find anything?"

"Let's say that the Chetwynds are not like the Zazakos family but we found some things that Old Tom, then Roger saved: old photographs."

"Well?"

"A few, the old sepia kind, showed Harlan standing horses."

"You'd think the Chetwynds would have saved more things. They have every trophy they ever won."

"Silver," Mercer replied simply.

"I used to have scrapbooks but when I left my first husband, a worthless worm if ever there was one but handsome, oh so very handsome, he burned everything before I could come back to move them. Even burned my hats. Spiteful and silly."

"Mother, that is the most I've ever heard you say about your first husband."

She half laughed. "I married in haste and repented at leisure. Back then, son, if a woman wasn't married by twenty she was an old maid."

"You were and remain beautiful. I bet you were besieged."

She loved hearing that and recalled, "Graziella and I had our gentlemen callers and I must admit, Graziella married better than

I. More sensible. But I learned." She inhaled. "How I learned. Your father, my third husband, like you, was a good, responsible man. My second husband was, too, but World War Two claimed him like so many." She held up her glass. "Might you fetch me another?"

He did as he was told, then settled again opposite her, flicking a speck of dust from his cashmere sweater.

"Son, how much did that cost?"

"The sweater?"

"I'm not looking at your shoes."

He stalled, then confessed. "Four hundred and twenty-five dollars."

"Mercer." Her voice rose.

"Mother, I deal with ultrawealthy people. I can't look unsuccessful. Failure has a scent, you know, and so does success."

"True." She nestled more deeply in her chair. "Tomorrow you will call the Lexington authorities, I have the number by the phone, and inquire about the dental records. If they have had time to compare. They need to hear from more than me and you have a voice that can get attention."

Mercer did not think he had such a voice but he knew an order when he heard one. "Yes, Mother."

She sat upright. "I want to know and I want to know what happened. I put this out of my mind and then it rushes back again like a swarm of hornets circling, or maybe a wind. I don't know." She waved her hand. "I can usually express myself but I find I become overwhelmed. Daddy died while I was so very young."

"I'll do my best."

Finishing her drink she lowered her voice. "A restless soul, painful and never good. We must lay those bones and that soul to rest."

He believed as did his mother and he, too, lowered his voice. "I wonder sometimes, I wonder about all those people killed in wars throughout time. Never properly buried if they were buried at all.

Are they out there wandering? There's so much we don't know, Mother, spiritual things, things that so many people would ignore today or think we were unintelligent for feeling this way."

"Son, the truly stupid people are the ones who think they know everything."

CHAPTER 11

Water sprayed off Mill Ruins's water wheel, thousands of rainbows flying with it. Saturday, February 8, welcomed The Jefferson Hunt Club members, hounds and horses, with pale sunshine and a temperature of 36°F by 9:30 A.M. This tempered by nine-to-ten-hour winds from the north northwest.

Her senses keen from having hunted since childhood, Sister knew the mercury would rise, but not dramatically. Desirable as that was, a tricky wind could bump up quickly. You never knew about winds cascading from the north northwest, sliding down the mountains, which at Mill Ruins lay twelve miles west. The view always delighted people the first time they beheld the old mill and the clapboard house, some of which dated back to 1730. This had been Peter Wheeler's home. Evidence of Peter's unique personality lingered among his beloved boxwoods, his curving paths laid out to "alleviate the boredom of symmetry," as he would counsel Sister. Peter had believed his tall paramour was overfond of straight lines, squares, and quadrangles. She was.

Presently, her Joint Master could be glimpsed in the stable, below tremendous oak beams holding it all together for close to three hundred years plus a few. Walter babied Clemson, his hunter, even though Sister would chide him, "You spoil that horse."

"Look who's talking" would come his swift reply.

Sister was a woman who couldn't live without close relationships to men. A few, especially when younger, were sexual but most unfolded like Peter's roses, revealing surprising depth of color. Men trusted her and loved her. She felt the same.

Fortunately, she also loved her girlfriends like Betty, Tedi Bancroft, and young women like Tootie, but for whatever reason she gravitated toward men.

As a Joint Master, Walter dealt with Sister almost every day, usually on the phone or texting. He'd traveled so much this hunt season from one medical conference to another that he'd missed a lot of the season. His specialty was cardiology and every day something new transpired in his field. He wanted to keep current so that his patients benefited from the latest procedures, as well as Walter's deep concern. Walter was called to medicine the same way that Sister was called to hounds and horses.

She always told him his life was worth more than hers: He saved people. Walter would reply that she saved them in a different way.

"Oh, this will take fifteen minutes." Atop her former steeplechaser, Matador, Sister laughed as she saw Walter run up Clemson's girth.

Walter needed to walk Clemson around for five minutes, slide the girth two holes higher, and this would go on until the girth was tight enough for him to mount. But Clemson knew the trick of blowing out his stomach so once Walter—tall, with long legs—was tight in the tack, the horse would exhale. His stable boy would crank it one more time and, of course, Clemson would shy away from the side being worked on, usually the left. He was a stinker.

He was also plated in gold in the hunt field so one endured the horsey hijinks.

Betty, driving the rig, pulled on the long side of the barn, where Shaker had preceded them with the hound trailer.

With a minimum of drama, staff mounted. Betty, Sybil, and today, Tootie, remained behind at the hound trailer with Shaker.

At least once a week Sister put Tootie out with a whipper-in. If a visitor or one of the hunt members needed a buddy in the hunt field, then Tootie was assigned to ride near them. The young woman also worked young horses for others when time permitted. They paid her for this so she earned more pocket money. At the moment, Sister had no youngsters but when she found some, Tootie would be perfect to bring them along.

As Sister rode Matador toward those already mounted, a riderless Clemson hurried up to her.

"What have you done?" She grabbed his reins, leading him back to the stable.

"Nothing" came the unconvincing reply.

Sam Lorillard with his coworker, Rory, hurried out to take Clemson.

"Did Walter fall off?" asked a concerned Sister.

"No." Sam smiled. "Dismounted for one more bathroom run. Clemson took off before I could grab his bridle."

"How come you're here today? I would have thought Crawford would be out."

"He's in Connecticut at Westover," said Sam. "He wanted to talk to someone face-to-face about curriculum. He's going to Miss Porter's, a lot of those expensive schools out of state. He's also contacting Andover, Exeter, Taft, Choate, St. Paul's."

"Got the bit between his teeth." She paused. "Good."

"Edgy took sick, called me so I came over. Walter needs some-one in the stable." Sam smiled.

"As do we all."

Edgy, the stableboy, had gotten his name for his bad haircuts, which the young man declared were "edgy" so he was ahead of the curve.

Sister rode back to the ever-growing crowd. All were in their formal turnout, as Saturday's rides were formal.

Vicki Van Mater and Joe Kasputys, in perfect turnout, waited with the others. Sister smiled and called to them as they had hauled their horses down from Middleburg, two and a half hours north.

The wind kept the pines rustling. Sister looked up to see the treetops bending. Just no telling what the day would bring. Like any day, she supposed.

Finally, everyone was up in the saddle. She used to just take the hounds and leave, but so many laggards created havoc trying to catch up that Sister now used the tactic of waiting while staring at them. Somewhat helped.

Henry Xavier, always called Xavier, Ronnie's best friend, was present today. Sister noted he had lost one hundred pounds since undergoing the operation to shrink his stomach. He looked almost as he did when he was a boy, when he and Ronnie and RayRay, her son, would ride out in high spirits. Xavier never lost his baby face, which everyone had attributed to the fat, but his face remained youthful without the fat.

Looking over these people, some of whom she had known since they were born, others for at least forty years, others just a year or two, she thought Fate had brought them together. This touch of philosophy or superstition evaporated when Parker, a young hound, looked up at her and howled.

She laughed. "Well then, folks, we have our marching orders." To Shaker, "Hounds, please."

"Come along," he called and hounds followed him over the arched bridge, past the huge turning water wheel that always star-tled horses unaccustomed to it, the *slap, slap* as well as the sight unnerving them. They headed past the mill, curved left on the wide farm road, patches of shimmering ice in the low potholes.

On other side of the road, two fenced fields beckoned. The original dry laid stone walls, rehabilitated by Walter, stretched a half mile down to the woods at the end of the pastures. At that point the fencing became three-board fencing, for who could af-ford new stone fences? Walter used what stone he could find to make jumps, but for keeping stock penned in, it was three-board—which was expensive enough. Those locust posts, if one could find them, cost a pretty penny. The left pasture ran easterly while the right was westerly and longer.

Sometimes hounds would pick up a fox behind the mill but not today.

"My feet are already cold," Mercer grumbled.

Phil counseled, "A hard run will take care of that."

"No, it won't."

"Okay, they'll still be cold but you won't notice."

As he said that, Pookah, Parker's sister, nose down, started trotting. Pansy, another hound from Sister's "P" lineage, followed right behind her. Within a few minutes the whole pack, twenty-five-couple strong this weekend, kept moving—but silently.

Hounds are always counted in couples, a practice going back thousands of years to ancient Egypt.

Sybil, on the left, picked up the pace as did Betty, on the other pasture.

Ardent, a hound with a deep voice, one of Asa's get, boomed out, *"Hot, hot, hot!"*

All at once it was as though someone put a blowtorch to the earth, for the scent lifted right off, filling those hound nostrils. Ev-eryone spoke in unison.

On the road, Sister trotted, then galloped. She wouldn't jump in at the coop in the middle of the field until she knew where the pack would head. It was just as easy to make the wrong decision as the right on a day like this but she made the right one today, for hounds took the coop instead. Flying over in tandem, one by one, they jumped the facing coop into the right field to fly straight for Betty and Tootie, who adjusted in hopes they didn't cross the line of the scent. If they did, two sets of hoofprints could only do but so much damage.

Hounds headed due west to the edge of the pasture where two jumps formed a right angle. Betty took the western one, landing on a well-cleared path. Tootie followed. Shaker was soon over, then the entire field.

Mostly hickory and oak, with branches bare, these woods provided good views. The occasional oak had the old leaves, dried out, still attached. A steady wind, about nine miles an hour, kept up a light rattling sound. In a few dry places sheltered by rock outcroppings, the leaves underfoot crunched, but by February all the exposed places had the leaves squashed down, turning into the beginnings of soil.

The fox, a gray called Grenville, led them to a steep incline down to a narrow but deep creek. Hounds clambered down, then swam the few yards across to the other side and struggled up. Old tree limbs hanging out of the creek bed gave the place a sinister air. Sister picked her way along the edge to the crossing, walked across, then moved out.

A true February run lasted one hour and twenty minutes until Grenville returned to his den not far from the old mill and not far from a red fox's den. Try as they might, the hounds had lost the scent.

As the trailers were nearby, a few people, winded, decided to retire.

Sister rode up to Shaker. "Let's go to Shootrough."

A twenty-minute hack down that same farm road took them all the way to the back of Mill Ruins, where there was once a large shooting preserve. Walter dutifully kept it planted with millet, Alamo Switchgrass, and stands of corn here and there. He himself didn't shoot but he liked feeding the birds and, of course, the foxes, too.

The minute the hounds cast into the millet, they roared through. For two more hours, hounds would find a fox, run it, lose it, find another. Many days in hunting, especially in November, are trying. Once out of the November doldrums, however, one can expect a good run or two. Usually the great runs are from mid-January to mid-March, with February holding pride of place.

Sister had no proof of this other than her own memory and the memory of other old foxhunters. Maybe they told themselves that to make up for the bitterness of February, but she swore by it, and now she hadn't enough breath to swear because she and Matador, her former steeplechaser, had just jumped a wide ditch, and took two long strides on the other side to clear a long line of boxwoods. Peter had planned these jumps and, of course, during his lifetime the boxwoods had grown. Being American boxwoods, they were looser than the English variety. She could hear the *swish, swish, swish* behind her.

A long, long expanse of pasture confronted her, and she could just see her whipper-in and the huntsman and pack. Everyone was flying and Sister thanked her lucky stars for riding a great horse. Other riders were pulling up. The pace had been too fast for too long for many riders. Sister thundered on, the panorama in front of her swerved right. A storage shed, a formidable seventy by forty, was on her right along a deeply rutted farm road. She stayed in the pasture, even as the pack was now out on the farm road, for Sister thought she knew this fox. She figured he would duck right into the shed, where Walter stored some seed as well as old pallets—always useful.

He did. Hounds dug at the side of the metal shed. They sang

out in both triumph and frustration. Even though they couldn't get to the den, they had put their fox to ground.

Shaker slid off Gunpowder, a Thoroughbred he loved, walked up to the entrance dug by the fox and blew "Gone to Ground." Hounds hearing this distinctive call, not like any other, wriggled in delight. He praised them. Betty and Sybil, now alongside the hounds, remained mounted.

Shaker swung back up in the saddle effortlessly, which Sister envied as it was no longer that easy for her. Tootie stood on the other side of the shed, just in case the fox popped out.

Walter had just ridden up to the scene. Clemson lacked the speed of Sister's Thoroughbreds, but what the horse lacked in speed he made up in good sense.

"Hell of a run," Walter breathed heavily.

"The best. Just the best." Sister looked down at those glorious hounds, full of themselves.

"We can do more," Trooper promised.

His brother, Tattoo, agreed. *"We can run all day. Really."*

Sister asked Betty, on one side of the pack, "Where's Tootie?"

"Behind the shed, just in case."

"Let's call her to us. Shaker, I think we'd best head for the trailers. What do you think, Walter?"

"I think if we continue I'll wind up with some new patients."

They laughed and headed for the mill, walking along slowly. Took a half hour, and the wind came up, as did an unexpected rain; light though it was, it was steady and cold. Snow can be warmer than a rain in the high 30°Fs or low 40°Fs. By the time everyone reached their trailers, they were happy to dismount. After wiping them down and then throwing on a sweat sheet, most put their horses on the trailer. The heavier blanket would be thrown over soon enough when the sweat sheet was taken off.

Phil said to Mercer as they walked to Walter's house, "Think there's any food left?"

"If not, we'll make those that came in early go to Kentucky Fried Chicken."

"That will take an hour." Phil knew how far the franchise was— too far when one is hungry.

Fortunately, the table was filled with hot meats, salads, corn bread, macaroni and cheese, jams, and far too many desserts. It did not disappoint.

Too tired to stand, people found places to sit, some even repairing to the old country kitchen. The bar got a good workout, too.

Mercer, Ronnie, Xavier, Phil, and Freddie Thomas, a very attractive female CPA, sat at the kitchen table.

Phil leaned toward the voluptuous Freddie. "May I get you another drink?"

"Phil, if I have another drink you'll need to carry me out of here."

"That's the general idea."

Xavier raised his eyebrows.

"I am shocked. Truly and deeply shocked." Freddie never was averse to male attention but then what woman is?

"Did you view?" Mercer asked everyone in general.

Seeing the fox, always a thrill, was believed to bring good luck.

"No, I was too far back. Halfway through the hunt, I knew Diva and I"—Freddie named her mare—"needed to rate ourselves."

"Yeah, me, too." Ronnie nodded. "We started out with a great run, and then it just never stopped except for the hack to Shootrough. What a day!"

They replayed the hunt. Kasmir stuck his head into the kitchen and smiled. Someone called his name and he closed the door.

"You know, I don't think anyone viewed because I never heard a 'Tallyho,'" Mercer said.

"You're right," Phil agreed. "I didn't either."

As the food settled a bit, warmth crept into their toes, and the liquor added to the high spirits. They chattered away, people coming in and out of the kitchen, some sitting for a spell. The breakfast would be remembered as fondly as the hunt itself.

Freddie had a question for Mercer. "I know you're a bloodstock agent, but I don't really know what you do. I mean, do you sit and study bloodlines on the computer?"

"I do, but I'm fortunate in being able to see so many horses now and over the years. I go to Kentucky about once every two months and I've added Pennsylvania and New York to the list. About once every two years I'll head down to Louisiana, too. You'd be surprised at how many good horses are down there. Florida, of course. Florida horses around Ocala have the advantage of limestone soils but no one has the advantage like Kentucky."

"Really?" she asked, interested.

"Don't get me wrong. Virginia can still breed great Thoroughbreds, along with some of our neighbors. You're sitting next to one of the best."

Phil slightly tilted his head to one side in acknowledgment. "Freddie, we now have so many supplements that we can give growing foals an advantage similar to Kentucky, but there they just turn them out. We have to spend extra money on supplements. You only get one chance to ensure a horse has strong, strong bones."

"I never thought about that," she said. "I just hop up on Diva and well, like I said, I never thought about it." Freddie smiled, then added, "What did people do before supplements?"

Phil leaned in closer. "Broad Creek Stables was started by my great-grandfather back in the 1870s in a state wrecked by the war, no young men, no money, amputees in the streets. It must have been awful, win or lose, too many damaged people. Well, I'm off the track, literally." He laughed. "But I think about Old Tom and then his son, Roger; they had to have had it really tough. But what they did and what Broad Creek did was to haul mares to Kentucky by train to foal. This way they got the same head start that a Kentucky horse did. We often used our own stallions and we built our reputations on them. Navigator being the first really great one. We'd bring the boarders back as yearlings or two-year-olds and so we got great bone in them."

"And my family was part of that, my great-grandfather and grandfather," Mercer interjected. "They loaded horses on the boxcars with stalls, traveled with them. Grandpa studied what was in Kentucky. He made suggestions to the Chetwynds that put Broad Creek Stables on the map, so to speak. My grandfather got Old Tom to purchase Navigator. I think Roger was studying at the University of Virginia then. Grandpa bought a few horses for himself. You know, a good horseman can usually survive. He might not always make money but that's the thing about bloodline research, I don't need to buy horses. My job, let's say you want to get into the game and you tell me you have twenty thousand to spend on a yearling. That's nothing, but I can set you up. Anyway, for a percentage, small, I will find you the best twenty-thousand-dollar yearling possible and since I have so many contacts, a lot of times I can get you a really good horse right out of the pastures. Avoid the auction. All I need is gas money, my computer, and my notebook. My overhead is low. Phil's skyrockets but his profits are greater when it all works. I can put you in a syndicate, too, but that's another story."

Freddie listened intently to Mercer. "You love what you do, don't you?"

"I do. My fear is that Kentucky will just blow itself up with this gambling mess." He then explained to her how one could only wager on horses at the tracks, nothing else.

"But why would that hurt you?" She reached for a napkin.

"Freddie, people will go out of business. Horses will be dispersed to states where the legislature invites horsemen and gamblers alike. That means a lot more travel for me and having to make more contacts. Not to brag, but I know just about everyone in Kentucky. You have a mare who was bred to a son of A.P. Indy, take your pick, she delivers a foal and I call and ask about the foal or I send an e-mail. I know who I'm talking to and they know me. Besides, I can read between the lines. And remember, Kentucky is the heart of the Thoroughbred business. Destroy that business and you really take something from America. It's part of our history."

"True enough." Phil agreed.

Feeling a bit sleepy, Xavier murmured, "Mercer can put you in a syndicate, too, like he said. You know, where a group of people own a horse together? This defrays expenses but allows people from all kinds of jobs to play. Some people love racing like we love foxhunting, but it's costly. Syndicates open the door for more people."

On and on they chattered until finally Freddie looked at the wall clock. "It's four o'clock!"

They all turned around to look at the big round wall clock. "Time flies when you're having fun." Ronnie smiled, rose from the table, clearing everyone's plates.

Once home, Sister, Gray, and Tootie took showers, then collapsed in the living room, fire crackling in the large fireplace.

Gray sipped his scotch while Sister and Tootie stuck to hot tea. They also replayed the day.

As though out of the blue, Sister said to Gray, "Honey, does your family keep scrapbooks?"

"No. Why?"

"Just wondered."

He swirled the scotch around in the heavy glass. "We weren't really a close family. My sister spent more time with Daniella, her aunt, my mother's sister. Dad worked all the time. Mom basically turned us out of the house to do whatever while she did whatever she did. A lot of housework, I think. We were glad to get out of that. One of us would come back bloodied. Sam and I fought like roosters. I don't know how we lived."

"Worked out." Sister smiled.

"Daniella might have family pictures but I don't think any of them were too close, except for her and my sister. Also Daniella had too many marriages. High drama. My sister's just like Aunt D." Gray still could be irritated by his sister. "I will admit my mother, Graziella, could get just as uppity about our dash of Italian blood but Aunt D can outsnob everybody. She met Eleanor Roosevelt once and ever after referred to her as 'My dear friend, Mrs. Roosevelt.' You get the picture." He rolled his eyes.

"I guess Mercer's a bit of a snob," Tootie blurted out. "He's fun, though."

"Yes, Aunt Daniella still casts her spell." Gray laughed.

Sister looked at Tootie. "Gray, let Tootie show you something."

Ten minutes later, in the den, Tootie showed him the Broad Creek Stable photo of Roger Chetwynd and the man who might have been Mercer's grandfather.

"What do you think?" Sister asked him.

"Could be. It's hard to tell from an old photo and sometimes we see what we want to see."

"Gray, why would Tootie and I want to see a family resemblance to Mercer?"

"You're right." He bent over to study the photo more closely. "Snappy fellow. No names on the photo. Well, yes, it could be Grandpa Harlan Laprade but"—he shrugged—"doesn't mean the bones with Benny Glitters or the watch belonged to him."

Curious about Gray's feelings, Tootie asked, "What if those bones do belong to your grandfather? You and Mercer have the same maternal grandfather."

"Like I said, we weren't close. I never knew him. He was long gone before I came into the world. And I hate to admit it but I am a little superstitious. I think you let the dead alone. I don't believe they should be disturbed. Whatever Harlan Laprade did, however he wound up underground with a horse and a dog, I figure he went into the afterlife with at least one friend, his dog. Just don't disturb the dead."

"Well, it's too late now," Sister replied sensibly.

CHAPTER 12

Kneeling in the birthing stall, Dr. Penny Hinson examined the newborn foal, male, who had struggled to his feet. At that moment, he looked as though he was on ice, with each leg in danger of sliding in the opposite direction. Didn't take the little guy too long before he pulled himself together.

Tootie Harris traveled with Penny on Mondays as the vet realized Tootie truly loved horses as did she. Hard to be a good equine vet without a bond of strong emotion for the animal. Sister gave her Mondays and Wednesdays off, sometimes Sunday and Monday, depending on what needed to be done in the stables or kennels.

Tootie hoped to become an equine vet and Penny, a good one, happily took the young woman along as a sidekick. Both stood in the stall while Phil Chetwynd stood outside.

"He's fine." Covered in blood, water, and manure, Penny stripped off her long, thin rubber gloves. Tootie wore them as well, along with heavy overalls, for the day was frosty. Penny tried to keep from introducing anything potentially infectious to a newborn. As it was, the little fellow would be breathing in air for the first time, along with some of the dust. Broad Creek Stables had immaculate birthing stalls, a ten-stall barn dedicated to this. Clean as it was, tiny particles of dust floated through the air.

With the newborn still wet from his journey, Penny looked him over carefully. "Phil, I think when he dries he'll be a blood bay, a true blood bay. Been a long time since I've seen one."

"You don't see them often," Phil agreed. "When sunlight hits that coat it's something, isn't it?"

Picking up gear, tossing gloves into a bucket, both women left the stall.

"How many mares are in foal this year?" asked Penny. "You had four foals last month and now this fellow. You're on your way to a full house."

"We're back up again, Penny," Phil said proudly. "When we last spoke I'd bred seven of my mares, three to my own stallions and four out of state. Sales prices are better, as you know, but the real issue is consumer confidence. If people think the economy is improving, they make it improve, know what I mean? Anyway, clients sent me five mares. Ignatius and I rejuvenated the old barn back on the northeastern quadrant. So far, it's been a good year, no problem births, no crooked legs either." He smiled, then glanced back in the stall. "That fellow is by Curlin. We paid good money for that stud fee. My fingers are crossed. 'Course the mare is topnotch, just topnotch. She raced sound for five years. Sound."

Penny remembered horses better than people. "I remember seeing her at Colonial Downs and then you took her up to Maryland for some races."

"Just a wonderful horse." Phil beamed.

They walked outside the foaling barn, a steeply pitched roof with a cupola, and a large copper weathervane of a mother and foal.

Broad Creek, like Walnut Hall and so many of the old glory establishments—whether they were in Kentucky, Maryland, New

York, Virginia, or South Carolina—had grown over the years. The various barns at Broad Creek with their building dates over the main doors, announced the years when the money was good. Anyone in the horse business or any business knows change is the one constant. Up, down, flat years, everything will happen to you sooner or later, but the difference with the equine world was the drama. Maybe this was because animals were concerned, creating a lot of emotion, or because the people who get into the business are gamblers by nature. Someone who wants a placid life doesn't breed Thoroughbreds. The lows can bring a man or woman to their knees. The highs make one feel as though they are soaring in Apollo's chariot.

From the 1870s to today, the Chetwynds had experienced it all.

Tootie noticed that the gorgeous Victorian main barn had the date in gold: 1877. The numbers had the flourish of those years. She looked around, seeing that two of the smaller barns also had that date. She made a note to check dates when she and Penny drove out, passing other structures.

Phil ushered the two women into his office. "Can I get you all anything to drink? A sandwich?"

"No thanks," Penny responded.

"No, thank you, Mr. Chetwynd." Tootie sat where he beckoned her to do so.

Phil took papers off his desk, along with some high-gloss announcements concerning stallions. He sat in a wing chair opposite the ladies, who perched on an old leather sofa. Decorated in 1877, the office maintained the ambience of that time. The two wing chairs and sofa had been re-covered once in excellent cowhide back in the 1930s. The walls, jammed with photographs of horses— horses even before Navigator—bore proof to the success of Broad Creek Stables. One wall held silver trophies and even silver Christmas balls, inscribed with horse names. The silver glistened; someone polished it regularly.

Tootie thought the task must take an entire day, which it did.

Phil rummaged through papers from The Jockey Club, handed a few to Penny. "Mercer and I go over this all the time. If you look at the pedigrees of our standing stallions—and I've run them back to the 1870s—you'll see, especially in those early years, many of the same horse names, which makes sense. There were not as many standing stallions in the country. At least I don't think there were. Hell, there weren't as many people."

Penny read the sire line on each certificate, the dam line going back three generations. She recognized names like Teddy, an early one, Rock Sand from 1900, Spearmint from Great Britain, 1903. Moving forward, she read the great Count Fleet's name, coming much closer to now. Lots of Forty Niner blood in 1987, Danzig, 1977, Lyphard, 1969 and, of course, Northern Dancer, 1961 and Mr. Prospector, 1970. She handed the papers to Tootie, who—while not as well versed in bloodlines—did recognize the names Northern Dancer and Mr. Prospector.

"Great ones," the vet said. "The mares are great, too. I always loved Toll Booth, just loved her name."

Toll Booth was a mare who was Broodmare of the Year in Canada in 1989. The Canadians breed some great horses, but then most all of the former British colonies do, whether you look at South Africa, Australia, you name it.

He laughed. "Penny, me too. I'm supposed to be a hard-nosed horseman, but I can be won over by a great name or a lovely soft eye. But, hey, I know you have calls to make. I'm curious. What I know about DNA is what the public knows: the double helix and all that. But is it really possible to determine ancestry from DNA? Equine ancestry?"

"That depends on what you really want to know." Penny folded her hands together. "If you're talking purely about genetics, yes. Mitochondrial DNA called mtDNA is inherited only through the female line and it doesn't change from mother to daughter unless there's a rare mutation. So it's reliable. You can trace the Y chromosome too but not nearly as far back as mtDNA; mtDNA is pretty amazing."

"What's the disclaimer?"

"Records are notoriously unreliable. *The General Stud Book* was published first in 1791, in England. We imported our blooded horses from England so it matters to us, as well. Anyway, sometimes people would change the name of a horse when it changed owners. Hence the unreliability."

"It is a mess." Phil nodded. "But even with that, if I know the mother of a horse, say Rock Sand, whose mother was Roquebrune, an English mare born 1893, then we would know, right?"

"Right," Penny said. "You're probably aware of the study at the MacDonald Institute for Archaeological Research at the University of Cambridge, which gets us closer to the true origins of the Thoroughbred."

"That's why I sat you down here and am taking up your time," Phil explained. "The conclusion of the study was that Thoroughbred foundation mares were not all Arabs, or what were called Turks in the eighteenth century. Turns out they were cosmopolitan in origin, with British and Irish native horses playing a big part in those foundation mares' bloodlines. As more work is done, and it certainly will be, could this throw our bloodlines into question?" He slouched back in his chair.

Penny smiled. "Not a chance, Phil. Don't worry. This is about foundation mares. Once we move into the middle of the eighteenth century, going forward into the late eighteenth century, blood representation is pretty solid. We have track records, literally, for those horses, as well as the records of their get."

Phil smiled in relief. "Well, I am a little too sensitive maybe, but Penny, people are so crazy now. I had a bad dream of someone suing Broad Creek Stables over a bloodline misrepresentation."

"Hopefully, you've had better clients than that over the years," Penny's mellow voice soothed.

"For the most part, but every now and then. I remember Dad found out a fellow he did business with was a crook. That's not exactly the same. But people are so quick to find wrongdoing or imagine it, and as more and more new people come to us—and of course, I hope they will—I feel Broad Creek has to protect itself more. Our country is run and ruined by lawyers, I swear it."

Penny burst out laughing. "I'll tell that to my husband."

Phil blushed slightly. "I didn't mean Julian, of course."

"Phil, put your mind at rest." Penny stood up. "You get more beautiful babies on the ground like the one I just delivered and you won't have a worry in the world."

Back in the big vet truck with Tootie, Penny headed toward Greg Schmidt's house out in Keswick. A highly respected equine veterinarian, sought after on many levels, he'd sold his business, thinking he would retire. Well, in a sense he had, but practitioners like Penny often asked for his advice.

"Dr. Hinson, that foal's eyes wandered," said Tootie.

"No, he doesn't have strabismus, which is a deviation of the eyeball's positioning. People can have it, too. But often a newborn's eyes aren't settled yet, so there's asymmetrical movement. This usually corrects itself in a few hours or at the most a few days." She slowed as a car pulled out in front of her without looking. "Idiot! Sorry."

"Does make you wonder." Tootie smiled.

"Nobody pays attention anymore. How's that for a sweeping statement? Oh, yes, while I'm thinking about it, foals are like human babies. The eye detects the information but the brain doesn't know what it is. A foal has to learn to understand what it's seeing, just as a baby does. It's a big world out there." Penny laughed.

"The thing that amazes me is how a horse remembers everything," said the younger woman, gazing at the beautiful pastures going by. "Once they see something, say an overturned bucket in front of the barn, they're going to look for that overturned bucket."

"Memory is fascinating. I was reading somewhere that memory evolves, at least for humans. It isn't set in stone. I'm willing to bet equine memory is more complicated than we now know."

Tootie perceptively remarked, "People remember what they want to remember."

"And forget what they want to forget." She turned left onto Dr. Schmidt's road. "And then something happens or they hear a song and boom, so much for forgetting."

CHAPTER 13

"Lime green. Good silk." Mercer in Brooks Brothers placed the tie back on the store's display, an eye-catching tie-wheel on a round imitation Hepplewhite table. "I like a little color." He looked at Gray. "You, on the other hand, have no imagination. You don't need one more regimental tie."

Gray held in his hands a lovely tie of olive with regimental stripes of thin gold next to wide maroon. "Mercer, I work in Washington in a conservative business. No one wants an accountant in a paisley tie, especially if that client is a senator."

"How'd you stand it when you worked full-time? I couldn't abide the boredom!"

"Same way you stand talking to people about breeding, people who don't know a thing. That's got to be boring, repetitious. It's part of the business, educating the client."

"Yeah." Mercer pounced on a gorgeous raspberry tie with small embroidered rampant lions in pale blue. "This would do well."

Gray reached over, taking it from his cousin's hands. "Would."

As Gray held the tie, Mercer stared at it. "Are you going to buy it?"

"Not if you are."

"No, I need something bold. Anyway, we couldn't both buy the same tie."

"Like two women buying the same dress." Gray laughed.

Mercer rolled his eyes. "Never." He checked his thin watch. "Where's Sam?"

"He'll be along. Crawford always seems to come down to the stables just as Sam's ready to leave."

"Tough nut, that Crawford."

"I steer clear. Actually my worst fear is that someday Janie will snap and kill him."

"We'd all cover for her," Mercer replied. "This salmon color, great for spring."

"Mercer, it's the middle of February."

"Spring is just around the corner."

Both men dressed well if a little differently. Their mothers, the sisters, drummed into them that you had only one chance to make a good first impression. And both women were clotheshorses themselves, loving the opportunity to dress husbands and sons. For them, it was having two fashion lives, male and female.

Gray walked over to a wall with square shelves, all of equal size, like a big bookcase. Shirts filled the squares, each one having a brass plate at the bottom, indicating neck circumference and sleeve length. Gray found the square with spread collars.

Mercer joined him. "Go ahead, buy a pink shirt."

Gray turned to him. "Mercer, I'm not afraid to wear pink or peach or sea green. But only for casual wear. There is no way I can wear a shirt like that with a suit in D.C. Now stop sounding like my mother or your mother."

"I could never sound like your mother," said Mercer, imitating Graziella's intonation, making Gray laugh.

Sam walked through the store's entrance, looked around, spotted them and walked over.

"Get hit up by Crawford as you were leaving?" Mercer asked.

"No. Tootie and Dr. Hinson swung by. Marty's horse has an abscess. I told Crawford I soaked Tonie." He named the horse. "As I've been doing for the last three days. It will pop soon enough. But Crawford has to have an expert's opinion, so he called Penny Hinson. He just came back from dragging himself all over the northeast to check curriculums. I'll give him one thing, he is indefatigable and, of course, it helps to have your own jet."

Gray and Mercer smiled.

Mercer appraised Sam. "You need a new jacket."

"No, I don't. I don't go out at night."

"Because you don't have any clothes." Mercer was half right.

The other half of the reason was that although Sam had stayed sober for years, nighttime carried the whiff of temptation.

"What I really need is a new pair of boots. Crawford says he'll buy them if I go up to Horse Country for the February Dehner sale."

Dehner, a boot company in Omaha, Nebraska, sent a representative to measure one's foot, calf, instep. The customer then picked the type of leather, the color, the cut, and type of sole. A new pair could run $1,000 plus with the extras and, of course, everyone wanted the Spanish cut, which was a bit more leather on the outside knee, making one's leg appear longer. Very elegant. Bespoke boots lasted for decades if one cared for them, which somewhat justified the price. When you're in boots for most of the day, comfort becomes important.

"Go on up, then," Mercer counseled.

"Guess I'd better."

Gray and Mercer bought their ties and Mercer bought two shirts he liked.

In the parking lot, Mercer slid behind the wheel of his Lexus

SUV and said to the brothers standing nearby, "Follow me. Lunch is on me."

The two brothers drove behind their cousin a very short way to a nice restaurant near Brooks Brothers.

Once seated at a booth, the two brothers waited for Mercer to speak as he had asked them to lunch, a rare occurrence.

"You all are quiet," the dapper fellow remarked.

"We're waiting for you," Gray replied.

Mercer launched in: "The funny thing about the body in Benny Glitters's grave is the little dog elicited more sympathy than the human. The story got a lot of play in the media in Kentucky but it received a mention on national media, too."

Sam was surprised. "It did?"

"You never watch the news," Mercer chided him.

"Well, I missed it, too," Gray confessed.

"It was there for one day, a brief splash. Anyway, I called the detective in charge. Granted this isn't a red-hot case, but because of all the attention they make a stab at it. I asked if I find any of my grandfather's dental records, will they compare them to the skeleton's teeth? He said yes."

"Mercer, do you have Harlan Laprade's records?" Gray asked.

"I wasn't half-assed about this." Mercer paused dramatically. "Mother called Peter Zazakos, whose father, grandfather, and great-grandfather were dentists. *Mirabile dictu,* they kept all the records." Mercer was almost jubilant.

For a moment, Gray and Sam said nothing, then Sam said, "I guess we should give him a decent burial in the Lorillard graveyard. That's where we're always planted. I know that's Grandpa Laprade. They should know shortly in Kentucky. There can't be that many murders in Lexington in February."

"One hopes not," Gray replied.

"Where's Auntie D in all this?" Sam asked, about Mercer's mother Daniella.

"Lashing me on. She's quite caught up in the drama." This was an unexpected comment from her son on Daniella Laprade, who at ninety-four retained most of her good qualities and all of her bad ones.

"She's used to getting her way." Gray's eyebrows flickered for a second.

"We can solve this murder." Mercer sounded so confident. "Mother says she knows in her bones. Those bones are her father and he was killed."

"Mercer, you've fallen off your perch." Sam used the old country expression. "Her, too!"

"No, I haven't. I can't say about Mother." He smiled. "Sam, you've got good research skills. Think of all those term papers you wrote at Harvard."

Sam got to the point. "Mercer, just what do you want?"

"I want you to research whorehouses in Lexington, especially the high-class ones. Lot of men with money to spend in Lexington. Times were good." He paused. "We know that the fancy houses of prostitution for the white boys often had a few drop-dead gorgeous ladies of color, Chinese girls, other women considered exotics. International trade." Mercer could always see the business angle of any transaction. "Might even be exciting. You know, his clothes were left folded in the laundry room."

"Maybe the killer was in a hurry," Sam suggested.

"Then why take off his clothes?" Mercer pointed a fork at Sam.

"That is a puzzle." Gray took a swig of his hot coffee.

"Well, I guess I could do it." Sam was a little intrigued.

"Gray, you investigate gambling parties," his cousin ordered. "Poker. Dice. Horses. I've got a hunch a wide net of gambling was part of this."

"Mercer, I think the dead should be left alone," Gray interjected quietly.

Quick to seize on something he could use, Mercer agreed

warmly. "Right, but Harlan Laprade is disturbed, so we might as well find out what happened. It would mean so much to Mother and to your mother, too, were she here."

Hard to argue against this. Graziella died five years earlier of an aneurism. She rested in the Lorillard graveyard.

Gray sighed deeply. "I'll see what I can do."

"Given our business, Gray, I expect you know every trick in the book, how to make money illegally, how to hide gambling wins and losses. That sort of thing. And people keep records, even if it's chits. They have to remember who owes what to whom."

"I'll try."

"Oh, the dog. It was a Norwich terrier. A vet looked at the skeleton. Didn't need DNA."

To change the subject, Gray asked, "You hunting tomorrow?"

"I am. After All is one of my favorite fixtures. It's perfect, really." He mentioned the Bancroft farm, everything arranged for foxhunting. Trails, jumps, creek crossings, all were maintained by the Bancrofts. People always liked driving through the covered bridge to arrive at the stables and thence up to the house.

"I'll be with Crawford," said Sam. "He's hunting down in Buckingham County tomorrow, a huge fixture, about fifteen thousand acres of pine."

"But Buckingham is Oak Ridge's territory," said Gray, referring to the hunt club that had the right to hunt there.

"Crawford is happy to spread his brand of contempt for others all around. Rules be damned. Sooner or later, the chickens will come home to roost." Mercer hoped Crawford would get his comeuppance.

Sam was envious. "You all should have a good hunt." Tuesday's hunt in what was known as The Jefferson Hunt's home territory would prove just that. For those who believe in prophecy, it would prove haunting.

CHAPTER 1 4

Comet, hunting on the Bancroft property, heard the trailers rumbling down the long gravel drive, then they rattled through the covered bridge at After All Farm. The covered bridge amplified the sound.

Comet, like all The Jefferson Hunt foxes, knew when a hunt was to occur. Not that he kept a fixture card in his den. He didn't need one. Every time Sister's trailers left the stables and the kennels, it was hunt day away from the farm. When humans wore their kit, hounds yipped with excitement in the kennels, and Sister's trailers stayed put. The hunt would be at the farm.

The only days that confused this healthy gray fox were when the trailers left the farm to go all the way around to Foxglove Farm on the other side of Soldier Road. If they had ridden up over Hangman's Ridge, then down into the often swampy meadow below, they'd cross Soldier Road and wind up at lovely Foxglove Farm, owned by Cindy Chandler. Sometimes they'd strike a line and then the red Foxglove fox would cross Soldier Road, the meadow, Hangman's Ridge, and shoot to Sister's house. So he was on Comet's territory. For whatever reason that fellow loved her house and had various ways to wiggle under it. Once the Foxglove fox leapt into an open window of the gardening shed. What a mess. The red fox was just thrilled with the damage he'd caused. Comet was less thrilled. What if it made Sister mad at all the foxes? He liked his treats she left out.

On this Tuesday, February 11, Comet felt confident he would be far ahead of hounds should Shaker cast down Broad Creek. He was three-quarters of a mile from the bridge. He listened intently. Human babble fascinated him. They uttered so many sounds; some high, some low, and their laughter especially fascinated him. Big bellow laughs, little titters; some people laughed like woodpeckers, *rat ta tat tat.* While Comet was too far away now to detect the titters, the low guffaws, he could hear big laughs and he could always hear a high-pitched sound. Thank God for the horn. He always knew where Shaker was.

Comet, full, for hunting had been successful, sat until no more trailers passed through the covered bridge. The youngsters in the pack, once scent was found, usually ran right up front. While this was not a blindingly fast pack, it was fast enough so that Comet, who owed much of his health to Sister's feeding and worming program, plus the fact that as a youngster he'd been trapped and given his seven-in-one shots, headed for Pattypan Forge. He, too, was fast, also having the advantage of more nimbleness. If they did pick up his line once the pack reached Pattypan Forge, they would become confused for a time.

Aunt Netty kept an immaculate den in the old forge. Occasionally, Uncle Yancy would visit. The old stone building—the stones square-cut, quite large—held scent inside on a moist day. Today, at nine-thirty, the mercury had just nudged up to 34°F and clouds hung low, ranging in color from dove gray to charcoal. The rawness in the air promised snow flurries. Scenting would be pretty good, so why not throw them off early?

Pattypan, abandoned for close to a century, had the additional advantage of being overgrown. The place was full of rabbits, always a plus in a fox's mind, and other foxes did come around thinking the same as Comet: game. Crows would hang around and a medium-sized barn owl lived up in the rafters, keeping to himself. He loathed commotion and if Aunt Netty and Uncle Yancy screamed at each other, this foxy fellow would tell Bitsy, the screech owl who nested in a tree hollow at Sister's farm. This was like telling the town crier as Bitsy, believing in a free press, more or less kept every animal current with the latest gossip.

Shaker blew two short toots that meant "Pay attention." This was really for the humans. Comet knew it was time to move on. He trotted along Broad Creek while a downy woodpecker clinging to a tree trunk swiveled his head to see the gray ghost below.

"Morning," the bird called.

"Morning," Comet called out. *"Good eats?"*

"Tree's a supermarket." The downy pecked to prove his point, extracting a cocoon that Comet could see in his beak.

As Comet moved on, Shaker moved out with twelve couple of hounds, a decent number, although Sister especially loved those days when she'd ride out with thirty couple. The sound remained in one's memory forever. But twelve couple allowed youngsters—and he had half his pack as young entry and second-year entry—to step up to the plate. One must develop future leadership among hounds the same as among humans. Both the Senior Master and the huntsman believed this and planned for it.

Betty, per usual, rode on the right, Sybil on the left, while Too-tie rode in the field with Felicity, who took Tuesdays off. The two had been classmates at Custis Hall, the prep school. Felicity needed a break from her curious, active child. The two school friends had ridden together all four years at Custis Hall. Felicity became preg-nant, graduated, then married, a surprise to all. Gray, Ronnie,

Xavier, Phil, Mercer, Kasmir, his old school chum, High Vijay, the Bancrofts, Walter, Ben Sidell, Ed Bancroft, the Sheriff, and Freddie rode out, along with a guest this Tuesday. The guest, a drop-dead gorgeous lady in her early thirties, perfectly turned out in rat-catcher, was visiting from North Carolina. The clothes for informal days were usually a tweed jacket, a tie, or colored stock tie. One had more room for personal expression wearing ratcatcher. Many men in the field fervently hoped this would be the first of many visits from Alida Dalzell. Plus she rode a stunning, 16H flea-bitten gray Thoroughbred/Quarter Horse cross. They were a vision.

Shaker headed down Broad Creek. The draw intensified the moisture. Even during one of those awful Virginia dry spells, awful when they occur during hunt season and not especially wonderful during hay season either, the scenting along creeks or around ponds and lakes might hold, if ever so briefly. Today a carpet of enticing odors curled into hound nostrils: rabbits, two bobcats, a gopher, a few minks, turkeys, turkeys, turkeys, and the lovely powdery scent of a woodcock.

"Oh, this is sweet." Giorgio closed his eyes.

"Bobcat. We'll get a fox soon enough," Cora counseled.

Dragon, who would jostle to take the lead, only to be put in his place by bared fangs and a snarl from Cora, smarted off. *"Giorgio, you wouldn't know a bobcat if he bit you in the ass."*

"No, but you'd know if I tore into yours." Cora shot him a dirty look, which the other hounds called *"the freeze."*

Dreamboat, emboldened with each hunt now, nose to the ground, concentration intense, moved faster. Then he trotted. Finally, sure, he lifted his head, let out a deep call, *"Gray fox."*

As though someone tossed a match into a tinderbox, *whoosh,* everyone spoke at once, everyone on.

Shaker blew "Gone Away." He and Hojo negotiated thick tree roots that had risen out of the ground with the freezing and thawing.

Some of those roots were best to jump, which the horses determined to do, to the surprise of some of their riders.

Many people in the hunt field like to set up for a jump, always a good idea, but terrain in central Virginia throws curveballs. Sit deep and take what comes. If you're tight in the tack, you'll be fine. Easier said than done, of course, and already two people popped off their mounts like toast.

Bobby Franklin, very glad he had Ben Sidell back there who took care of stragglers, kept the last horse in First Flight clearly in sight.

A light snow now fell like a lace curtain, adding to the extraordinary beauty of the wide creek, ice edging the sides, the conifers dusted with white.

Well ahead, Comet had taken the wide right path through the woods to Pattypan Forge. Hounds followed and just as the wise fox planned, hounds threw up at the forge. There were too many smells, including fox.

Threw up is the proper term for losing scent and literally throwing their heads up.

Aunt Netty, in her den inside, suffered no worries.

The pack blasted into the forge.

"Over here. Over here." Tattoo dug so fast at Netty's den that two rooster tails of dirt flew behind his front paws.

Diana stopped for a moment. *"Tattoo, she's an old nag. Let's find someone who's running."*

From the anteroom of her den, Aunt Netty cursed, sounding like a wail from a sepulchre. *"How dare you, you domesticated toad poop!"*

This so shocked Tattoo that his jaw dropped open. He stopped digging.

"Come on, Tattoo," Twist, his littermate, advised.

Shaker and the field held up outside as hounds worked inside. The riders sported a mantle of light snow.

"I've got the line," Pansy cried.

"I've got a hot one, red, red hot," Dreamboat bellowed.

Cora checked first Pansy's line, then Dreamboat's. Hounds knew, thanks to all their schoolwork, that one should stay on the hunted fox but a red-hot line is a red-hot line. Cora thought to hell with it. They'd chase the hotter line.

"Come on!" The fabulous hound rallied the others, for the pack was just about to split.

Already flying out of the back of Pattypan Forge, Dreamboat was now followed by the entire pack. The underbrush made the going rough and the humans had to run upwind, southerly, that day, on a narrow deer trail until it intersected with a somewhat wider riding trail, not very wide but wide enough to gallop without smashing your kneecaps.

Sister, on her beloved Rickyroo, eleven years old, almost twelve, knew that sure-footed though he was, the snow could be slippery and it was falling faster. Hunting in a falling snow, one of life's great pleasures, made her glad to be alive.

Most hunts wouldn't go out in a deep snow because it's not sporting. The fox can't run well should he be out. While hounds have to surf a deep snow, they plow faster than the fox. Hard on the horses, too. On the other hand, if a crisp coating lays on even a deep snow, a fox can fly along, whereas hounds slip and slide, break through, cutting their pads. But this snow, flakes large, twirling medium to fast, ground now covered with a thin sheet, this was perfection.

Ducking a few low limbs, Sister lost sight of Shaker but thanks to a blast on the horn every now and then, she knew where he was headed. In a quarter of a mile, the bridle path intersected two roads making a turkey's foot. Right, left, or center, those were your choices.

Which one would the fox make? Uncle Yancy, ever so clever, didn't bother with the path. He slid under thick brambles, and catapulted onto the ruins of an old stone wall to run atop that for a bit. Hounds struggled in the nasty undergrowth but once they reached the stone wall they hopped up, as had Uncle Yancy. All twelve couple tried to get atop the stones, but some had to settle for walking beside it.

Walking frustrated them because they knew the older codger was gaining ground.

Betty, on the right, could no more get into that thick cover than anyone else. Tempted though she was to dismount, she knew better. Unless someone is in trouble, stay up, always stay up. Sybil, on the left side, had a little bit easier time as she was on a deer trail with fallen trees. Fortunately the crowns of the blown-over trees had smashed into other trees so she jumped tree trunks, easy to do on Kingston, bold and smooth.

Sister emerged onto the turkey-foot intersection. Shaker to her left headed fast toward the Lorillard place. Hounds, all on, hit the "hallelujah chorus."

Edward and Tedi rode in Sister's pocket with Kasmir not far behind. They allowed a decent distance but were right up there. Sister had offered the guest, Alida Dalzell, the honor of riding up with her but the beautiful woman demurred, saying she didn't want to slow down the Master.

As it was, Alida wouldn't have slowed down anyone but she didn't want to seem to take advantage and the only person she knew in the field was Freddie Thomas. As she had invited her, Alida rode with Freddie. As some riders were slowed a bit by the snow, the two women began to creep forward. This was not a violation of protocol. For those men whom they passed, this was a delicious experience; Alida, up in the irons, rode at such pace, her rear end well out of the saddle.

Little by little, Sister and First Flight were closing the gap between themselves and the hounds, whom they couldn't see but could sure hear. Ahead of them, Shaker could now see his tail hounds. Betty, finally able to move along, had crossed the turkey foot, taking the straight road where she knew a narrow trail would cut off toward the Lorillard place. Sybil wove through the debris-strewn path to emerge at an old, still-sturdy shed. If she kept going, she would shortly reach the edge of the front pasture at Sam's farm.

Just as Sybil galloped to the front pasture, Uncle Yancy shot into it, going straight for the graveyard, which rested a distance from the house.

Sybil took her hat off, pointed Kingston in the direction of the fox, and as the pack and then Shaker came into sight, she shouted "Tallyho!" That done, she quickly hopped the fence into the pasture, veering wide left, hoping to get up to the side of the pack as she, like Shaker, ran behind.

Jumping a tiger trap into the pasture, Betty had heard the "tallyho" so she kept to the right with extra vigilance. The last thing she wanted to do was turn the fox, nor did she want to lose the pack.

Shaker, on the road side, flew around to the right, jumping the same tiger trap that Betty had just cleared. Seeing this from a distance, Sister headed straight for it once she, too, got off the road.

By now Uncle Yancy had glided over the neat graveyard stone enclosure, reached his den, and ducked in. No one saw him duck out to creep to the Lorillard house, where he slipped under the back mudroom, climbed up into it, pushed back the rags, and jumped from one thing to another until he was on the top shelf, warm, a bit winded, and quite happy. Really happy, since he could hear the hounds blabbing outside.

The pack leapt into the old graveyard and found the den. Not wanting to jump into what he considered sacred ground, Shaker dismounted, throwing the reins over Hojo's neck. Perfect gentleman that he was, Hojo watched the proceedings inside the graveyard.

"Leave it. Leave it," Shaker ordered.

One doesn't want hounds digging at graves, even if there is a den there. The huntsman blew "Gone to Ground." As he did so, Mercer—unable to control his excited horse, Dixie Do, who pulled like a freight train—passed the Master. Sister and the field watched the show.

Dixie headed straight for Hojo, came close to the patient huntsman's horse, swerved for a moment, and took the low stone wall to stop hard in front of Shaker. That Mercer stayed on was a miracle.

"I do so apologize, Shaker." Mercer couldn't say much else.

"Happens to us all one time or another. Best you apologize to the Master."

One never passes the Master.

Mercer turned the now tractable Dixie Do toward the field, Sister in front, the whippers-in to the left, removed his cap, and bowed his head.

A moment's silence followed, then Mercer quipped, "Sooner or later we'll all end up here."

CHAPTER 15

"*N**o one could quite believe it.*" Diana talked to Inky through the kennel chain-link fence. Hound and fox were quite comfortable conversing this way. Good fences make good neighbors.

"*We were too astonished to speak,*" the hound continued. "*We looked at him, looked at Shaker. Everyone shut up. Mercer apologized.*"

"*Bet Uncle Yancy is still laughing.*" Inky admired the old red fox and his wily ways.

"*What a setup he has.*" Diana knew the old boy could get into places, then disappear.

"*Getting cold again.*" The beautiful black fox looked up at the cloudless night sky. "*When it's clear, the stars seem bigger, don't they?*"

"*They do.*" Diana fluffed her fur.

The two canines—one wild, one domesticated—chatted a little bit about other creatures, and celebrated the seasonal lack of bugs, one advantage of the cold.

"*I'm going back to my den,*" said Inky. "*I built up a lip on the northwestern side and it's even warmer than before.*" Inky paused. "*Do you know where you're hunting from on Thursday?*"

[4][4][4][4][4][4][4][4][4]

"No, but it won't be around here. Sister never likes to overhunt a fix-ture if she can help it." Diana headed back to the kennels to curl up with her roommates, warm with all those bodies and deep bedding.

Inky hurried to her den in the apple orchard, happy to go home after eating the treats left for her in the barn. She liked talking to Diana—a most sensible animal, in Inky's estimation.

Inside, Tootie, tired after the day's run, checked her e-mails on Sister's computer. Felicity loved the hunt as did Parson, her horse. Val, Tootie's old Custis Hall roommate, had e-mailed her from Princeton, decrying the lack of good men to date, a common theme with Val.

The next message she read, then re-read. Within a minute she was furiously scrolling through information online. After, she walked down the stairs, stopped in the library, then headed to the kitchen.

"Sister."

"Yes, madam," Sister teased her as she sat at the table, polish-ing her boots. "If I don't do this after hunting, I wait until I really resent it because I need clean and shining boots."

"I cleaned mine, too." Tootie took one of Sister's boots, polish evenly applied, and began brushing the well-worn leather.

"Thanks, sweetie."

"Dr. Hinson e-mailed me about bloodlines. Actually, she started with the Przewalski horse from seven hundred thousand years ago. We know the animal's DNA, isn't that something?"

"It is."

"Anyway, she said I should investigate the Turn-To line, espe-cially the mares of El Prado, Sadler's Wells, and go back to Turn-To. She said I can never know enough. If I want to be an equine vet I should know the most important sires and mares for a lot of differ-ent breeds. She said start with Thoroughbreds as the records are good."

"Be specific. What do you mean about mares?"

"I mean the mothers of those great stallions."

"And did Dr. Hinson tell you those Turn-To mares, out of his line, have real toughness, can go long and hard without injury?"

Turn-To lived from 1951 to 1973.

"She did." Tootie smiled at Sister, always admiring of how much she knew about horse and hound bloodlines. It was people's bloodlines that the Master didn't care to study although by now, at 73, she's seen, in some cases, up to five generations of humans from one family.

"Dr. Hinson knows her stuff. She's right to get you to study more than, say, the skeletal system," Sister said.

Tootie then told her about the call at Broad Creek Stables, how lovely the foal was and then the discussion with Phil.

"Never thought of that, I mean lawsuits over bloodlines. Once the Jockey Club started having Thoroughbreds tattooed in 1947 I should think that would have cut down on unethical representatives of Thoroughbreds."

"Some letters and numbers can be altered," said Tootie. "A *T* can be made to look like an *F*."

"Well, yes. I would think Phil has few worries. His stallions and mares have produced good foals, good runners, for close to a century. The Chetwynds are both lucky and smart. Takes both in the horse business."

Though tired, Tootie polished with energy. A slick shine gleamed on the old black boots.

"Did you know that Hail to Reason's dam?" Tootie named one of the great horses of the twentieth century. "Nothirdchance raced ninety-three times in six years and went on to breed?"

The mother of Hail to Reason clearly evidenced stamina and soundness.

"Well, I didn't know that name but I did know that Turn-To bred a lot of tough mares to compensate for his unsoundness. From his line we got Hail to Reason in 1958, Sir Gaylord, so many great horses."

"How do you remember all that?"

"Honey, it's easy to remember what you lived through, and I was a horse-crazy kid. Still am. If you want an interesting project, given that you were over at Broad Creek Stables, check the pedigree on Navigator, the horse that put Broad Creek on the map long before even I was born." She laughed. "Hey, that's a good shine."

"So Turn-To bred tough mares and produced tough mares who then produced tough foals, regardless of sex?" Tootie asked.

"When it all went right, yes, and luckily it went more right than wrong. You know breeding higher vertebrates isn't exactly like breeding Mendel's pea. Seems to me there's a lot more variety."

"I guess. Oh, Dr. Hinson sent all the research stuff to Phil Chetwynd. I mean since he asked her about DNA and stuff. Does that ever happen to you?"

"What? I don't know but so much about genomes and DNA."

"Sorry. I meant sometimes do you get obsessed about something and you can't let it go? You have to find everything about it?"

"I do. I only wish that when I was young I had done more research about some of the men I was attracted to. Would have saved a world of trouble."

They both laughed.

Then Sister said, "Actually, Tootie, physical attraction isn't logical so I don't know if the research would have prevented my mistakes, and wisdom comes if you learn from your mistakes. You'll notice some people make the same mistake over and over."

"Kind of like they've got one foot nailed to the floor and spin in circles."

"One way to put it."

"Sister, is Mercer gay?"

Sister looked up from her boot. "No, why?"

"Well, he's never married. He's kind of emotional."

"I'm not sure emotional stuff has anything to do with it. No, Mercer never married because his mother never released her claws. Daniella would have destroyed any woman he did marry. No one was ever good enough."

Sister picked up the boots, putting them in the mudroom. The two house dogs and Golly slept on the floor, the kitchen being warm.

"You know, I think that's the best shine my boots have ever had. Thank you." She looked down at the threesome. Raleigh the Doberman let out a long sigh.

"You'd think they'd hunted today." Sister laughed.

"What a day." Tootie smiled.

It was and it wasn't over yet.

The Chetwynds, Phil and Cheri, hosted a small dinner party for seven people: Kasmir, Alida Dalzell, Freddie Thomas, High and Mandy Vijay, and Sybil Fawkes. Mercer's account of his disgrace added to the high spirits. This followed his story about his presumably murdered grandfather; he was certain it was his grandfather, given the history: Harlan's horse transport by train in the old days, the slate memorial, Mercer's mother's many axioms for a happy life, which could be reduced to "Have a bad memory."

Mercer was at his best. As another round of after-dinner drinks enlivened the proceedings in the high-ceilinged living room, Mercer piped up again. "Phil, can I go through Broad Creek's account book and files from the twenties? Just in case I find something?"

Phil thought for a moment. "What you'll find is mildew, but sure. Just put everything back where you found it."

Next to Mercer on the sofa, Alida said, "What a fascinating story, your trip to Kentucky, the freezing fog and sleet storm and then finding a body."

Phil smiled. "It was an unforgettable hunt, pretty much as today's was."

Sybil leaned toward Mercer. "You got off lightly."

"Sister was in a good mood." He sighed happily.

Thinking out loud, Alida said, "Maybe there's some kind of symbolism about your grandfather and his dog being buried with Benny Glitters."

Phil was curious. "Symbolism?"

"He rode to heaven on a horse," Alida responded.

"Or the other place." Mercer shrugged.

"No, Mercer, that will be you." Phil lifted his glass to Mercer. They all laughed, lifting their glasses, too.

CHAPTER 16

A stiff breeze swept across the front of the main Broad Creek Stables barn. Patches of snow dotted pastures facing north. Otherwise, the mud-brown landscape offered no promise of spring, not even an early crocus.

Phil stood next to Sister and Tootie while Phil's manager, Ignatius, trotted a yearling.

"Let-down hocks aren't going to be a problem foxhunting and they might not even be a problem racing." Phil pushed his gloved hands into the pockets of his down jacket, as he focused on the hind legs. "But racing, as you know, can be hard. I'd rather not see him end up there." He broke into a smile. "He'll have a wonderful life as a hunter."

Sister replied, "Conformation is always worth studying. We've all seen horses with less than perfect conformation who were fabulous winners. Seattle Slew for starters. Ignatius"—she smiled at him—"hold him up a minute."

Sister walked over to the colt with Tootie. Phil stayed put. The older woman touched the youngster on the neck, ran her fingers down his neck, then over the muscles on both sides of his spine. He didn't flinch, nor did he move away from her. She continued over his hindquarters, felt his stifle, then stepped back. She returned to his front, knelt down and ran her hands, gloves off, down each leg, then picked up a hoof. The colt stood calmly. She moved to the rear, picked up the hind hooves.

Coming back to his head, she reached into her pocket and pulled out a delicious peppermint, which he happily ate off her palm. She liked that he had been handled, had ground manners. Quality was already there: bone, a wonderful sloping shoulder, a good frame. He would muscle up naturally if he came to Roughneck Farm, and with no steroids.

She never asked Phil if he used steroids or doses of growth hormone. They were illegal but not that hard to get. Walking up and down hills, running around the huge pastures, gave youngsters a solid foundation. At three, a horse would begin to learn his trade. Sister rarely hunted a horse until the animal was four. She preferred five. Like people, some mature more quickly than others, but she believed in bringing a horse along slowly, no drugs. Usually the horse told her when he was ready, and she listened.

This handsome one looked at her with a large soft eye, nickered, and was rewarded with another peppermint.

"What's his name?"

"Midshipman."

"Your Navigator line then?"

Phil nodded. "Yes, so you know he has stamina."

"I do." She patted him on the neck, offered one more peppermint.

Ignatius returned Midshipman to his field.

The horses at pasture had large three-sided run-in sheds, backs to the wind. They were warm enough. Phil always had them deep in straw. Once in work, they would get their own stall, plus plenty of turn-out in the pastures.

After Midshipman thundered across his large paddock to join his friends, Phil waited as Ignatius brought out another three-year-old. Sister carefully watched the colt move. He was fluid.

"Okay," Phil called. "Trot him right toward the Master."

Ignatius did, then turned and trotted the horse about 16.1 hands away from her.

"Tracks well," Tootie said low.

By this she meant his legs didn't flay out to the side, nor did he have an odd way of moving. As Sister would say, "Has a hitch in his giddy-up."

Then Ignatius slowly trotted the horse in a circle in each direction.

After this, Sister checked out the colt just as she had with Midshipman.

"So, Phil, you gelded him."

"I did. He's sort of a number-two guy, you know? I figured he'd be better off gelded with other geldings. We broke him, worked him on the track, and truthfully, he's slow."

She laughed. "Your slow isn't my slow."

"Exactly." He laughed, too. "Both of these boys have good minds, manners. No one is afraid, rolling their eyes, avoiding people. They're curious. When I mentioned these fellows to you I was way wrong about their ages. Both are three years old."

"What do you want for them?" asked Sister.

"Come on into my office, get out of this cold and we'll talk."

Sister glanced at Tootie. They briskly followed Phil through the stable and into his wood-paneled office. How good it felt to be warm.

"Sit down, ladies. Anything to drink?"

"No. Don't butter me up, Phil. Oh, what's the three-year-old's name?"

"How do you know I wasn't offering you coffee or tea? I know liquor won't work." He smiled genially as he peeled off his coat.

"The three-year-old's name is Matchplay. He's got that Wimbledon blood if you go back a bit. He's pretty easygoing."

"Okay. How much?"

"Well, I've put time and money into the boys. They're sweet guys. I'll send them over. You live with them for a month. If you like, Sister, how about two thousand dollars apiece?"

"Phil, that's generous."

"Not so generous, Sister. With the economy the way it is, you can't give away horses. I try to help out the Thoroughbred Retirement Fund, as I know you do, too. It's depressing but I figured you'd hit it off with these two. They're your kind of horses. Mostly I'm trying to get back what I put in. I'll never recoup the stud fees but two thousand dollars covers food, trimming, and shots."

"I appreciate that. Let me think it over. I'll call you tomorrow."

Before she could rise, she heard a heavy thud from the secretary's office next door.

"Dammit!" Mercer's voice grumbled.

A woman's voice could be heard, Phil's secretary. "Mercer, sit down. I'll pick it up."

Phil rose. "Excuse me a minute." Opening the door between the two offices, Phil stuck his head in the other one. "Are you mistreating Georgia?"

Georgia's voice carried. "Mistreating me. He's a pain in the ass. Look what he's done to my office."

"Oh, Georgia, I have books spread out," said Mercer. "It's not that bad. I'll put everything away."

"Phil, why did you tell him he could go through records from the early years? I could strangle you."

Phil laughed. Mercer and Georgia could be heard laughing, too.

Sister couldn't stand it so she got up to position herself in the opened door. "Georgia, strangling is too good for him. Did you hear what he did on the hunt yesterday?"

"I did and Sister, you were too kind to him. Should have thrashed him with your whip. Or tied him to a tree."

"We could still do that," Phil offered.

"Yeah, yeah." Mercer sat down at the small second desk. "Well, Sister, I've been busy, so before you all sit in judgment of me"—he stared hard at Georgia—"I found the cost of Benny Glitters's slate slab, the bill for the engraving, and the bill for shipping. And, best of all, the cost of Harlan Laprade's travel to Lexington, Kentucky, with the memorial slab."

Phil folded his arms across his chest. "Anything else?"

"I was looking for lodging."

"Mercer, obviously Harlan went to the house of ill repute," said Phil. "I really doubt my grandfather would note that in the official records. He wouldn't put in a rate for lodging, I just know it."

"Oh, hell, Phil, none of us know what our grandfathers would countenance. I just wanted to see what the slate cost. For giggles, I went to the old studbooks—on the computer, of course—and pulled up Benny Glitters's pedigree. Blue chip. Too bad he washed out at the track."

"A lot do."

"Yeah, but Domino for a sire?"

Phil listened. "Mercer, you'd better put everything back in its place. If you don't, I have to hear about it from Georgia."

"You can hear about it now." She threw a paper clip at Mercer.

"Oh, Georgia, you just want my attention."

"I've got it."

Phil closed the door. "I must have been out of my mind to let him root through the old account books and files."

"Phil, Mercer can talk a dog off a meatwagon." Sister laughed.

"Yes, and I had imbibed entirely too much wine." He sighed. "I suppose I hoped he would wear himself out with this research stuff; 1921 was a long time ago and he isn't going to find anything to help him solve what happened. And for all we know," Phil whispered, "Harlan Laprade may have deserved it. He inflamed someone's anger. I'm not going to say that to Mercer, and I sure won't say it to Daniella. She orders him about. She orders me about."

Sister couldn't help but laugh, which made Phil laugh, too. "There are people who leave an indelible impression."

Phil's eyes brightened. "She used to swing a cricket paddle at us. Oh, yes, she'd come to the barns because we'd usually be here after school and she was ready for any manner of boyish wrongdoing. Neither of us liked school. We went to different ones, of course. I don't know whose was worse, mine, which was private and cost Dad an arm and a leg or his, public." He frowned. "Another trip down Memory Lane. I've heard so much about Mercer's family, now I'm doing it. Hey, let me get Georgia to run off the pedigrees of Midshipman and Matchplay."

Phil opened the office door again and Sister and Tootie heard, "I haven't done a thing. Stop checking up on me."

"This has nothing to do with you. Georgia, run off the pedigrees of Midshipman and Matchplay."

The sound of a chair being rolled could be heard, then Mercer appeared in the door frame.

"Sister, aren't those two good-looking horses?" he asked.

"Yes, they are."

"I admire you for looking at young horses. Means you think you'll live a long time." He ducked back into the office before she could say something.

Driving to the farm, Sister smiled as Tootie read the pedigrees. "I hope I'll live a long time."

CHAPTER 1 7

Alone red-tailed hawk watched from high up in a pin oak. Hounds worked diligently below, scuffling and snuffling. High winds postponed Tuesday's hunt to this Saturday. They were glad to be out. No fool, the hawk knew hounds might stir a mouse, who'd zip out from under leaves. Presto, lunch.

Dragon moved ahead of the pack. The wet leaves had packed down but an enticing delicate hoof stuck out from under a deep layer of decaying leaves. The large, powerful hound nosed over, inhaled deeply, yanked the deer leg out from under. The foreleg, still jointed, dangled from his jaws. Tail upright, he circled the pack, tempting them with his treasure.

Sister fretted over anything that brought a hound's head up when working. Deer carcasses, what was left of them, lay in all the fixtures, although some more than others.

This fixture, Mousehold Heath, had more than others because the Jardines, a young couple, both worked during the day. Poachers made good use of their absence. The terrible thing about poachers is sometimes they would wound a deer but not be able to track it and kill it, for fear of getting caught. The poor animal suffered for days, weeks even. In other cases poachers were trophy hunters, would take the antlered head, leaving the remains. Of all the misdeeds of irresponsible hunters, this enraged Sister the most. When so many are hungry, to waste food, to not share, to her it was an unforgivable sin.

Well, Dragon's prancing wasn't unforgivable, but she hoped he'd pay for it soon and he did. Sybil swept up upon him.

"Leave it," the strong rider ordered.

He slunk away and that did it. She popped her lash, catching him right on the rump.

Ever the dramatist, Dragon howled. *"I'm being murdered!"*

His sister, disgusted, walked right by him, nose down. Didn't look up.

Nor did any other hound. At one time or another, Dragon had offended every four-legged creature out there. He did, however, get back to business.

Rain started. Even with your tie tight around your neck, water would slide down your back. The mercury, hanging at 43°F, intensified the effect.

As it was a Saturday hunt, February 15, everyone endured it.

"We've been out here a long time," complained Twist, one of the second T litter, a year younger than the first.

"Keep trying," Cora encouraged her. *"Sometimes in bad conditions, you'll hit a line."*

"In this stuff?" wondered Thimble, Twist's littermate.

"Oh, come on now, Thimble, you've hunted in the rain before," Ardent, older, teased her.

"I don't remember it raining this hard," the elegant tricolor replied.

Within five minutes, the rain bumped up from a light steady patter to a barely-can-see-your-hand-in-front-of-your-face downpour.

Sister would hunt through any weather but she knew few people felt as she did. She was ready to turn back to the trailers when Pickens, a young entry, spoke.

The older hounds checked it out and within a flash, every hound in the pack roared.

Sister was on Lafayette, who surged. He was one of her best horses and best friends. Between them, they had twelve years of friendship, as she had bought him when he was a two-year-old.

The footing would deteriorate rapidly but at this moment it wasn't too bad. As the rain soaked in, it would get ugly.

She couldn't see Betty or Sybil. The only reason she could see Shaker at all was his scarlet jacket. If anyone behind her had a mind to turn back, the incredible music changed their mind.

"Whoeee!" Shaker called out. He then blew "Gone Away," which is a bit different than calling hounds to a line. However, the rain rolled into the bell of the horn so this call sputtered.

He kept calling. Hounds kept speaking. An obstacle would loom in the rain just in time for one to see it. The pack, then the people, threaded through an old wooded patch—huge trees whose bark turned dark with the rain. The sight would frighten anyone with an active imagination.

The red-tailed hawk returned to his nest. Most animals had the brains to seek cover. Not the foxhunters. Even Thimble—running hard, scent strong—became oblivious to the lashing rain.

Way ahead, the fox ducked down into a creek with deep banks. A tree, half its huge root system hanging out over the creek, contained a half-hidden entrance to the den. Within a minute, she was snug in the back of this cavern. Plus she had other entrances and exits.

Hounds reached the creekbed, threw up for a moment.

"You can do it," Shaker urged them.

Much as they didn't really like each other, Diana and her brother worked well together. In tandem, the two worked past the line, returned to where the scent last held.

"She jumped in." Dragon looked down and as he did so, his sister had launched herself into the swiftly running creek.

He followed her, both of them swimming against the current. The entire rest of the pack poured over the bank. The drumming of the rain now had the counterpoint of the separate splashes of hounds.

Diana reached the thick tree roots. She could hold on with both front legs, her nose pressed to the roots. *"She's in here!"*

Other hounds joined her but when the current would carry them downstream, they'd swim back. Cora wisely found a place where she could scramble up. Everyone but Diana followed. They all worked around the wide trunk at its base.

"Found another den opening!" Twist cried out.

Thimble, Twist, Taz, Pookah rushed to it. Digging wasn't much use, so Trooper stuck his head into the small opening.

"Do you know how stupid you are?" a squeaky voice sassed.

"Huh?" Trooper was surprised.

"Stupid. Stupid. Stupid. Do I need to repeat myself?"

Diana finally gave up her post, clambering up with the others. She, too, cocked her head at the den opening.

"The vixen sassed me," Trooper informed her. *"Rude. So rude."*

"Stupid!" The fox was now enjoying this. *"I'm high and dry and you all are wetter than muskrats."*

On the opposite side of the bank, Shaker put his horn to his lips, playing the three long notes. "Come on. Come on. Well done."

"Nothing much we can do," Cora counseled.

Last to follow the others back into the creek, Trooper threatened, *"You're lucky we're leaving."*

"Don't let me keep you." She emitted that foxy puff of air, a laugh.

Trooper now felt insult added to injury. He did join the others though, and Shaker turned back.

It took everyone twenty minutes to pick their way back to the trailers because the surface on some of the hillsides began to give way, and horses slipped. Other spots proved fine—better drainage perhaps.

Back at the trailers, as always, people wiped down their horses. Because of the unremitting downpour, they put them on the trailers, haybags in place.

"This is so heavy," Sister said as Betty helped pull off the Master's sodden jacket, heavy even when dry.

Sister grabbed one of the terry-cloth towels she kept in the trailer tack room where the three women crowded together, tried to dry off. Tootie shivered.

Betty, ever maternal, ordered, "Honey, take off what you can. I always bring a gear bag with extra clothes in our sizes. I even have a pair of jeans."

Through chattering teeth, Tootie began to peel off layers of soaked clothes. "I didn't think it was supposed to get this cold."

"Rain in the low forties. Always a killer." Sister wiped down her torso, grabbed a sweater from her gear bag, slipping it over her head.

"You're not going to keep your breeches and boots on, are you?" Betty sternly intoned.

"Well," said Sister.

"Take them off," Betty ordered. "You have jeans in your bag. Just put them on. The Jardines aren't going to care that the Senior Master shows up for the breakfast in jeans. Come on, you'll catch your death."

Tootie took the clothes that Betty handed to her as she was fussing at Sister. "Catch your death," said Tootie. "A strange phrase. Makes death sound like a baseball."

Sister sat on the little carpet covering the lower ledge in the cramped quarters, taking the socks Betty offered her. "Warm socks. Listen to that rain!"

The aluminum trailer amplified the hard rain.

"Maybe we need water wings." Now in dry clothing, Betty inspected Tootie. "Umm, the jeans are a tiny bit big on you, but not so bad that you could fit another person in there." She rummaged around in her bag. "Here, use this belt."

Finally dry, warming up thanks to dry tweed jackets, the trio looked at one another.

Sister thought for a moment. "Rain comes from Zeus, right?"

"Lightning bolts and thunder sure do." Betty pulled down Big Ray's old golf umbrella from a ledge above the hanger rod. "Sister, this thing has to be thirty years old."

"If it keeps us reasonably dry while we make a run for it, fine. I never saw any reason to throw it out."

"All these years, I never really paid attention. Just looked like an umbrella tucked up there with your helmets." Betty then burst out laughing. "Ray was a terrible golfer."

"If he'd changed his pants, he would have improved his game." Sister could still hear her first husband cursing after a misdirected shot.

Tootie hugged herself; her tweed jacket was thin.

"He wore these corduroy pants with embroidered crossed golf clubs," Sister reminisced with the others. "I swear that ruined his game."

Sister and Betty laughed, remembering Ray. Betty opened the door to peek out, then quickly shut it when rain blew into her face.

"Can you see anything?" Tootie asked.

"Obviously not."

"Well, we have to try. Everyone else is in the same boat." Sister pushed open the door but the wind pushed it back.

Putting her shoulder to the door, she forced it open, nearly tumbling out onto the now soaked ground. With difficulty, she held the door as the other two hopped down. Betty quickly put the umbrella over their heads as the wind slammed the door shut and Sister made sure the latch caught. She was already wet.

The huge umbrella blew inside out as they hurried toward the

Jardines' small house, other people also braving the mess to get there. Once inside, everyone sighed, shook water off. Betty didn't leave the umbrella open but leaned it against the umbrella stand, more or less ruffled.

Bobby greeted his wife; everyone was talking. The Jardines—young, happy with each other and their tight little house—buzzed everywhere at once. Jim put more logs on the fire in the kitchen and in the living room.

Everyone gravitated toward anything hot.

After a half hour, the food worked its magic, as did the drinks. Scattered throughout the living room on furniture, on the floor, chat filled the entire house.

Back to back on a large hassock, Phil and Mercer talked to those close to them. Sister, being Senior Master and a lady of some years, was offered a seat on the sofa by Walter, who stood up.

Walter said to Sister, Phil, and Mercer, "Shaker was smart to stuff the hound trailer with straw. They're as warm as we are."

Sister nodded, then said to Phil, "How about if I get those two horses Monday, weather permitting?"

"Sure."

Leaning against Phil's large frame, Mercer bragged to Sybil, Tedi, and Edward how he had written a letter to *The Blood Horse* about the gambling issue in Kentucky and how he squarely placed the blame on unscrupulous Indiana people paying off equally unscrupulous folks in Kentucky.

Phil turned his head. "Mercer, those boys play rough. Like the hound with the deer leg, leave it."

Mercer didn't reply but shrugged.

Sister remarked to Mercer, "Phil has a point. Excuse me while I find my whipper-in."

"See you next hunt." Phil smiled as Sister walked through the people, many slightly damp as she was herself.

"Betty."

"Mmm." Betty swallowed quickly. "Got me with my mouth full. These biscuits are light as feathers."

Sister held up her hands palms outward. "Don't tempt me. You know breads are my downfall."

"You've been the same weight since I've known you and that's over thirty years. I'm the one that has to worry." Cheerfully Betty picked on herself because she had once gotten heavy and worked hard to lose it.

"Will you drive the rig back to the farm?"

"Yeah, sure. Where are you going?"

"Riding with Shaker and the party wagon." She cited the hound conveyance. "Need to review some things with him. Breeding ideas. Stuff like that."

Once back at Roughneck Farm, Sister in the kennels with Shaker, Betty and Tootie in the stable checked everyone over, as did Sister and Shaker. After finishing chores in the kennel, Sister ran to the stable for the rain continued.

"Hey. Everyone okay?" Sister called as she slid through the small opening in the big double doors.

The swirling rain even managed to fly through that small opening.

Betty noticed. "If this keeps up there will be flooding."

"You're right about that and then tonight it will all freeze. Boy, I hate that." Sister watched Tootie put a heavy blanket on Lafayette. She noticed Tootie checking the big clock inside the barn. "Date?"

Tootie smiled. "No, but I wanted to drop off my paper for Dr. Hinson and she said she'd be working a little late today, but it is already five-thirty."

Sister looked into each stall, water buckets were filled, and a nighttime flake of hay had been tossed in just in case someone got the midnight munchies. "Come on, we'll take you over. Everything looks fine in here."

"Good idea," Betty agreed. "I can pick up that wonderful paste she mixes up. Stuff heals surface wounds in no time. I put it on those thorn scratches I got a week ago and all gone." She held up her hand. "Thorns cut right through my glove, too."

Sister inspected. "Penny never stops thinking of ways to make life better for horses. As for you, well, she'll be happy about that, too, but not as happy as if it were a horse."

The three of them laughing, they shut off the lights, walked through the tack room and paused for a moment.

"Let's go in my old yellow Bronco. A lot easier to see in this weather," Betty suggested sensibly.

Making a dash for it they scrambled into the large SUV, Tootie in the second row of seats.

The clinic, about twelve miles from Roughneck Farm, would take longer to reach in this weather. Betty, a conservative driver, sometimes drove Sister crazy because she always thought Betty drove too slowly. Today, she was glad of it and actually kept her mouth shut.

Twenty-five minutes later the large curved Westlake Equine Clinic sign appeared in the Bronco's headlights.

Pulling into the parking lot, Tootie exclaimed, "Good. She's still here. The truck's here and the lights are on."

"We'll wait for you." Sister, damp for half the day, was beginning to feel it.

"I need my magic cream," Betty said as she cut the motor.

Sighing, Sister replied, "Well, if you two are going to get wet again I might as well join you."

Even though the three of them wore Barbour coats, best for horsemen, the lashing rain found its way down the back of the collar, hit their faces, and a bit dribbled onto their fronts, a trickle sliding down their hunt shirts. And the rain was so cold, a few degrees above sleet.

LET SLEEPING DOGS LIE

Tootie, the fastest, reached the door, holding it open for the others.

The front office was empty, tidy and clean as always. A light shone out of an office in the hallway, polished except for some muddy bootprints that looked as though the wearer had slid on the floor.

"Dr. Hinson," Tootie called, pulling her paper from under her coat.

"Are you writing a term paper?" Betty asked.

"I'm practicing." Tootie smiled. "It's my bloodline research on the Turn-To line."

"Penny," Sister called, then said in a lowered voice, "Maybe she's in the bathroom."

After waiting five minutes, Tootie pushed open the low door separating the public space from the large receptionist's area, her desk, computer, files on the other side of the divider. That area, too, was neat and clean.

Tootie walked down the hall and entered the door with the light—Dr. Hinson's own office.

"Dr. Hinson?"

Sister and Betty, each of whom had gratefully sunk into a waiting-room chair, stood up as they heard Tootie running down the hall.

The young woman's face registered shock. "She's dead!"

Both Sister and Betty shot down the hall behind Tootie. As they entered the roomy office, Sister noticed nothing amiss except for Penny Hinson, head on the computer keyboard, arms reaching toward her computer.

A single hole in her back, slight powder burns on her shirt, bore testimony to how she was killed.

Hands on her face, Tootie sobbed.

Sister put her arms around the young woman, as did Betty.

The two older women looked at each other and Sister released Tootie. She picked up the office phone and dialed 911.

After reporting this dreadful discovery, Betty walked Tootie out to the lobby. Sister followed.

Sheriff Ben Sidell was close by, as he kept his horse at After All Farm. He reached them in fifteen minutes. He'd called his team immediately, but upon opening the clinic door he was glad they'd be behind him. He wanted to get statements as quickly as possible, so Sister and Betty could get the distraught Tootie home.

They each recounted what had transpired.

Tootie cried, "She never hurt anyone."

In a gentle voice, the sheriff counseled her. "Tootie, sometimes terrible things happen to very good people. This could be a robbery. My team and I will have to go over everything. She was a special person with a gift for healing, and you made her happy because you hoped to follow in her footsteps."

Tootie nodded as Ben touched her shoulder.

Sister leaned toward him. "I used the phone in her office. If you take fingerprints mine will be on it. The papers on the floor are an exercise Penny wanted Tootie to do. She dropped them when she saw the body. Betty and I left everything as we found it."

Betty added, "There were muddy prints into her office and in the office. We walked all over them adding our muddy prints."

Ben smiled tightly and nodded. "I'll take that into account. You all can go now. I know where to find you."

Tootie, face puffy from crying, whispered, "I will follow in her footsteps, Sheriff. I will."

"I know you will," he replied with feeling.

CHAPTER 18

The constant drumming on the roof of Westlake Equine Clinic added to Sheriff Ben Sidell's dismal task. Three hours after arriving, Ben, along with his best officer, Eli Mason, stood at Penny's desk one more time.

Eli reviewed what they found. "The force of the shot rolled it forward just a bit." He kneeled down to point out the tracks in the rug.

"Right." Ben stood beside the chair. "She was working at her computer, not worried, *bam,* she slides forward slightly, slumps over, head on the keyboard. Since the bullet wound was in her back, she had to have been forward a bit in her seat. Whoever killed her had a clear shot, stood close to her."

"The bullet didn't exit, so my guess is it's flattened on a rib."

Penny's body had been removed but both men had been able to intensely focus on the scene and the victim before the ambulance took her away.

"Save your guesses, Eli. The autopsy will tell us that. And I guarantee you the gun isn't registered."

"Everything in here is neat. No drawers rifled through. The petty cash is undisturbed." Sporting a fashionable three-day-old stubble, Eli rubbed his cheek. "Her guard wasn't up. She knew her killer."

"Most likely. The question is, what else did she know?"

"Vets cast a wide net. She works on horses, sees the barns and owners everywhere. No telling what she stumbled into if she did."

"There's always that, the odd moment when the wrong person notices something at the wrong time, but veterinarians deal in drugs. There is a black market for equine drugs, just as there is for human drugs."

Knowing next to nothing about horses, Eli raised his eyebrows.

"There are the obvious drugs," explained Ben. "The painkillers, some of which people take, but there are also far more lucrative drugs for an enterprising person: steroids, any performance enhancing drug, even growth hormone. Some of these substances can be cooked up in labs here, some in other countries and smuggled into the U.S. like any other contraband. It's an enormous market."

"But surely there are ways to detect illegal substances, just like for human athletes," Eli asked.

"A clever distributor, someone who comes and goes without attracting attention, could easily sell, deliver the goods. Could be a vet, a trainer, anyone others are used to seeing. There isn't the societal pressure to test animals that there is for people, with some exceptions."

"What exceptions?" Eli cracked his knuckles.

"Show jumping. Racing, especially racing. A crooked track vet could be useful. I can't imagine Penny being part of a drug ring, distributing stuff. Then again, Eli, you never really know, do you?"

"That's the truth. So let me get this straight. You pay for the drugs. They are delivered. But there has to be someone on the take who does the testing at the track."

"Pretty much, but there's a market besides the track. Anyone breeding horses who wants them to muscle up early might use steroids or growth hormone—both of them controlled substances. The horse looks mature, looks well muscled and impressive early. The muscle gains stick but the downside is the joints aren't fully developed. Easier to sell a well-muscled youngster. Many kinds of equine discipline might benefit from steroid use. Rodeos don't perform drug testing. Nor do most jumper shows or cross-country shows. Now some of those have vet checks, like endurance rides, to make sure the animal is okay, but that's not the same as testing for steroids. There's money to be made, a lot of money, but especially on the tracks."

"Would a clinic legally carry them?"

"Most will have some controlled substances because they do have useful applications. Just like for people."

"So this clinic would have, say, steroids?"

"Yes. When we talk to her senior partner, we'll ask him to unlock cabinets, show us their supply and the tracking system." Ben crossed his arms over his chest and looked out the window. "This rain just won't let up." Then he focused on Eli, now standing on the other side of the chair. "Westlake serves a few breeding Thoroughbred barns, dressage, jumper barns—everything from a big operation like Broad Creek Stables to someone like me, who owns one horse and loves that horse like crazy."

"So your horse might be prescribed steroids?"

Ben nodded. "Maybe for an unusual illness. Foxhunters wind up with leg injuries, a tendon problem, an abscess in the hoof, maybe even an abscess in a tooth. Or we might see West Nile virus, things that call for specific medicines. Unfortunately, there are many problems for which there really aren't good medicines. But a hunt horse would rarely be put on a controlled substance. Penny gave me joint supplements for Nonni, a little equine aspirin when Nonni needed it."

Eli smiled. "I have a lot to learn."

"We all do," said Ben. "Like you, I have my hunches. I leave the medical investigation to those with that skill, but you and I have to think of all manner of things, no matter how odd. The only clue we have right now is that Penny probably knew her killer and trusted him or her."

"We have her computer." Eli cocked his head in its direction. It was still turned on, a letter to a magazine on the screen.

"She'd been reading *The Blood Horse*, Mercer Laprade's letter. When our team goes through the computer, they'll find accounts, all manner of barn calls, patient notes, magazines, professional newsletters. Getting back to hunches, my hunch is that Penny stumbled onto something."

"Could be it has nothing to do with being a vet."

"True." Ben sighed deeply. "She was a good woman and a good vet. You didn't know her but those of us who did trusted her with the lives of our horses, which is like trusting someone with the life of a family member." He held up his hand. "I know that sounds silly to someone who doesn't own a horse."

"I have Joker, that counts." Eli smiled.

Joker was a cat so fat he should have been named Two Ton.

"Counts." Ben looked around. "Let's go through each room one more time. We could have overlooked something, especially me, since I know the victim. No matter how experienced you are, when someone you like is murdered, it gets you."

They opened the closet door in Penny's office. Clean overalls hung on a hook, along with two lab coats. A pair of work boots and a pair of Wellies sat on newspaper, caked with mud. Leaving her personal office, the two men walked down the hall, turning into each partner's room. There were three, counting Penny. They opened a supply room. The drug closet was locked. When her senior partner arrived, they'd tackle that.

Penny's unlocked truck had been searched by the first team on the scene. Very neat, Penny even had a tray in her truck where small items like pens, notepads, and Scotch tape were organized in the center console. The large medicine cabinet on the back of the truck was locked, but the keys were in the truck so that was investigated, too. Pretty much, she carried what every equine vet would carry on a call: lots of elbow-length, thin rubber gloves, syringes, clenbuterol, magnesium-based drugs for joints, horse tranquilizer, and a metal box with scalpel and other tools. Occasionally, Penny had to operate on the spot. For this she carried a large canvas sheet and a plastic one, also. She had items for bacterial infections, vials with antiviral meds, many of them new to the market. She had thread to sew up wounds, needles for same, and she even carried a small steamer, which she used before she would operate. She'd wipe her scalpel with antibacterial fluid, then steam it for a second. Penny was nothing if not thorough. Her X-ray equipment, plates, and heavy lead-lined gloves—all very, very expensive equipment— were neatly tucked into the truckbed medicine cabinet.

Establishing a veterinary practice wasn't cheap, nor was maintaining it to the highest standards. To Ben, it was clear that Penny cut no corners.

The two men walked back down the hall to the inviting lobby and receptionist's long desk.

As they watched the deluge, waiting for Westlake's senior partner, Ben softly said, "Had she lived, I think she might have gotten elected to national office in her profession. She was so bright, so forward thinking and she truly cared about horses. You know, Eli, the media harps on all the bad actors out there regardless of profession. There are so many good people doing their job, helping others, helping animals. Educators, doctors, carpenters, you name it. Good people. She was one of them."

Eli thought. "You are, too, Sheriff."

. . .

Sister, Gray, and Tootie, along with Raleigh, Rooster, and Golly, felt the warmth from the library's fire. Sister's favorite room, the library always felt peaceful, but especially on a difficult day. Photographs, some from the 1880s, reposed in polished silver frames. Sister was surrounded by her family, most gone. Sometimes she'd look at a photo of herself at thirty and wonder, "Was I ever that young?"

A wonderful photo of Sister—in a white evening gown dancing with Gray in his evening scarlet—sat on the corner of the desk, a testimony to the present.

They'd eaten a light dinner, discussing what had happened to Penny with surprise and sorrow. Now they listened to the crackle of the fire, inhaled the fragrance of the applewood burning with seasoned oak.

Gray read the paper: "The western bypass is like malaria. It keeps returning with exaggerated symptoms."

A proposal for a western bypass around the heavily traveled north/south 29 corridor had been batted about for thirty years plus. With it came studies, meetings, outrage, presentations from those in charge at the state level, and innumerable environmental studies. It went on and on. So far, the public had been able to stop the bypass from being constructed.

"Gray, this will be going on into the twenty-second century, I swear. Tootie, your grandchildren will be fighting it."

Tootie looked up from her book and smiled, but tears filled her eyes.

Gray noticed, rose, going over to her. He sat on the edge of her chair. "Honey, I'm so sorry. It was just a terrible shock."

Tootie cried harder now, so Sister fetched a box of tissues and sat on the other chair arm.

"How could something like this happen?" the young woman sputtered.

"I don't know." Sister handed her a tissue.

"I expect Ben Sidell will eventually root it all out," said Gray. "He adored her. Well, we all did." His voice carried his own sorrow.

"Is it always like this?" Tootie's voice wavered.

"Like what?" Sister asked.

"Is life so sad?"

"Sometimes, yes, but you get through it," Sister said.

Raleigh came over, putting his head under Tootie's hand.

"They know. Animals always know." Tootie cried a bit more.

"They do," Gray agreed.

"I bet there's an animal that knows who killed Dr. Hinson." Tootie dabbed her nose.

The rain streaked across the windowpanes.

"Maybe so." Sister put her palm on Tootie's smooth cheek.

Tootie looked up. "Maybe this is about an animal."

Gray and Sister looked at each other, then Tootie.

Sister said, "It's possible. Let a little time pass, perhaps things will fall into place."

CHAPTER 19

U ncle Yancy watched the somber group of humans make their
way to the Lorillard cemetery. Yesterday two men had dug a
neat rectangular grave, flinging mud over their shoulders. Sitting
on the back stoop they had not noticed him, but today, the thirty-two
people arrived. Uncle Yancy needed to hide. From under the front
porch, the view was clear. Human behavior interested the older fox.
Sometimes he thought he understood it, other times he found it
very mysterious.

Mercer pushed his mother's wheelchair, sending specks of
mud onto his trousers. At the front of the stone-walled cemetery,
the wooden gate with a cross cut into it was open. Plain yet aesthet-
ically perfect for the place, the tombstones, some over two hundred
years old, worn smooth, stood in neat rows. No tombstone was huge
or gaudy. Some graves were covered with slate like Benny Glitters's
grave. Harlan Laprade's grave would rest at the end of the middle
row, next to his wife. Graziella Lorillard, sleeping forever, would be
next to her sister when that time came.

Gray and Sam's sister, Nadine, walked on the left side of Daniella Laprade. Both women, wrapped in furs against the cold, emitted streams of breath from their mouths. The ground, frozen since last night, forced people to take care where they put their feet.

After Kentucky authorities had confirmed the skeleton as Harlan Laprade's, Mercer, his mother, and Nadine—who now insisted upon being called Chantal—had chosen Friday for the bones' interment.

Most of the mourners were hunt club members who had taken off work. Phil Chetwynd walked to the right of Aunt D, as he called Daniella Laprade, thanks to the long association of the Laprades with the Chetwynds.

The service included a reading from the Old Testament, one from the New Testament, an invocation, and a prayer for the peace of the soul.

Sister thought Friday a bad day to bury anyone. In some parts of the United States and Europe, executions were held on Friday, considered to be the Devil's day. Of course, she kept this to herself. Gray had enough on his hands. Gray and Sam's sister had flown up from Atlanta to be with Aunt D, who she loved more than she had her own mother. Nadine also intruded into decisions her male relatives had made without her.

Mercer had picked a funeral director to receive Harlan's bones, plus the dog's bones sent from Kentucky. The authorities saw no reason to keep what was left of the fellow. This was an old crime. Like any urban area Lexington had more pressing ones, not that Lexington considered itself urban. Cincinnati was urban, Louisville was urban, Lexington was beautiful. They had a point.

Nadine wanted a regular casket. Mercer, Sam, and Gray balked. A child's casket would do, for there wasn't enough to put into a large casket. The savings would be considerable.

She screamed, "You are rearranging your grandfather's bones to save money?"

So Mercer and Gray had then split the normal-sized casket

costs. Sam had driven to Arvonia, Virginia, in Buckingham County to pick up a beautiful piece of slate donated by Bill and Carolyn Yancy from their slate quarry. Then Sam, who barely had two nickels to rub together, paid to have the thick slate engraved with name, date of birth, and date of death—or, as close as they could approximate Harlan's date of death. Ever sensitive, Sam also added under Harlan's name, "His beloved dog sleeps at his feet."

Nadine was one step ahead of a running fit. This in front of Daniella, ninety-four, whom Nadine had supposedly come to comfort. Earlier, the screaming, tears, and outpourings had taken place in Daniella's living room, with the old lady present.

After twenty minutes of prime-time emotion, Daniella bellowed, her voice strong, "Shut up, Chantal. The boys have paid for everything. You haven't paid a red cent. Furthermore, Phil has arranged for a catered lunch in the home place and the hunt club has paid for all the liquor. Shut your big flannel mouth."

In a plaintive voice, Nadine warbled, "I paid for my plane ticket."

Now, Harlan's remaining daughter and grandchildren stood beside his grave. The men bowed their heads. Not one of them looked at Nadine while she dabbed at her eyes with a lace handkerchief. She handed one to Daniella, who clutched it in her begloved hand.

After the service, the assembled trod back to the house, spotlessly clean, as Gray had hired a cleaning service for their place. Not that it was so bad, but Sam worked long hours and Gray shuttled between D.C. and central Virginia. Also, they were two men— enough said.

At the front steps, Sister paused, sniffed. Eau de *Vulpes vulpes*. Ah, yes, the graveyard fox, which was how she thought of Uncle Yancy. Filling her lungs, a small smile at the corners of her lips, she stepped into the center hall.

After having been lifted up the stairs by all three of "the boys," as she thought of them, Daniella reposed by the living room's roaring fireplace, fruitwood lending a wonderful aroma to the gathering.

Nadine helped the nonagenarian out of her coat. The elderly well-dressed lady could walk with two canes, but the wheelchair was more reliable. She was loath to give it up. Nadine wasn't the only drama queen in the family.

As Nadine hurried upstairs to hang her aunt's coat, Daniella, hair white, close-cropped, crooked a finger at her son. "Bourbon," she ordered.

"Yes, Mother."

"A double."

"Yes, Mother."

"No cheap stuff, you hear me?"

"Yes, Mother." Mercer sped to the kitchen, where Gray and Sam had set up a makeshift bar the night before.

Behind the bar, Xavier said, "Nice service. The slate was impressive. A lot of people here."

The last act of the burial had the two gravediggers, in black suits, lift up the slate to lay it exactly right over the freshly dug grave. It was still to be filled in but the slate covered it for the mourners. Mercer had wanted people to see it. With the help of the generous Yancys, Sam had done a good job.

"If slate was good enough for Benny Glitters, it should be good enough for him. Thanks." Mercer took the drink, hastening back to his mother.

Without a word, she grasped the offered libation and tossed it back. Handing him the empty, she ordered, "Another double with a chaser of ginger ale. I want old-fashioned ginger ale. The stuff that bites your tongue. I need more than a water chaser today."

The boys knew her habits and her favorite brand rested under the bar with her name written on it.

Mercer reappeared in the kitchen. "Another double. A ginger ale chaser," he told Xavier.

"Mercer, there's not a lot of your mother to absorb this. Want me to lighten it?"

"Hell no. I would wheel her back here, drop a siphon in the Woodford Reserve, and she'd suck it right up. You'd never know the difference."

"I don't remember her drinking so much when we were kids."

"Because we were drinking too much ourselves. Didn't notice." Mercer laughed, taking the drinks, one in each hand, to again attend to Mother.

Sister was talking—well, listening actually—to Daniella. She smiled weakly as Mercer approached.

"I tell you, that man could do anything with a horse. Had an eye, could calm the most fractious." The crotchety old woman paused, then said loud enough for Phil, standing near her, to hear, "And our family built the business with the Chetwynds."

On cue, Phil turned. "Good luck for both families."

"Not for my father, ultimately." She swallowed half the bourbon, then downed the ginger ale.

Mercer watched wordlessly. "Mother, I'll be right back but I need a drink myself."

Chin jutting upward, she appraised him. "I'll expect you back here shortly."

"Yes, ma'am."

Turning her face up to Sister, voice low, Daniella said, "I told my nephews to make Artillery Punch. Just knock people out. You need it after a funeral."

"Excellent advice, Daniella."

And indeed, an enormous punch bowl borrowed from the Bancrofts contained a lethal concoction.

With Phil kneeling to chat with Daniella, Sister walked over to Mercer.

"You are very good to your mother." She recounted Daniella's description of Harlan as an expert horseman.

Mercer burst out laughing as they reached the bar. "She has a vivid imagination. She was small. I doubt she remembered much of Harlan. No way. I expect she listened to her own mother. Me, I just nod my head."

This made Sister envision a bobblehead doll in Mercer's image. She put her arm through his for a moment. "You have much to bear."

He shrugged. "We all do in our own way, don't we?" Xavier handed Sister a tonic water with a lime wedge and a stiff bourbon for Mercer, who, eager to change the subject, said, "The attorney general for Kentucky ruled that Instant-Racing is a pari-mutuel game. Good. But the Kentucky Supreme Court passed the buck, excuse the pun, and wouldn't make a ruling on the legal status of Instant-Racing. So it's been bounced to the Franklin Circuit Court. That will be a circus, all the pros and cons argued before the bench." He looked straight into her light hazel eyes. "You know, Sister, it's the same old, same old. Doesn't matter the issue."

"There's a lot of truth to that," she agreed.

A brief interlude at the bar allowed Xavier to listen. "Mercer, what's Instant-Racing?"

"An electronic racing game that the racetracks will run and they set the take-out. See, it's gambling but it's not casino. Indiana, as you know, has really put the hurt on Kentucky and the Kentucky legislature—well, don't get me started. You all read my letter to *The Blood Horse.* Anyway, it will put money in the coffers." Mercer wished he hadn't used that word—too close to coffin.

"If it gets through the Franklin Circuit Court," Xavier remarked.

"Yeah, there is that. But it's not a bad idea, you know?" He heard his mother bellow out his name. "Back to it."

Sister and Xavier glanced at each other just as Kasmir walked in.

"Master, I can only wonder what's next," he said.

"Kasmir, we're on the same page there. First the discovery of

Mercer's grandfather. The watch. I will forever see that finger in the dirt and the hint of gold from the watch. Mercer was determined to prove it was his grandfather and he did."

Xavier chimed in, "And now Penny Hinson."

"A supreme shock," Kasmir murmured quietly.

"These events are unrelated, of course, but still, two murders almost a century apart," Xavier said, then they all paused, for Nadine's voice from the living room was so loud even Uncle Yancy under the front porch heard her.

"Don't you call me that! Don't you dare call me that, you worthless drunk!" Nadine spit into Sam's face.

Gray stepped between them as Mercer tried to shield his mother, who observed with disdain.

"Our mother named you Nadine," Sam shouted back. "What is this Chantal shit? Everyone in this room knows who you are."

"Sam, come on. It's the wrong place, the wrong time." Gray grabbed his brother's elbow, hauling him back, whispering in his ear, "The bitch isn't worth it. Don't give her the satisfaction of getting under your skin."

Mercer bent down. "Mother, I see your glass is empty."

She handed it to him with one hand, but held him with the other. "Don't go just yet." Then she looked up at Nadine. "Chantal, comport yourself. Today is a day to honor my father, your grandfather. I don't want to hear another cross word." With that, she nodded to Mercer, who headed for the kitchen.

Nadine burst into tears, left the room, and could be heard thumping up the stairs.

In the kitchen, Xavier, having gotten the drink ready just in case, handed it to Mercer.

Mercer wordlessly took it, hurrying back to the living room. He feared what his cousins might do next, especially Nadine, who trouped down the stairs again.

All eyes upon her, Daniella handed the immediately empty

glass back to her son, and hoisted herself up on her canes. Phil hurried over to help steady her. No one made a peep.

"Mom?" Mercer whispered.

Ignoring him, she addressed the gathering. "This has been a disturbing time for our family. My father is at peace but we are not." Taking a long pause, she, too, raised her voice, "Revenge. I want my father avenged."

Mercer said nothing. Then Phil gently lowered her back into the wheelchair. He whispered to Mercer, "Let sleeping dogs lie."

A shiver crept down Sister's spine. On the contrary, she thought: Give the Devil his due.

CHAPTER 20

The day after the proper burial of Mercer's grandfather, The Jefferson Hunt met at Orchard Hill, the farm on the northeast corner of Chapel Cross. Sister and Walter had recently secured an additional farm, also large, which abutted Orchard Hill to the east. Named Tollgate, as before the railroad came through there was a tollgate there, it now had new, more sporting ownership. The club could hunt through first Orchard Hill, then Mud Fence, then Tollgate. Put together, the fox and hounds could run over three thousand, five hundred acres, not an enormously large fixture but certainly an ample one for Virginia.

As always, Saturdays drew the largest number of riders, this February 22 being no exception.

George Washington, one of the best riders of his generation, a passionate foxhunter with his own pack of hounds, was born February 22, 1732, so this was always a special day. Washington's huntsman was a slave whom he respected greatly. General Washington was the only Founding Father, and indeed one of the few men of his generation, who freed his slaves upon his death. Men, both

— 160 —

North and South, owned other human beings then. Sport brings people together no matter what the century and in many ways, no matter the circumstances of those who pursue it. In Washington's day, the chance for hard riding, beautiful vistas, and catching up on all the news afterward at a breakfast created closeness. No phones, radio, television, Internet—back then, you learned what was afoot from your neighbor or perhaps a broadside. Newspapers were few and far between in our country's early days. People always want to know the latest news. Then as now, spicy scandal is cayenne for conversation. And again, then as now, foxhunting enlivened the blood, causing some people to forget the restraints of monogamy.

Sister noticed Alida Dalzell, again Freddie Thomas's guest, in the field. Sooner or later, a Jefferson Hunt man would lose his head over that woman.

Addressing the group before taking off, she cited our Founding Father's birthday and simply encouraged them, "When you drink the water, don't forget the people who dug the well." With that, a nod to Shaker, and "Hounds, please," they headed due east.

Cora with Diana led the pack. Twenty-two couple hunted today, for the temperature promised good scenting. The clouds covered them like a gray blanket, the frost was melting, and the mercury at 36°F promised to climb into the low forties. The breeze was tolerable but shifty. In central Virginia the winds usually come down from the northwest. If wind blows from the south, often it brings moisture from the Gulf of Mexico. Rarely does it blow steadily from the east, a slashing easterly wind meant a storm off the sea, the true nor'easter.

A little gust bent over broom sage. The untended fields at Orchard Hill were reverting back to the yellowish-tan broom sage. Bad for pasture but good for cover.

A gray fox named Gris heard and saw the trailers so he prudently moved toward his den, about four miles east. A young fellow, he had not yet found a mate, so he had roamed a bit out of his territory. Earl, the red fox on Old Paradise, secured one vixen, but Gris knew there was a girl out there just for him.

Right now there was a pack of foxhounds looking just for him. They trotted through Orchard Hill briskly, no scent, not even feathering. Crossing the railroad tracks, they climbed a small bank into Mud Fence.

"How about if I steer toward the right?" Diana suggested. *"The tree line ought to yield something."*

Cora, nose down, said, *"I'll move that way, too, but you be furtherest out. We don't want Shaker to think we're skirting."*

Huntsmen from the British Isles, often strict about skirting, will call a hound or have a whipper-in push them back. They want the pack more tightly together. Often huntsmen from the old countries aren't familiar with American hounds when they first arrive on our shores. They want to hunt them like an English pack. But American hounds exhibit independence just like American humans. If they trust you, even if they go into woods and you can't see them, they will come back. Some English and Irish learn this lesson, others do not, but most of our cousins on the other side of the Atlantic learn how very, very good those American noses are. Golden.

Highly intelligent and driven, Diana put her nose down, following the line of the woods. She could detect woodcock scent and squirrels, which were everywhere. She passed over a bobcat line and wasn't interested. Then she picked up rabbit, promising because often rabbit scent or the rabbit himself can lead to fox scent. Same with turkeys. The only thing better would be a cornfield with lots of leavings or blackberry bushes in late fall. In February food becomes more scarce and all animals forage in wider circles unless humans feed them. She passed over deer scent, keeping on the rabbit line that faded, it being a very light odor. Disappointed but determined, she continued on, then stopped at a large fallen tree trunk. She leapt onto it, following a definite fox scent.

"He's been here and not long ago!" Diana sang with excitement.

The entire pack trotted her way, many of them following as she walked on the tree trunk. What a sight!

Then Diana jumped off, barreling straight into the woods. Everyone followed, hounds beginning to open.

Long snaky vines dangled from trees and the underbrush. These slowed the horses but the hounds found ways under or through them.

Betty, per usual, on the right, had ridden down to the east/west tertiary road to run along the grassy strip. Behind her and across the road, the fire station receded quickly as she clipped along.

Sybil rode along the edge of the woods as Shaker went straight in along the field. Sybil, a complete whipper-in, possessed game sense, which she was well rewarded for as Gris popped out fifty yards in front of her. She counted to twenty, for one must always give the fox a sporting chance, and then called at the top of her lungs, "Tallyho!"

Shaker didn't hear her but hounds sure did. They trusted Sybil but also knew to keep on the line. Field members could tallyho golden retrievers, cats, sundry animals. With Dreamboat alongside, Diana did not rush to Sybil. They kept on the line, which veered to the north and intensified.

Within two minutes of Sybil's sighting, the pack burst out of the woods, followed by Shaker, then the First Flight.

Shaker called, encouraging them on. Hounds lived to hear their huntsman's excitement. So did the horses and humans. Next, Bobby Franklin blew out of the woods, with Ben Sidell close to him.

A bystander would see the panorama unfold with human riders in the same dress they donned during the reign of William and Mary. For some viewers this was a step back in time. And if they could overlook the attire, they could even step all the way back to

Homer's time. Hunting on horseback has been consistent for millennia whether the quarry is chased by sight hounds or scent hounds.

Scarlet coats dotted the subdued winter landscape. The horses added more color: bays, chestnuts, a few grays, cream-colored horses, and even a paint or two. Each animal was groomed to perfection, coat shining, tack clean but not for long, as a bog lay straight ahead on both sides of a quirky little stream that widened, then narrowed.

Gris knew scent better than hounds. Naturally, he dashed through the swamp—not so difficult for him as he weighed about seven pounds. He could hop from fallen branch to moss-covered tree trunks, usually avoiding the water. Hounds blew in and sank right up to their bellies.

"My coat is a mess!" Twist grumbled.

"Stop being a priss!" ordered her littermate, Thimble. *"Next you'll want your nails painted."*

Hounds knew about canine beautification from the TV in the kennel office. Occasionally Shaker or Sister would allow small groups in while they did chores. The hounds especially like advertisements featuring animals. A certain Pedigree food ad was their current favorite.

The struggle of the hounds to slog through the bog was nothing compared to the horses. They had to blast off their hindquarters, leaping up, then drooping down—tiring work. They crossed the stream only to hit the bog on the other side. Everyone emerged with slick gray hindquarters, for the gray muck flew upward. People wore mud on their faces, coats, and, of course, every pair of boots in the field was now slimed up.

Once out of this, they flew straight into Tollgate with its new fences, new gravel on the farm road, and new equipment sheds.

Sister saw an unfamiliar figure fly by riding a gorgeous steel gray Thoroughbred. The horse made Sister recall Buddha, a gray racing Thoroughbred some years back.

"What the hell?" She couldn't help herself and then she saw over the rise Crawford's pack of hounds in front of this woman. The black and tans were in front of her but out of sight until they charged up over the swale.

The woman had the sense not to blow her horn. She would only spoil a good run. Sister noted that. Whoever this was, she knew hunting and was a lovely rider.

The interloper sailed over a seven-board coop. Sister soon followed. She always thought a jump existed to keep stock out or stock in and you only needed one big enough to fulfill that function. The new owners of Tollgate—three-day eventers—built big jumps for training. She thought they were at a show this weekend. Sister was grateful, for she didn't know how they would take this impromptu joint meet on their land.

Hounds stopped. Cast themselves. The woman, perhaps midthirties, her face already a bit weatherbeaten, but she had good features, rode up to Shaker.

"I'm terribly sorry, sir. They came to your horn."

He nodded. "You must have just been hired by Crawford Howard."

"Yes, sir. I'm new, but Sam Lorillard went over maps with me. I know this is off-limits. I truly apologize."

"God help you." He smiled. "Come on, girl. Stick with me. Your hounds will hunt with mine."

As hounds, now forty couple strong, all opened, she had little choice. Crawford's Dumfriesshires, not as racy as the Jefferson hounds, nonetheless hung right in the middle of the pack. What a vision, black and tans with Jefferson's tricolors.

Hounds circled in the front meadow and hurried behind the spruced-up house. Sister did not follow too closely because she didn't want to tear up what was lawn. She circled at the edge just as the pack dove back into more woods.

This run lasted for an hour and a half, but the pack had switched from Gris, who dropped them. Hounds knew. The humans did not, but the gray, clever fellow had ducked into a den where a red fox had been while that fellow had also been out courting.

Now both packs, screaming, headed back through Mud Fence, back through Orchard Hill, past Chapel Cross itself, and crossed the road west of the Gulf station to tear through Old Paradise.

As the two huntsmen reached the old tobacco barn, far away from the main barn and the ruins of Old Paradise, Crawford Howard, his wife, Marty, and Sam rode toward them. When their pack had flown out of their hearing, they had been trying to find it again. Sam had followed Shaker's horn but the huge loop somewhat confused them.

Beet-faced, Crawford rode toward the two huntsmen now calling hounds back.

Marty spurred her horse to come alongside him. "Honey, don't fire that girl. Please don't. It was her first time out and our pack heard the other hounds. We couldn't, but they did."

"Goddammit!"

"Crawford." Her voice became stern. "It takes a long time for a pack to trust and know its huntsman. She needs the summer to work with them and don't you dare embarrass me by cussing her out. Do you hear me? Gentlemen don't cuss women in Virginia!"

Only Marty could speak to him like this.

His color began to fade. He slowed Czpaka.

Sam prudently rode behind.

Very close to him, Marty leaned over. "You be civil or you won't get any for a month."

This threat reached him. "All right."

"I love you. I will not let you make a fool of yourself. Give this girl time."

He took a deep breath, rode up to Shaker. "I see you've met my new huntsman, Cynthia Skiff Cane."

Shaker inclined his head toward the woman. "She rides like a Valkyrie."

Skiff blushed. "I'm sorry, sir." She addressed Crawford. "I—"

Crawford interrupted, Marty right by him. "No need. What I want to know is how did they hunt?"

"Well," she replied.

Mindful of the situation and having dealt with Crawford for years now, Shaker added, "You've done wonders with them, sir. They hunt as a team."

Marty inwardly sighed relief, grateful to Shaker.

A mud-splattered Sister rode up. "Good to see you, Marty, Crawford, Sam. How I wished you'd been with us. I think we picked up your main barn fox but somewhere on this hill we lost him. What a run."

Marty immediately replied, "One of these days we'll just put them together."

"Indeed." Sister said this in a welcoming voice. "Kasmir has put together a wonderful hunt breakfast at Tattenhall Station. Please come. We'd love to have you."

"We'll be there as soon as we get the hounds and horses up." Marty beamed. She missed her old Jefferson Hunt buddies.

Riding back to Old Paradise, Jefferson turned in the opposite direction toward the train station, and Crawford knew he was out-numbered.

Marty said, "Honey, I'm proud of you and you know I'm proud of our hounds."

"They did sound great coming up the hill, didn't they?" He felt somewhat vindicated.

"Did, and I think this girl will work out. She's a gentle soul and the hounds like her, as does Sam. I trust his judgment." Marty smiled at him.

True to their word, Crawford and Marty came to the breakfast. Sam and Skiff took the hounds and horses back to Beasley Hall, Crawford's estate.

Kasmir, warmth itself, greeted the Howards when they walked through the door at Tattenhall Station. Gray zipped to the bar along with Ronnie Haslip, who knew Crawford well. Actually many of them did, as he used to hunt regularly with The Jefferson Hunt. Gray had a drink in Crawford's hand in about three minutes.

"Scotch on the rocks, as I remember."

"Thank you, Gray."

"Marty, your vodka tonic." Ronnie gave her a drink.

Kasmir clapped his hands. Gray whistled and the large noisy gathering fell silent. "Join me in a toast to our first joint meet with our neighbors."

"Hear! Hear!" Phil Chetwynd raised his glass.

After that, even Crawford enjoyed himself as everyone did their best to say something nice to him. They all liked Marty, so that part was easy.

Mercer, once he had Crawford's ear, wanted to know more about the Thoroughbred ridden by Skiff. "The gray?"

"Son of Holy Bull."

"Ah, Crawford, you do have an eye. I always wondered why you didn't get into the game."

"Mercer, I learned long ago the way you make a million dollars in racing is to start with ten million."

Although he'd heard that line, sadly true, for decades, Mercer laughed. Crawford relayed that he'd heard the burial was special and the slate memorial had a tribute to the dog. Mercer, of course, replayed every detail from the pogonip hunt. On his second scotch with a plateful of food, some of it Indian, Crawford listened.

Freddie came up as Mercer left. "Good to see you and looking so well. May I introduce my friend from North Carolina, Alida Dalzell."

Of course she could.

Food, drink, and the company of a beautiful woman put Crawford in an excellent mood. Marty didn't mind a bit. She was in the middle of people she liked and had been terribly upset to leave when Crawford had yanked out his support when not chosen as Sister's Joint Master.

Younger, less egotistical, Walter had been the right choice. He would guide The Jefferson Hunt in the spirit unique to it. He lacked Crawford's fortune but his other qualities ensured careful leadership. Walter was also the outside son of Sister's late husband, Ray, which she didn't know until shortly before she had chosen Walter. Walter's father, if he knew, ignored this, and had raised Walter as his own, which emotionally, he was. Truly, let sleeping dogs lie.

Even as a boy Walter had reminded Sister of Big Ray in so many ways. She never thought about Walter being his son. Why would she? But it made her feel good to have part of Ray with her. Sister thought monogamy a good idea but difficult to achieve. Ray conducted his affairs with discretion as she did hers. The marriage had thrived. Everyone finds their own way.

Walter was now chatting with Crawford, good politics on the Joint Master's part.

Kasmir spoke with an animated, delighted Alida. She laughed until the tears came to her eyes.

"I hope you are not returning to North Carolina soon," said Kasmir. "We have so little hunting left but the end of the season is often the best." His liquid dark eyes shone with kindness.

"I," she paused, "Mr. Barbhaiya—"

"Oh, please call me Kasmir. I insist."

"Kasmir," she pronounced his name with a lilt, "I'm on a leave of absence. I won't bore you with the details of my work but I'm thinking it through. Anyway, if Freddie will tolerate me for a bit more I would like to hunt, but I've only one wonderful horse."

"I have a stableful, all bombproof. Sister has taken very good care of me. You come take your pick."

"I can't impose upon you like that."

"You must. Dear lady, I have made a fortune. I lost my wife to cancer and she was my heart and soul. I moved here to be close to the Vijays; High and I went to college together." He abruptly stopped. "Here I am talking about myself. The point is, why have something if you don't share? To see you ride my horses would make me happy and I think it would make my horses happy, too. You'll do a better job than I do." He laughed.

She touched his hand. "You flatter me, but I would love to ride your horses and you aren't boring me."

With that they both sat down in a railway pew and couldn't stop talking.

High noticed his friend. Kasmir looked enchanted, enlivened even. Sister noticed, too.

Ben Sidell and Mercer discussed the old murder since Mercer couldn't distance himself from it. But then, having your mother cry for revenge in front of everyone kept it all front and center.

Gray handed Sister a brownie. "Sugar, chocolate. What more could you want?"

"Just you." She kissed him on the cheek. "Well, I'd better do my duty." With a deep breath, she walked over to Crawford, now talking to Betty and Bobby.

"It's good to have you here." Sister smiled at him. "And before I forget, I'll e-mail you my suggestions for natural science changes at Custis Hall."

Betty and Bobby left them alone.

Crawford recounted some of Mercer's tale.

"It was bizarre," she said.

"Well, Mercer feels sure he can find out the whole story." Crawford put down his plate on the long table. "Why bury a man with a horse and his dog?"

"Solve that and I suppose you solve the crime."

Crawford shrugged. "Obvious to me."

Sister leaned a bit forward, curious, for he had a unique mind. "What? Who killed him?"

"Why he was killed?" Crawford shrugged again. "The horse, of course."

CHAPTER 21

Pookah was a small weedy hound, a throwback, for her sister looked a proper American hound. She ate her kibble from the trough. Fortunately, the kennels had a small kitchen where Shaker and Sister could heat up foods and keep medicines in the refrigerator. The two humans had worked together for years. Given the cold and the long run, they decided to warm some chicken broth, along with gallon bottles of corn oil and canned food for hounds who needed a little help keeping on the pounds. A hound or horse can burn off weight quickly with hard hunting. So can people.

Master and huntsman watched the young gyps gobble everything. At the hunt breakfast, Sister hadn't gotten to eat much and was still hungry. She opened the fridge, pulling out a power bar.

"How can you eat those?" Shaker grimaced. "They taste like cardboard."

"Well, they do, but if I eat a candy bar it's too much sugar. Once we're finished here, I'll heat a little lasagna. Gray made some last night to soothe his nerves. He makes the best lasagna."

"Crazy days," Shaker acknowledged. "Hearing Daniella holler

for revenge, I don't know. Does that sort of dramatics ever solve anything?"

"I don't know, but I guess for her it would." Sister peeled back the bar's foil wrapper, taking a small bite. It did taste like cardboard.

"Thimble," Sister admonished the dog as she had bumped her sister Twist to grab more food.

"She takes too long," complained Thimble, but she moved back to her spot. *"If she doesn't eat it fast, I will."*

"Chatty Cathy." Sister laughed. "You know, most times I'm glad I don't know what they're saying. It's probably something like 'Here comes that old dame again.'"

"I would never say that," said Twist, lifting up her elegant head. *"I love you."*

"Me, too," came the chorus from the youngsters.

This made both Sister and Shaker laugh.

"That huntsman can ride, can't she?" Sister admired competence in all pursuits.

"Yes. She seems nice enough. You were smart, well, you are smart, to invite Crawford and Marty to the breakfast."

"I will kill him with kindness," said Sister. "My mistake in the past was to let him anger me. I confess I should never have socked him at the Masters Ball in New York City. Even if he had it coming."

"Oh, that was years ago." Shaker wished he'd been there.

"He'll never forget."

"Sister, that man probably never forgot the first time his own mother insulted him. I call it injustice collecting."

She took another bite, hungry as she was. "Mmm. A big ego. As long as you tug your forelock, he's fine, and you know, Shaker, he earned that ego. The man built an empire, starting with strip malls in Indiana and branching out from there. Only Kasmir exceeds him in accomplishment. Sure, the Bancrofts are rich, but that's inherited wealth, and I hasten to add, they use it wisely. Edward managed the family company for decades so he didn't sit on his butt and collect dividends, yet it isn't the same as starting from scratch and building an empire. That takes guts, faith, and incredible energy."

"And luck." Shaker crossed his arms over his chest.

"You're right about that." She smiled, covering the bar with the foil wrapper.

Pookah watched every move. *"If you're done with that, would you mind if I chewed it up?"*

Noticing soulful eyes turned upward to her, Sister looked at the power bar. "Sweetie, if I give you this there will be a nasty fight. However"—she walked back into the kitchen, grabbed a handful of little meaty chews, returned, and sprinkled them all over the broth-drenched kibble—"More treats."

"You spoil those hounds."

"And you don't?" She poked him. "I can't eat this thing now, but maybe I will later."

Shaker half closed his eyes, shook his head. "Boss, how would you feel if I contacted what's-her-name?"

"Cynthia Skiff Cane, she goes by Skiff."

"Right. I have a hard time remembering names. Anyway, if she needs anything I'll do what I can. I like her. She must have whipped in somewhere. I don't recall hearing of her as a huntsman and I know pretty much who's who."

"Go ahead. I don't know who she is or where she learned her stuff either. Anyway, it is in our best interest and her best interest to try to get on even terms with Crawford. You know, he still hasn't named his outlaw pack. I would have thought that would have been the first thing he did when he broke away from us."

Hunts are forbidden to rent land but one hunt may lease a fixture or territory to another hunt. All the rules can get confusing.

"Don't know. But you all can't have the same territory. No

way the MFHA will abide that and he doesn't rent territory from us."

"But if he did, that bugaboo might be laid to rest. I support the MFHA most times, and the times I think they've gone over the top, I just shut up."

"The truth is, Sister, Virginia can do whatever she wants. The entire state can walk away from the national organization, and the threat for others of being excommunicated if they hunt with us won't work. People will still come here. This is the center of hunting in the United States. No one can break that power."

"Give Maryland her due." Sister loved the Maryland hunts.

"I do, but Maryland would be neutral, just as she was during 1861 to 1865."

"Shaker, it's a small state. They have no choice." Sister did her best to keep things on an even keel.

"So you've thought about it?"

"A secession?" Sister laughed. "Well, I suppose any Master in Virginia has had it cross their mind if something upsets them, but I think we can always work things out, whether it be with the national organization or Crawford."

"He won't join the MFHA."

"I know. I'll consider that problem later. Right now I want, if not harmony, then accommodation. His pack has joined ours three times. Once, a fine mess, a couple of years ago, and twice this year. We need to think this through and your idea of getting to know Skiff is a good one. Right now, I just want to finish out the season on a happy note."

"Been a good season."

"It has, thanks to these children." She indicated the hounds.

"Wait, wait until we're in our prime like Diana," Pansy bragged.

"We can give everyone a rest tomorrow, then walk out Monday," said Sister. "I wish this cold would break. Going down into the teens again tonight. The electric and propane bills are thirty percent higher than last year. Thank God for wood-burning fireplaces and the stove in the basement. By the way, how's your stove doing?"

"Fine. Heats up the cottage and I can keep the thermostat at fifty-five degrees."

Shaker lived in a clapboard cottage not far from the kennels and stables. He could walk to both places, which saved gas. Living arrangements and often a vehicle were usually part of a huntsman's employment package. Every hunt differed to some degree, the richer ones able to offer more, but The Jefferson Hunt covered the basics. Also, Walter, thanks to his being a doctor, had a decent idea of the insurance coverage changes and how to adjust for Shaker.

"I'm going to head up to the house," Sister said. "You hunted the hounds beautifully today and you handled a strange woman riding up to you and Crawford's pack with your usual aplomb."

"He needs good whippers-in." Shaker identified one of Crawford's main problems, a problem for most hunts.

"That's just it," she said. "No one can work for him without jeopardizing their position with the MFHA. You aren't supposed to hunt with outlaw packs any more than you are supposed to work for them. Which is why I like your idea of finding out a little bit more about Miss Cane," she said, taking her leave.

From the front office, she stepped into cold air and a setting sun.

Raleigh and Rooster greeted her as she neared the house.

"I've been so lonesome without you." Raleigh leaned on her.

"Me, too. I've been bored." Rooster jumped straight up.

Opening the door to the mudroom, bigger than the one at the Lorillard place, she hung up her barn coat and scarf. After taking off her lad's cap, she opened the door to the kitchen.

"What a heavenly smell." Gray had heated up the lasagna for her. She grabbed the bootjack by the mudroom door, pulling off her boots. "Oh, I do like taking my boots off in a warm room. Doesn't hurt as much."

Gray bent down to check the glass door on the oven. "Almost ready."

"Honey, have I told you I love you?"

He grinned. "I can never hear it enough."

"I saw you eating a big plate at Tattenhall Station." She removed her vest, tie, and titanium pin, which she fastened through a buttonhole.

"And I saw you didn't. People don't let you sit down and eat."

"Gray, it's always that way. I don't even notice anymore. At least I get a drink. Where's Tootie?"

"Reading *Handley Cross*." Gray named one of Robert Smith Surtees's novels from the nineteenth century. "She needs a distraction."

"I envy her reading it for the first time. Kind of like the first time you read *Gulliver's Travels* or *Huckleberry Finn*."

He placed the plate of lasagna before her, a drink, too, then sat across from her as Golly wove between the chairs. Golly operated on the principle that humans were clumsy. Be prepared. The dogs sat, ears up, hoping for a morsel. Not the cat. Trusting her lightning reflexes, she'd snare anything that fell from the table.

"Quite a day," said Gray. "Crawford and Marty actually enjoyed themselves."

"Marty especially." Sister savored the delicious pasta. "She's such a good person."

"She is," he agreed.

"Things settling down?" she asked, changing subjects.

"In the sense that neither Sam nor I have to deal with Nadine, yes. She's with Auntie D and flies back to Atlanta tomorrow. She doesn't want to see us any more than we want to see her. I'm glad it's over. Or almost over. Mercer's taken up his mother's cudgel, so to speak."

Sister told him what Crawford had said. "Preys on my mind."

Gray crossed his ankles under the table, leaned back in his chair. "You know, it does. Whoever killed Harlan knew about the memorial slate, knew the grounds of Walnut Hill, and obviously knew Harlan and his proclivities." He sat up, folding his hands on the table. "It's possible that someone also knew his schedule, argued with him, and a fight at the whorehouse did him in."

"Is. It's also possible that Benny Glitters knew something about Harlan."

"Vice versa." Gray now tapped his fingers on the old kitchen table.

Finishing up, she put her plate on the floor so the dogs could lick it, while handing a piece of lasagna to Golly. After this, she washed her hands and the dish.

"Gray, I'm about to abuse you."

"Really?" He started to unbutton his shirt.

Laughing, she put her hand on his shoulder. "That, too, but right now I need you at the computer. You can do anything."

Smiling, he replied, "If I can't there's a whiz kid upstairs who can."

In front of his big screen in the library, Sister asked, "Get Benny Glitters's breeding."

Didn't take Gray long. "Domino the sire, the mare was by Hastings."

Sitting next to him, she said, "Man o' War's grandfather, Hastings. An excellent pedigree. See if you can get Benny Glitters's racing record."

That took a little longer but finally, "Here. He started out pretty good."

"He did, ran third in his first race, then two seconds, and then didn't place. So they retired him. You'd think he would have been learning, gotten better. As far as we know, based on what they knew at Walnut Hill, he retired sound."

"Maybe he just didn't like racing," Gray posited.

"Possible. Such a pity with that pedigree. Few if any would use him as a stud, given his race record."

"Anything else?"

"Not right now. Thank you, honey. Something doesn't ring true for me. I can't put my finger on it."

"Janie, horses wash out at the track all the time. Plenty of them have successful sires."

"I know, I know, and some like Secretariat sire okay sons but great daughters—great broodmares, who in turn sire winners. But I'm going to call Ben Sidell. You can listen." She sat down at her desk and called. "Ben. Sister."

"Wonderful day," said the sheriff. "Wonderful breakfast."

"It was. Forgive me, but I'm going to intrude on your case. Sort of."

"I'm all ears."

"Do you have Penny's home computer?"

"We do. Her husband gave it to us. Didn't have to ask."

"Shall I assume there's nothing amiss?"

"It's what you would expect. Clients, ailments, treatments on the office computer and her personal computer is crammed with e-mails from friends and some research. Lots of stuff on wildlife but nothing that would set off an alarm."

"Will you do me and maybe Penny a favor?"

"Of course I will."

"Have your tech person sweep through for bloodline research. Before Penny's murder, she became interested in the Przewalski horse."

"Never heard of such a breed."

"Well, you won't see one in the hunt field. It's an ancient feral horse, one hundred percent wild, and it is at least seven hundred thousand years old. We have the genome, the oldest one we have up to now anyway. It's far older than any genome we have for humans."

"Where did they find this?"

"In the permafrost in the Yukon. Found a foot bone. This animal is the ancestor of horses, donkeys, zebras. Somewhere between 72,000 and 38,000 years ago the line split and one line became domesticated horses. The other remained feral."

"What do you think is the connection?"

"DNA. As an equine vet, Penny would be interested. But if you find she was looking at any pedigrees, especially of current horses or Benny Glitters, the horse in the tomb, maybe if I look at them I might be able to help discover why she was killed."

"You think her murder is related to the one in Kentucky? The one in 1921?"

A long, long pause and then Sister said with conviction, "Actually, I do. Something tells me this all goes back to Benny Glitters."

CHAPTER 22

In the distance, Sister saw Comet lounging on the foundation ruins of Roughneck Farm's original house built after the Revolutionary War. Although the air remained quite cool, the sun shone and the elegant gray fox, winter coat luxurious, warmed in its rays. Most mammals know enough to blunt wind, and Comet sprawled on a flat lintel stone that must have once graced the door of the small stone place. Over time, with more money, the original inhabitants—a husband and wife, both British subjects—built the summer kitchen, which still stood at the big house. They also built the core of the big house. Stones intact or fallen provide domiciles for foxes, skunks, minks if they felt like it, plus skinks, snakes, and other sharp-eyed creatures, although not all at once of course. With Comet in residence, no other medium-sized or small mammal would live there. He would make certain of that.

Walking hounds with Shaker and Tootie, Sister saw him about a football field away.

"Hold up," she said quietly, pointing out the reposing fox to Shaker and Tootie.

Shaker put his horn to his lips, blowing two sharp toots to get the attention of the hounds with them.

Comet lifted his head. *"Oh bother!"*

"Two toots?" Young Pickens sat wondering.

Dragon sat also. *"Listen, kid, I don't know why two toots, unless Shaker wants our attention for something or just to get us to stop. Don't worry about it."*

Worried, the youngster asked, *"But what if I hear two toots in the field? What do I do?"*

Cora put Pickens at ease. *"That's Shaker's way of telling you where he is if we can't see him, or he's fallen behind."*

"Oh." The satisfied hound rose as Shaker, Sister, and Tootie walked forward.

Shaker always loved viewing a fox. "I expect he would have heard us in plenty of time, but a sunbath might dull the senses. Every now and then he'll give us a merry chase, just like the black vixen in the apple orchard but I swear, if they see us walk down to the barn or the kennels in hunt kit, they repair to their dens. I find that so unsporting," he joked.

"Maybe they find us unsporting." Tootie smiled.

"I expect they find us crazy." Sister laughed, for she loved foxes, had spent a lifetime observing them. "We go out in most all weather, we run around, they are either running in front of us or watching us from a vantage point. They know every trick in the book and we keep falling for it."

They walked another half mile to the base of Hangman's Ridge, turned back, puddles still frozen, strips of snow deep in crevices, lining the north side of any kind of rise. But it felt so good to be outside. A little slip and slide only added to the adventure.

Back home, hounds waited in front of the big draw pen to the side of the kennel office. Shaker called each one by name. When that hound came forward, he swung open the tall door to allow the hound inside.

Once inside, everyone received a treat. Again, each hound's name was called when boys were separated from girls. Tootie then walked the girls to their various runs while Shaker led the boys.

Like any hunt, The Jefferson Hunt divided animals by sex to ensure no fights because the boys could tell when a girl was coming into season long before a human. This made for a happy atmosphere and no kennel fights, plus there were no unintended pregnancies.

Shaker and Sister studied individual hounds, knew hound families, and when possible, tried to hunt with other hunts to observe their hounds in action. One of the glorious things about The Jefferson Hunt was that six excellent hunts fell within an hour or hour and a half radius. And if willing to travel longer, one could hunt with another fifteen crack hunts. Sister loved watching other hounds, closely observing staff work as well. Seventy-three she may have been, but she was always learning, and one thing she was sure of was that she would never know it all.

The rumble of a huge diesel engine caught their attention.

"Oh, it's the horses from Broad Creek," said Sister. "Shaker, do you need Tootie right now?"

"No. We're done."

"Come on, girl." Sister walked outside just as the stable's big rig turned in the large circle before her barn.

"Ignatius, how did they load?" she asked.

"Good. Phil's had us working on it, they've had some natural horsemanship lessons. Once they understand what you want, they are pretty willing."

"If you need a hand you tell me, but you know what you're doing." Sister appreciated a good horseman and thought it best always to get out of the way.

"Where'd you like these two?"

"Let's put them in this smaller paddock here. Stretch their legs a bit. Tootie and I will bring them in to their adjoining stalls in an hour."

Ignatius walked up the rubber-covered ramp, slipped the butt bar, and untied the slipknot, bringing Midshipman off first, which set Matchplay to screaming.

"Don't leave me! What's happening?" the flashy chestnut whinnied.

Midshipman neighed back, *"It's a pretty place. Don't worry."*

"Ignatius, I'll hold this fellow so you can get the other one," said Sister. "No point in more stress."

"Righto." He bounced back up, yanked the slipknot. It was a good thing he had the lead rope securely in hand because Matchplay didn't back off the trailer. The athletic gelding leapt backward, Ignatius hanging on.

Sister couldn't help but laugh. "Well, if I ever have to jump backward, I believe he can do it."

The sensitive horse quickly nuzzled his buddy, being instantly reassured.

"Tell you what, they are both athletes, but this guy . . ." He glanced up at Matchplay. "Quick, quick, quick. Once he's in work, I bet you he could turn under you in a skinny minute. Good you've got a long leg."

Sister led Midshipman, Ignatius took Matchplay, and she responded truthfully, "Ignatius, that long leg is attached to a seventy-three-year-old body."

"You ride like you've always ridden." He flattered her but it was mostly true. Sister was tough.

"You are kind." She changed the subject. "Tootie will be working with these fellows and Sybil Fawkes will come over."

"Sybil's good. I used to bug Phil to use her to catch ride but he wanted men." Ignatius mentioned the practice whereby young people or journeymen jockeys ride whatever is available at a stable. Often those horses were difficult.

"I can understand that since most jockeys, whether on the flat or over fences, are men. Some good girls get in the game now. I don't know what the percentage is but it's all to the good. I figure a good rider is a good rider."

"Me, too, but you know how Old Man Chetwynd used to grumble about a horse being woman-broke."

"Yeah, I know. He'd point the finger at me and complain, 'You're too soft on them. Too soft.'"

Tootie opened the gate to the paddock. Sister and Ignatius walked the two horses in, turned them to face them, then slipped off the halters. That fast, they wheeled around to run. Why walk when you can run? Same with children.

After five minutes of this, with the humans watching, the two snorted, slowed down, then stood and looked at the other horses in the larger paddocks and back pasture.

Lafayette, the senior horse, called out, *"You two listen to me. You are lucky to be here. No biting. No kicking. You are at the bottom of the totem pole. You hear? And furthermore, don't you dare hurt our Sister."*

"I'll take a chunk out of you if you do," warned Matador.

"They're fine." Sister put her hands in the pockets of the old flight jacket. Even with gloves, her hands got cold fast.

"Phil's got all the paperwork—you know, all that stuff, transferring ownership from Broad Creek to you."

"I do."

He climbed back up in the cab, grabbed a folder already a little greasy, and handed it down to her as he stepped down.

"Jockey Club papers in there, too." Phil had registered the two horses with the national organization.

Sister flipped it open. "How about that? He went all the way back to the foundation stallions. Past breeding papers in here. That's helpful."

"Phil never does anything halfway." Ignatius grinned. "Plus those foundation stallions put Broad Creek on the map."

"Yes, they did. Well, Midshipman goes back to Navigator, which makes sense. Do you remember a 'chaser Broad Creek once ran, called Bosun's Mate?"

"Could jump the moon, turn on a dime, and give you a nickel's change." Ignatius grinned.

"By now, Broad Creek has to have used up every naval term imaginable." Sister smiled back.

Ignatius pointed to Midshipman's pedigree and his Jockey Club name, Nelson's Midshipman. "This is the sixth generation with a Midshipman in the name. Oh, the farm's gone through them all."

"Easy to remember." Sister handed the paper to Tootie, who read it.

Ignatius put his forefinger on Matchplay's papers. "Goes all the way back to Spendthrift."

"Becomes an addiction, studying bloodlines." Sister took the paper back from Tootie. "We can study these in the house. Ignatius, wait up a minute. I have the check for Phil."

As she trotted into the tack room, the place where years fell away and memories flooded in, Ignatius and Tootie chatted.

"How do you like it here?" he asked.

"Mr. Donaldson, I love it. I'm learning so much."

"Tootie, call me Ignatius. I think the last time I was called Mr. Donaldson was when I sat in the recruiter's office just out of high school. Navy." This was said with pride.

"My father was in the army. He always said it made a man out of him," Tootie responded.

"Sure did for me. And now women can go in and do something other than nursing and personnel. Even when I was young, I thought that was kind of narrow."

"How did you wind up with horses?"

"I grew up here. I learned a lot in the navy, saw a lot, but then I wanted to marry and see my kids grow up. So I came home and

Phil hired me. I knew a little bit about horses. Learned a lot more. Ah, here comes the Master."

Sister handed him two envelopes, one with Phil's name on it and one with Ignatius's name. It is customary to tip anyone who shows a horse at a breeding establishment and customary to tip anyone who delivers a horse for you.

Ignatius, naturally, did not open his envelope. Sister had a blue chip reputation for doing right by people.

"Oh, hey, I almost forgot. I was standing here flapping my gums." He reached up, placing the envelopes on the seat of the truck, then dashed to the back of the trailer. "Present from Broad Creek."

"That Phil." Sister shook her head.

Phil had sent Matchplay's and Midshipman's winter blankets along. It is customary to send a halter with a sold horse but as blankets can cost upwards of $300, depending on make and style, this was quite a gift.

Ignatius smiled broadly. "He says nothing is too good for the Master."

As Ignatius drove off, the two new to-be-foxhunters watched the rig.

"I don't want to do that again," Matchplay declared.

"What, worm?" Aztec called over the fence.

"Get on that machine," the young Thoroughbred answered.

"Kid, you've got a lot to learn." Keepsake laughed.

Midshipman prudently said nothing.

Back in the house, the two women hung their coats in the mudroom, eagerly stepping into the warm kitchen.

"Some days I feel colder than others, even if the temperature is the same," said Tootie.

"Weird, isn't it?"

The two sat down to pore over the pedigrees. Gray came into

the kitchen and Sister told him the two geldings had arrived. He sat down at the table with them.

"Would you all like anything hot to drink?" Tootie offered. "I'm still cold."

"Sure," Sister said. "Surprise me."

"Me, too." Gray allowed Golly to jump onto his lap. "Just got off the phone with Ben. He asked for you to call him."

"Ah. I will after"—she turned her head—"the hot chocolate."

"He asked me to recommend a forensic accountant. Not from the area."

"I suppose you can't mention the case."

"Actually, I can. Ben wants someone to go over Penny Hinson's books—anything relating to billing, accounts receivable, and cost of supplies."

"Someone not from here?"

"Well, it is better, and I recommend Toots Wooten in South Carolina. She won't miss an errant comma." He smiled. "Being an accountant in some ways is consoling because you do find answers in black-and-white. The problem is when you start thinking life is black-and-white."

Tootie placed three mugs on the table. "Real milk."

"Perfect." Gray appreciated real hot chocolate.

Sister held the mug in her hands as Gray said to her, "I've been thinking about Benny Glitters, what you said the other night, and I don't think we should tell Mercer. For now."

"He'll run to his mother with it?" Sister's voice lifted up.

"Yes, then who else will he tell? And God only knows what Aunt D will do."

Sister spoke to Tootie, "While you were reading Surtees after the hunt, Gray and I pulled up Benny Glitters's pedigree. He is Domino's son. Then Gray got his race record. Started out pretty good, then back of the pack—pretty much what we'd heard his story was."

"Doesn't Mercer know all that?" Tootie inquired.

"He does, but Crawford said something at the breakfast, kind of an offhand remark. He said it wasn't the human in the tomb that mattered, it was the horse."

This startled Tootie. "That's strange."

"This is me—not Gray or anyone else—but I have a feeling I can't shake. Penny Hinson's murder is somehow connected to all this."

Tootie said, "How?"

"Well, that's the question, isn't it? Let me call Ben back." Sister rose, walked into the library and dialed.

Whenever possible, Sister used a landline. If the government wanted to, they could put on a tap like in the old days, but all the new technology—cell phones and computers—attracted them more because more people used them. Also, they were easier to hack. Corporations could spy on one another, too. It wasn't that she had anything to hide, it was just that she was of a generation that valued privacy.

"Ben."

"Good of you to call," the sheriff said. "You asked for any bloodline research on Dr. Hinson's computers. She had the breeding for all of her patients—I guess I call them patients—who had breed registrations. In the case of a backyard horse, she listed the parents if the owners knew. But she did have all the breed registrations and she also did research as you mentioned concerning the, I can't pronounce it—"

"Przewalski, forget the Pr, say it like a Cz."

"I expect the only way to speak Polish right is to be born to it," he replied good-naturedly. "Penny had looked into that; she'd investigated gene splitting. Her research was what one would expect of a woman of her intelligence and dedication. But nothing that shouts out 'danger.' "

"Ben, any signs of clients with a drug addiction? Not that she would be dishonest, but sometimes clients can order drugs they don't really need, even needles, and then they sell them."

"No. There are bills for needles and 'bute. But again, nothing that would indicate abuse. Let me get back to her DNA research for a minute. Again, I don't know about any of this, but is it possible to manipulate DNA?"

"In theory, yes. In practice, not so easy." Sister inhaled. "You're thinking, can someone duplicate the DNA of a great stallion and not pay the stud fee? Get DNA from a son or daughter? Well, it wouldn't be an exact duplication, but when you consider that some stud fees soar well over $100,000, the motive is there."

"It occurred to me."

"Again, in theory, yes. In practice, no. It's still too complicated. Too few veterinarians would be able to do this and ultimately, they could fall under suspicion."

"So one would need to be highly specialized for that sort of trickery?"

"For now. In time these things will be simplified, like using stem cells to cure some conditions in horses is specialized, but more and more veterinarians can now do it. Also, Ben, all this takes a fair amount of investing in the technology. But something's there. Something is right under our noses."

He breathed deeply. "If only I had a hint as to what she had or knew that was so valuable or dangerous. But then again, Sister, Penny's murder may not be related to her profession." He paused. "But I'm on your train. I think it is, too."

After that call, Sister walked back into the kitchen. "I have an idea. Let's find every photograph we can of Domino, his sons and daughters, and Benny Glitters."

CHAPTER 23

Aztec picked his way over timbered acres; an inviting snow-covered pasture beckoned the horse to the western side. Hounds drew through the slash. This last Tuesday in February proved that February was actually the longest month in the year, with grim, cold, sleety, snow-filled days. However, fox breeding was in full swing so frozen toes or not, a true foxhunter gladly mounted up.

Soldier Road ran east to west, with Hangman's Ridge on the south of that paved road. When Sister hunted from Cindy Chandler's farm, Foxglove, the ridge loomed as ominously as it did from her farm on the other side of the high, long, flat former execution ground. Driving toward Charlottesville on Soldier Road, one would arrive at Roger's Corner, a clapboard convenience store at the first crossroads going east from the Blue Ridge. Traveling west, if you drove a four-wheel vehicle you'd eventually come to dirt roads but you could snake your way up and over the Blue Ridge Mountains, finally reaching a two-lane paved state road between Waynesboro and Verona. A turnoff on the left side of Soldier Road would take you to Route 250, a much easier passage over the Rockfish Gap.

All along this Appalachian chain, rounded by time, gaps allowed inhabitants before colonists to travel east to west and vice versa. However, the Native tribes on either side of the famous fall line engaged in killing, capturing, and harassing one another, so little traffic took place.

The fall line runs roughly southwest to northeast, traveling northward. The angle, not acute, allows a sense of direction even for those born without this sense. Then again, if you can see the mountains, you always know where you are. However, you can't see them from the fall line where the state of Virginia lowers to the Atlantic Ocean many miles away. There the soil changes, the land flattens out. The three great rivers—the Potomac, the Rappahannock, and the James—enriched those flat lands. Even heading west, the alluvial deposits were generous.

On the east side of the line lived the Algonquin-speaking tribes; to the west were Sioux speakers.

Sister often thought of different peoples colliding—be they Indian or European, and then the later importation of Africans. Somehow out of bloodshed, truces, broken truces, and the superior technology of the Europeans, Virginia became what she now saw, a state of breathtaking beauty laden with natural treasures.

Like Aztec, she peered over the slash to the pasture beyond, distinguished by snake fencing, an inviting yellow clapboard house circa 1816, a true white stable and a red barn in the distance. She was excited. She had wanted to hunt this new fixture before the season ended mid-March. Close Shave was so named because survival there had been a close shave.

She'd hunted since childhood and had been a Master for close to four decades. She knew not to rush into a new fixture, throw up jumps everywhere. You needed at least a year to study the land and your foxes—or perhaps coyote—as Close Shave sat hard by the mountains. Once a Master and huntsman had a grasp of the fox's running patterns, jumps could be put in the best places to keep close to the fellow. Naturally, the foxes figured this out but by that time, the humans knew the territory well enough to compensate for the latest clever ruse.

Today's field, just fifteen people, did make it a bit easier. A large field on a first day can be as difficult for staff as it is for the field.

Mercer, Kasmir, Freddie, Alida, Phil, Tedi and Ed, Walter, Cindy Chandler, Sam Lorillard, Ronnie, Xavier, Tootie and Felicity, and Gray, all wore their heaviest coats, and were eager to see the new territory. Staff had ridden it at the end of the summer and once again mid-fall to get their bearings. Cindy Chandler had secured this place for the club, as it abutted the westernmost part of Foxglove. Like Tollgate, it was owned by new people; middle-aged, neither Derek or Mo Artinstall rode. Cindy, charm personified, shepherded them to social-club functions, sent a personal invitation to the panorama of Opening Hunt while giving them glorious coffee-table photograph books of foxhunting. They had such a good time, they gladly gave permission for the club to ride across their land.

Cora stopped at a large walnut. The timbering in these parts had been select cut, and were pine only. *"Damn, this is a tough day,"* said the hound.

Diana touched the same spot. *"Old. But if we fan out, maybe this line will heat up."*

Ardent, also in her prime, inhaled. *"A signature. A calling card. I say we'll get lucky. Come on, girls."*

Trident grumbled behind these three to Trooper. *"I really get sick of the girls thinking they are better than we are."*

"Me, too!" Trooper agreed.

Thimble, sweet but not always as astute as one would wish, piped up. *"We have more drive. Shaker and Sister always say that."*

The two males whirled toward her with angry faces, and the sweet girl dropped her ears and eyes.

"Sorry."

Dasher, an older male, coming up behind this little knot, cheerfully said, *"Hey, who cares what anyone says? If there's a fox, we'll find him."*

Hounds spread out. Reaching the snake fencing, they jumped over, continuing to search through the pasture.

Dreamboat, right up with Diana and Cora now, pushed toward a brook, not really wide enough to be a creek. On the western side of this fast-running water were rock outcroppings. Blue ice frozen from the crevices stood like a wall. These deep gray rocks, a few two stories high, contained larger crevices, suitable for housing critters. The rocks continued on for forty yards, then abruptly stopped, giving way to firm ground in heavy woods.

Dreamboat flung himself into the brook.

Diana trotted to the edge of the brook as Dreamboat crawled out under the rocks. *"Cora, he's on a roll."*

He was, too. Dreamboat had finally come into his own, out from under the shadow of his aggressive brother, Dragon, who'd been left behind at the kennel that day.

Sister and Shaker found out the hard way that when you assemble your pack for the day's hunt, you had to select with care. Not every hound would hunt with Dragon. Maybe they should have drafted him out, but he was brilliant. Sister always thought of this as her batting lineup for the game. Dragon was Number 3 while Diana was Number 4 when together. Apart, they did better and both could be number 4s, no jostling for position.

Cora hit the water, too. Within two minutes, the twelve-couple pack worked on the rock side of the brook.

Tails feathered. Hounds moved faster. Noses touched the ground, lifted up a moment, then touched again.

"Let's boogie!" Trooper shouted with glee and off they ran.

From their exploratory rides, Shaker knew where a nice crossing was. He quickly got over. Betty and Sybil found the going a bit harder because once over the water, they needed to find some kind of deer trails. The undergrowth was almost impenetrable, easily as bad as Pattypan Forge.

Sister followed Shaker. That summer, the club had cut a big cross through the woods, a trail large enough for horses and one that terminated on each of the four sides of the large woods.

In front of the hounds ran twenty wild turkeys. Hounds ignored them. A few horses found the sharp-eyed birds unnerving.

The lead turkey, an old turkey hen, cast a hard, bright eye at Aztec, the imposing horse leading the field.

"Mind your manners. I can fly right up in your long face."

"Bother," exhaled Aztec, who saw turkeys in the pasture often.

"Pauline, don't start something," the turkey immediately behind the lead turkey advised.

"This is our territory. These creatures need to be put in their place." Pauline flickered her long tail, but she did scurry away just a bit faster.

X-man, a green horse ridden by Sam Lorillard, snorted. *"What if they all fly up? I hate that sound."*

Sam would ride Crawford's green horses with The Jefferson Hunt to season them. As it was his day off, Crawford felt he was getting free labor although he was loath to admit a day with Sister helped a horse more than a day with him.

Nighthawk, Kasmir's beloved best mount, advised X-man, *"They have brains the size of a pea. Ignore them."*

"I resent that. You're the peabrain." The last turkey at the rear of the line clucked as she hurried to catch up.

As the line disappeared in tall grass their movements reminded Sister of that old dance the Turkey Trot, except that the turkeys did it better.

Right after the turkey parade, a confused squirrel paused for a moment, then prudently shot up a tree.

Far ahead of the field, hounds continued their cry, but the line was fading. They lost it at the edge of the woods.

"Dammit!" Trooper cursed.

The racket disturbed a barred owl, now awake and crabby. The golden-eyed bird looked down at them from her hole in the tree trunk.

"Vulgarians," she issued her verdict.

The vulgarians, confused and irritated, sought the line in a 360° radius. Finally reaching the hounds, Shaker held up to watch. Anyone can thrill to their pack in full cry but to watch them work was Shaker's joy, and Sister's as well. Given the narrowness of the passage she stopped fifty yards behind him, but some of the hounds worked back toward her.

The huntsman allowed them ten minutes, deemed it futile, and called them to her.

Sister looked behind her. "Huntsman."

Shaker yelled out before people tried to back into the mess. "Master, just turn around and go out. Let's get back in the pasture."

When they reached the pasture, hounds cast again. They tried for another hour but to no avail.

Not about to brave the cold, Close Shave's new owners waved from the kitchen windows when the field rode by. Shaker took off his hat and Sister tapped hers with her crop. The field followed suit.

A stiff wind rolled down the mountains. Clouds backed up on the crest.

Shaker blew hounds back to him and rode up to Sister. "I think we're done. This will be a very good fixture."

"Yes, it will. God bless Cindy Chandler. We've got some work to do, but that's hunting, isn't it?" Sister smiled, and turned Aztec as they walked back to the trailers.

A small tailgate marked the first hunt at Close Shave. Derek and Mo Artinstall allowed the club to tailgate in an old well-built, six-stall empty barn. Putting on a hunt breakfast was a great deal of work. Sister and Walter would never ask for such a gift from a landowner. In fact, they were happy to use the barn. Somehow it fit the spirit of the group. Out of the wind, director's chairs and card tables set up, people were warm enough in their coats, some changing to down jackets for the tailgate.

Taking Tuesdays off, Walter had bought a variety of Woodford Reserve bourbons, each having been aged in different casks. Ribbons in hunt green colors adorned the necks of the bottles. These stood open on one card table with a large card, hunt scene on the front.

"Everyone, sign the thank-you card to celebrate our first hunt at Close Shave," said Walter. "I'll drop this off at the Artinstalls when we're finished."

One by one people came up, removed their gloves, blew on cold fingers, signed their names.

"How did you like Mumtaz?" Sister asked Alida.

"Ravishing. The mare is one of the best horses I have ever ridden." Alida glowed.

Kasmir joined the two ladies, bearing two cups of bracing tea. "Would you all like a spike with that?"

Sister kissed him on the cheek. "You're spike enough, Kasmir. Alida gave Mumtaz a good ride."

"Ah, my girl needs a good rider. I bump along," he demurred modestly.

"Kasmir, you're a wonderful rider." Alida complimented him honestly, for he was.

"A wonderful man." Sister dearly loved Kasmir, praying as did everyone who was drawn to him that he would find happiness.

Mercer signed the card, then joined the others. As it was a small field, most everyone crowded around the Master and staff.

"Why don't we all sit?" Sister invited everyone. "I don't know why but my legs are tired."

Those who brought their director's chairs pulled them over. Always organized, Walter had carried bales of straw on the back of his truck, plus a few in his trailer. He'd placed them around the chairs and everyone gratefully sank onto canvas or straw.

Phil remarked, "It is funny how you can ride hard one day, no aches. Not much another day and you're shot."

"Low pressure," Freddie Thomas offered.

"Well, a nip of spirits should pick up everyone's pressure." Mercer held up his plastic cup. "Say, whatever happened to our stirrup cups, the ones with fox heads?"

"Mercer, no one is carrying stirrup cups to a meet unless it's a joint meet or a high holy day," said Tedi Bancroft, who always found Mercer amusing.

"We need more elegance," Mercer declared with conviction.

"Oh, Mercer." Sam shrugged. "You've been saying that since grade school. Since you discovered Hubert de Givenchy."

The crowd laughed.

Phil offered a toast. "To Mercer, first flight of sartorial splendor."

"Hear! Hear!" They all agreed.

People wanted to amuse Mercer, especially those who had been at his grandfather's somber reburial. No one could forget Daniella and most knew how demanding she was of Mercer.

They chattered among themselves.

Seated across from Phil, Sister smiled. "Remind me to carry a director's chair."

He wiggled on his straw bale, too. "Sticks right where it hurts, doesn't it?"

"By the way, thank you for the extensive pedigrees for Matchplay and Midshipman. I enjoy reading pedigrees. Going back through the names brings back memories."

"Yes, it does," Phil agreed enthusiastically. "I suppose most everyone measures their life by music, sports, books, movies, special occasions. For us, it's horses, great runs."

"That it is. Gray, Tootie, and I were looking at photographs of old horses. It's interesting how some sires leave a stamp, and others not so much. Given Midshipman's line, of course, we went back to Navigator. A very nice-looking horse with what was then thought of as a lackluster pedigree."

Mercer leaned forward. "Proved them wrong."

"I think it was the Ca Ira blood, the old French Thoroughbred who was Navigator's sire," Phil said. "No one knew much about him."

"Ca Ira." Kasmir popped up. "An eighty-gun frigate, French, that had the misfortune to battle Lord Nelson."

"How do you know such things?" Alida was impressed.

"Going to school in England helped." Kasmir smiled. "You do learn everything about Admiral Lord Nelson."

"You did. I bet the others all forgot it," Alida teased him.

Phil referred back to the photographs. "Hard to tell too much from those old pictures but you sure could see the good cannon bone on Ca Ira."

"One doesn't think of the French when one thinks of Thoroughbreds, or Germans either," mused Gray.

"Given that those people had been at war with one another for centuries, that makes sense. Never give the other country credit," Alida remarked, which made most of the others realize she was more than beautiful.

Phil asked Sister, "Must have been a scavenger hunt finding old photographs?"

"Anything is easy when you have Tootie and Gray. Put them in front of a computer."

Tootie said, "It kind of started with Przewalski's horse. Dr. Hinson told me I needed to study the evolution of the horse. That led to DNA." She paused. "Dr. Hinson was so smart and she told me that one really breeds to families more than individuals. She said you needed the right mix. A horse like Benny Glitters from a great family is as rare as Mr. Chetwynd's Navigator. Dr. Hinson said horses usually breed true. Well, she said people do, too."

"She was right," Phil agreed. "I'll miss Penny. A terrible loss, both as a vet and someone who could see the big equine picture."

Mercer nodded in agreement. "No date set for her service?"

"Not that I know of," Sister confirmed.

"Medical Examiner. Takes time," Sam replied simply.

"Well, how many suspicious deaths can there be in February? They can't be that backed up." Mercer put an entire chocolate chip cookie into his mouth.

"Who knows?" Freddie raised her eyebrows. "But you do associate violent crime with hot weather. At least, I do."

"All the more reason to be a white-collar criminal." Sam laughed. "Not seasonal."

"Do you ever think that Crawford made his fortune illegally?" Phil asked.

"No. Not for one minute," Sam responded instantly.

"Umm." Phil changed course. "It's good of him to let you hunt with us on Tuesdays."

"It's usually my day off," said Sam, "but he is pretty good about it, especially if I bring along a green horse. Some learn more quickly than others. The trick is to be consistent."

"Sam, I still say Crawford needs to get into racing." Mercer ate another cookie, a pang of guilt accompanying the pleasure.

"He's not going to hear that from me." Sam tired of Mercer nudging him, always nudging him.

Phil stood up to look out the large glass windows in the closed barn door. "Windier."

Cindy Chandler got up, too. "This is the winter that refuses to end, isn't it?"

Sam and Gray talked to Mercer a bit more as the group started to break up.

"I'll fold up the tables, put the bales back on your truck so you can go drop off the bottles," Phil offered. "Otherwise, you'll be here for another half hour."

"Thank you." Walter smiled.

"Mercer." Phil called to his old friend to help him.

People removed their plastic food boxes from the card tables. No food was left. Mercer and Phil folded the card tables as the others folded their chairs.

Kasmir and Alida walked outside to his trailer. She thanked him again for allowing her to ride Mumtaz.

"Will you be hunting Thursday or Saturday?" He paused. "Of course, you will. You can ride Kavita Thursday and Mumtaz again on Saturday."

"Kasmir, I can't take advantage of you like that."

"You're not. My horses need to go out."

"Mumtaz is gray. Did you ever read Tesio?" She named the great Italian breeder of the first half of the twentieth century. "He thought grays a mutation."

"Yes. Tesio and the Aly Khan are worth study. But I don't agree with the mutation theory, do you?"

"No. But then I look at paints and pintos, color horses. I don't really know too much about their backgrounds but they aren't as refined as Thoroughbreds. Thoroughbreds don't come as paints. Although I bet there's one somewhere out there." She cupped her chin for a moment in her gloved hand.

"Bet not." Kasmir held up five fingers for a five-fingered bet.

"You're on."

They batted this back and forth, each becoming colder by the moment.

Freddie called from her truck. "Alida!"

"All right," Alida called back.

"I'll bring your horse Thursday."

"Kasmir, allow me to come to your stable. I can tack up my own horse. That way I'd get to know her a little bit."

"Well—"

"Really, I like doing my own grooming and tacking up."

"All right. Perhaps—Mmm, the fixture is forty minutes from my place—perhaps an hour and a half before the first cast?"

"I'll be there." Then with a mischievous glint to her eye she said over her shoulder, "I respect your opinion, but I think mine is better." She burst out laughing.

He laughed, too, slipped into the cab of his truck, and the tears came. His late wife would say that to him constantly.

"Thank you, my love," he whispered.

CHAPTER 24

"S he kept good records," said Mercer. Asked by Ben Sidell, he reviewed the pedigrees of horses on whom Dr. Hinson worked.

Also asked by the sheriff, Sister sat next to Mercer at Penny's desk at the Westlake Equine Clinic. "Ben, certain strains in all the breeds carry problems. Penny was wise to know each horse's background if she could."

Mercer turned from the screen to Ben, in the chair next to him. "That's one of the problems with what I call backyard horses. Often Old Jose is bred to Sweet Sue because the owners think they're a good match. They have no idea what they're doing."

"Isn't there hybrid vigor among horses as well as people?" Ben smiled slightly.

"Yes," Sister answered. "We don't need to know names, but I'm assuming nothing in Penny's records points to crime. Or misuse of drugs?"

"No," said Ben. "But I don't know pedigrees like you two do. And what struck me is the amount of research she put in during the last month of her life," he added. "Could have been just a notion, as you Southerners say."

"Oh, come on, they say it in Ohio, too," Mercer shot back.

"Sister, what do you make of this fellow here?" Mercer pointed out a Quarter Horse cross.

"Poco Bueno blood, if you go back four generations. A very good Quarter Horse line. The dam, his mother, was that line and the sire, you know well, a chaser son of Damascus."

"Right." Mercer tapped away on the computer keys.

"And?" Ben asked.

"Whoever bred the gelding used two very good lines, sturdy. They looked for a mating they could afford. Ben, very few people could have afforded Damascus's stud fee when he was alive. So this person knew his or her stuff, and wanted an appendix, a Thoroughbred/Quarter Horse cross. You can find good blood if you look hard enough at a reasonable price, and anyone breeding an appendix horse would do just that."

Ben rubbed the flat of his palm on his cheek for a moment. "Do either of you have any idea why Penny would have studied all this, plus all her research on equine DNA?"

"Again, to see if a condition she was treating could possibly be passed by blood," Sister repeated. "Things like the inability to sweat, or hip problems—you'd be surprised what can show up. It's only in the last twenty years, really, that some of these conditions can be pinpointed genetically. Prior to that, a lot depended on a horseman's memory."

"And honesty," chirped Mercer, always quick to find a financial motive. "If a yearling looks fabulous, moves well but, you know, is a little screwy, how many sellers will tell? I worry a lot more about mental states than, say, a slightly crooked leg."

Sister crossed her arms over her chest. "Ben, you know her client list, we don't. Did Penny have any pedigree research not connected to her clients?"

"No."

"What about going back to the beginnings, like Eclipse or Matchem?" Mercer named two foundation sires of Thoroughbreds in the United States.

"Matchem 1748, right?" Sister was thinking.

"Right." Mercer then added, "Eclipse 1764."

"You can go back that far?" Ben interjected, amazed.

"Very often, you can," said Mercer. "Sometimes further. For instance, we know the names of some of Charles the First's horses in the royal stud long before the English started their stud book." He leaned back in the office work chair, stretched out his legs under the desk. "For instance, Navigator, the great founding stallion at Broad Creek, goes back to Matchem, whereas Broad Creek's two other founding stallions from the 1880s, Limelight and Loopy Lou, eventually trace back to Eclipse."

"What about his new stallion, St. Boniface?" Sister asked. "Phil is very shrewd about stallions."

"Goes straight back to Ribot 1952, which will finally get you back to Eclipse." He swiveled his chair to face Ben again. "Any breeding establishment tries to go with the percentages. If a stallion has been able to throw a high percentage of Grade One stakes winners, naturally, you push him forward."

"That's where I differ." Sister sat upright. "I pay more attention to the mare."

"Well, true enough but a mare produces one foal a year, if she catches," said Mercer. "Whereas a stallion can cover many mares. It's all numbers or, as I like to think of it, the economy of scale."

"So Broad Creek has great blood?" Ben, not versed in pedigrees, was interested.

"Kept the farm alive through thick and thin but the funny thing is, no one gave a fig for Navigator before he started to breed," Mercer told them. "He goes back to Matchem but his immediate sire, Seneca and his grandsire, Naughty Nero, so-so. No one paid much attention to the horse but Old Tom Chetwynd said, 'Hell, let's try him.' So he bred a couple of in-house mares. Those foals started winning at age three and every crop after that, there were a high percentage of winners. If you go back far enough, you'll find Australian 1858 in Navigator's pedigree, and finally you get back to Matchem. But you never know."

"Old Tom bred to his own mares?" Sister was very curious.

"Initially he did," said Mercer. "He loaded the dice and put Navigator to a few of his best. It was his only chance if the horse had any quality at all."

"Why didn't they race him?" Ben asked.

"As you know, Broad Creek has its own training track and I guess Navigator's times were slow. I don't know. Long before my time. Even Phil doesn't know. You never ever know. A lackluster runner can produce wonderful foals. Some stallions produce great colts, others great fillies or broodmares. Some horses run better on turf than dirt. It's roulette, genetic roulette."

"But study helps," Ben said.

"Sure." Mercer flicked a few more pedigrees on the screen. "Sister, you know more about Warmbloods than I do." He named a larger, heavier horse than a Thoroughbred, a horse much used for show jumping.

"Not a lot." She peered at the screen. "Holsteiner. Lovely." Then she smiled at Ben. "When I was a girl and even unto my forties, no Warmbloods. No horses of color in the field either. By that, I mean paints, palominos, et cetera. Because all you saw were Thoroughbreds. Anyway, the Warmblood craze started here in the 1970s. The old line is: When you start a hunt, you're glad you're on a Warmblood, when you finish you're glad you're on a Thorough-bred."

Mercer filled in the blanks. "Warmbloods are calmer but they don't necessarily have the extraordinary stamina of a Thoroughbred. However, if someone gets their horse-hunting fit, the animal can usually last at least two to three hours, depending on the pace."

"Crawford rides a Warmblood, a lovely animal," Sister informed Ben. "Okay, we've sat here and blabbed on. Why are we here, really?"

The sheriff turned his hands up, then let them drop. "Because I'm in the dark. I can't see even a pinprick of light in Penny's murder, so I'm trying anything."

"Like whether she knew someone was breeding a horse with a passable flaw?" Mercer inquired.

"That was one idea."

"Ben, that would certainly be an issue in terms of veterinary expense for an unsuspecting buyer but a lot of possibilities may never occur," said Mercer. "Your mother may have diabetes, it may be in her family. Doesn't mean you'll get it. We go back to percentages. And the stud fees are really an issue only in the Thoroughbred world. Other breeds are less expensive, the fees."

"And Penny couldn't prove wrongdoing," Sister added. "She could only note to a buyer, if asked to vet the horse, what those possibilities might be."

Ben grasped the issue. "Still, it could be a sales killer."

"Yes, but you take a field hunter. A vet comes along who vets the animal as though he is going to race. That's a real sales killer." She laughed.

Mercer, too, said with amusement, "You take someone new to horses, the vet comes along and points out every tiny flaw and the person panics, just panics. No sale. The key phrase for a foxhunter is 'serviceably sound' and some vets can't do it. They are terrified of lawsuits. It's like just about any other profession these days. There's someone waiting in the wings to point the finger, bring a suit. I'm amazed any business ever gets done."

"Well, I don't think it's quite that bad but what Mercer says is true," Sister agreed. "But what he isn't saying is that a vet can be paid off."

This shut the other two right up.

"What?" Ben's eyebrows shot up.

Sister frowned. "A vet can pass a horse with a serious flaw if given enough money under the table. Some do. Corruption appears in all lines of work, Ben, even law enforcement."

A long pause followed this, then Ben, voice low, "Do you think Penny could have been party to that? Let's take Broad Creek Stables, since they are the biggest Thoroughbred breeder here. Do you think Phil would have given her money under the table?"

"No," both replied at once.

"But it happens," Sister calmly repeated the idea. "When a couple of hundred thousand are at stake, a lot of folks with shaky ethics wobble."

"Not Penny," Mercer loudly defended her. "And not Phil. You have two of his youngsters. Look at how sound they are. They just aren't that fast and furthermore, Midshipman doesn't want to race. On the other hand, I am willing to bet he will love hunting. It's more natural than running around an oval."

"I don't mean to imply that Phil paid off Penny," said Sister. "It's a kind of conjecture. A payoff would only be worth the risk if large sums of money lay on the table. And buyers for Broad Creek Stables horses usually have their own vets anyway, because the best of those animals are sold at Keeneland or Fasig Tipton." She named two sales venues of high quality.

"I see," said Ben. "So Penny wouldn't be used?"

"No," Sister replied. "She might be consulted here before the animals are shipped. Kind of an insurance policy. But she wouldn't be a candidate for that kind of dishonesty. Nor would she have done it."

Both men nodded in agreement.

"I looked at the drawings she had of horses," said Ben. "You know, where the vet marks a problem. She was thorough." He could read the illustration because when he bought Nonni, he was given one by the vet, who happened to be Penny.

"Ben, I don't think we've helped you one bit," Sister said sorrowfully.

"Actually, you have. You've helped me understand where other kinds of crimes could be hidden. First, I was thinking about drugs. And then seeing all her research, I wondered if there was some kind of tie-in, something I wouldn't know because I'm not really a horseman. I'm just a rider. You two were born into horses. I wish I knew what you forgot." He smiled.

As Mercer turned off the computer, Sister pointed to the screen. "Hey, turn that back on a minute. Go to the DNA stuff."

Mercer did and she quickly read as he moved the text along for her.

"Forgive me. But now I'm curious. We know Midshipman goes ultimately back to Matchem."

"Right." Mercer looked at Sister.

"I want to run a DNA test and we'll see how it works," Sister said. "Maybe if I go through the process, there might be something in Penny's research that resonates. It's worth a try."

Ben shrugged.

"Who can you use?" Mercer could think of a lot of good vets.

"I'll tell you after the research. If word should leak out, it might look bad for Penny and Westlake. You know how people jump to conclusions and it might not be so good for the vet either, as he or she will be bombarded by a lot of people who stick their noses in other people's business."

"Not me." Mercer smiled sheepishly.

She fibbed. "Never gave you a second thought."

"So you don't think Penny's sudden interest in pedigree and DNA was just a notion?" Mercer posited triumphantly.

"No, I don't." Sister held up her hand to quiet him. "But I don't know why. A hunch."

CHAPTER 25

Midshipman stood in the cross ties in the center aisle of Sister's barn. Tootie was pulling his mane, a standard grooming procedure endured by horses though not especially liked by them. Two ropes with clips, each affixed to the side of the aisle, helped the horse stand still as the clip fit on his halter. They were literally cross ties.

Rickyroo was watching from his stall. *"You got a lot of mane, boy,"* the old horse said.

"Oh, just give him a buzz cut," Keepsake teased from the neighboring stall. *"He'll look like a marine."*

The youngster remained quiet. He knew the older horses were giving him the business, one of many tests they would throw at him. The other horses demanded more patience from him than the humans.

Nearby in his stall, Matchplay whinnied. *"No one's touching my mane."*

Lafayette snorted, *"Let me tell you something, son. You landed in a great place. These people know horses and they take care of us. You shut up and learn to take care of them."*

Matchplay's nostrils flared. Having been nipped once over the fence line by Matador, he thought better of sassing back to an older horse.

Sister came up to Tootie, opened a Ziploc bag. Tootie dropped a bit of pulled mane into it with the root bulbs attached.

"That should do it." The Master returned to the tack room where Betty and she cleaned tack. Under hanging tack hooks that looked like grappling hooks, two buckets of warm water, clean sponges, saddle soap, and even toothbrushes had been laid out on towels.

Working on a bridle with a simple eggbutt snaffle, Betty said, "What's better than a heated tack room with a little kitchen?"

Sister smiled. "A bigger tack room with a bigger kitchen?"

"More to clean," Betty replied.

"I haven't done too good a job here." She looked down at the tartan rug. "All those years I polished the floor. Finally put this rug down and it is easier to vacuum than wash and polish but boy, it shows every single mud bit."

"Hard, hard winter. Ice. Mud. Snow. Sleet. And sometimes all in the same day. Have you noticed that on some of our fixtures, the footing is better?"

"Yes, I have. Time to break out the soil maps and review them all." Sister dipped a washrag into the warm water, then wrung it dry. "I wonder if I should put the mane hairs in the fridge?"

"No, why?"

"Things keep better if they're cool."

"Doesn't matter. Are you taking the mane to Greg or is he coming here?"

"He'll be by later. I miss seeing him. He travels so much now since he sold the practice."

Greg Schmidt, DVM, had sold his veterinary clinic with the idea to retire. In a sense he did retire, but his reputation meant people would call and beg him to speak at a conference, or to please just look at this one horse, et cetera and so forth. Despite not wanting to bother him, Sister had always relied on his superior judgment, discretion, and marvelous common sense. He was the only person she trusted to run a DNA test on Midshipman. It wasn't that most working vets were gabby, but something might slip out. She would take no chances. Greg was a deep well.

"Every now and then I dream about traveling like him," said Sister. "Cutting back on the responsibilities. I'd like to see South Africa and Namibia, Botswana. I've visited almost every former British colony but not those places nor India. Wherever the British were, there are good horses."

"Is this your revenge on the Empire speech?" Betty lifted one eyebrow like an arch actress.

Sister shook her head. "No. But I believe all of us once under the British flag have a great deal in common."

"Even India?" Betty was quick.

"Don't know. I haven't been there, but India is the world's largest democracy. And they inherited that incredible British civil service."

"You read too much," Betty teased her.

"Not enough. And who's talking? Of course, you stuff yourself with those hideous romances." Sister then spoke in a breathy voice. "She noticed his rippling chest, his piercing green eyes, the black two-day-old stubble. Her heart beat faster."

"Sounds good to me. Maybe you should try writing one of those. Boost your income."

They laughed just as Dr. Greg Schmidt, early, walked into the tack room.

"A two-day-old stubble," Betty repeated, bent over laughing. "Love that!"

Greg, always a good sport, ran his hand over his cheek. "I'm getting lazy."

"Don't pay any more attention to her than if she was a goat

barking," said Sister. "Greg, our Betty Franklin, a seemingly intelli-gent, levelheaded woman, has become intoxicated by romances and all the male heroes sport stubble."

The retired vet beamed. "So I'm in good company."

"Always." Sister handed him the Ziploc. "What a good boy that horse is. Didn't fuss when Tootie pulled his mane. She's now giving Midshipman the Roughneck Farm day of beauty."

Greg peeped out the window in the door that opened into the center aisle. "You know, he reminds me of Curlin, who stands at Lane's End Farm. One of the most beautiful Thoroughbreds I've ever seen."

"Lane's End." Betty said the establishment's name in such a way that confirmed its exalted status.

"Some of those farms in Kentucky are incredible," said Sister. "The knowledge is generations deep. Think of the Hancocks," she added, mentioning a prominent family.

Greg—Ziploc between his forefinger and thumb—leaned against the saddle rack. "Well, you know better than I that once upon a time Virginia and Maryland boasted horsemen of many generations."

"What is it they call people who leave to film outside of L.A.?" Betty paused. "Runaway production. That's it. Well, we've sure seen it here in the racing world."

"The Chenerys left. Ned Evans died. The late Clay Camp fi-nally left Virginia for Kentucky. What a brain drain." Greg stated a bare truth. "People who come here now aren't racing people. It's three-day eventers, show people, foxhunters, of course, and great as all that is—clean money, no pollution, all that good stuff—still, it's not the same as racing. Racing brings millions into a state. Right now the equine industry brings one-point-three billion dollars into Virginia. Just imagine what that figure would be if the old days re-turned?"

"Greg, I think of it a lot." Sister wiped down the bridle with a clean dry cloth. "When people ask me how do I feel about getting old, I say, 'Wonderful, because I lived through some of the best years this country and the horse world ever had. I'm lucky.'"

"I caught some of that when I moved here from California." The tall, silver-haired man looked at the bridle Sister was cleaning. "Who are you hunting in an eggbutt snaffle?"

"Aztec," Sister replied. "He has such a sensitive mouth, I don't need much."

"I've always liked that bit. When you started hunting, Sister, I bet people rode in double bridles."

"Plenty did. The bit sewn into the bridle. I still use bridles, English, with the bit sewn in."

"Greg, you know what a stickler she is," said Betty. "I change my bits. Sister sniffs when she sees me do it and tells me I can afford the true hunting bridle."

"I do not." Sister defended herself.

"Ha. I once saw you tell a man he had his garters on backward."

"Well, Betty, he did. I considered the correction an act of kindness."

"Eagle eye." Greg smiled at Sister. "Well, ladies, I'd better head home. Called the lab. Not much going on. You'll have your DNA results quickly. Week at the most."

With his hand on the doorknob, Sister asked, "Greg, did you ever talk to Penny about pedigree research? Equine genome?"

He thought for a moment, looked down at the plaid rug, then up. "One of the biggest arguments I ever had with Penny was over just that. She showed me the papers on some appendix crosses, gave the history of the horse, which I knew, then compared them to some of the Thoroughbreds she saw."

"She saw a lot of horses," Betty added noncommittally. "More once you retired."

Greg smiled. "She swore that a lot of Thoroughbreds were

turning into hothouse flowers, the stamina and bone being bred right out of them. She wondered why the Jockey Club didn't wise up and allow judicious outcrosses." He frowned. "Penny, I said, 'Never. Never. Never. Never!' Well, we got into it. I said the problem wasn't the Thoroughbred, it was the people who breed them. If someone knew what they were doing, they could and would breed a strong horse. I believe the Thoroughbred is the greatest athlete ever. She couldn't believe I was that conservative; I think her word was conservative. Better than jerk, I suppose."

Greg smiled at the memory, then continued, "But Penny was young, remember. She hadn't seen many of the old-style Thorough-breds, heavier cannon bone, you know what I'm saying. I laid into her about paper breeders, people who look at bloodlines but not the horses. That and the real problem is writing racetrack conditions so inferior horses can make a buck. There's a race for every possible horse, especially inferior ones. She blew up at me. Whew!" He spiraled his forefinger up in the air.

"How long did it take before she spoke to you again?" Betty wondered aloud.

"Not long. She apologized for losing her temper. Penny had such a good heart. She cared so much for horses and it pained her to see so many leg injuries. For West Nile virus, stuff like that, we have vaccines, but fragile legs, there is no cure. That's breeding," Greg remarked with feeling.

"She did have a good heart." Sister's tone softened. "Greg, I have a feeling that her death is tied up in all this, even though there's no way that woman would ever be party to anything shadowy."

"No, never," Greg rapidly agreed. "Penny was straight up."

"And because of that, if she found wrongdoing, I think she would have blown the whistle," Sister said.

"Yes, she would." Greg looked at the mane hairs in the Ziploc.

"Sister, I'll get right on this. I won't send it to the lab. I'll drive it down."

As he left, Sister knew he followed her line of thought, most especially what she didn't say.

Betty, too, had a vague sense. "Jane, what are you getting into?"

"I don't know."

"Be careful. We have no idea why Penny was killed or who did it, obviously. But if you blunder into something, well—"

Sister lifted up another bridle. "They have to catch me first."

"Don't be a smart-ass."

CHAPTER 26

Clytemnestra, mean as snakeshit, big as a house, glowered as the trailers parked at Foxglove Farm. The heifer's son, Orestes, now larger than his mother, evidenced a much sweeter personality. Nonetheless, if hounds traveled through their back pastures, the field certainly did not. No one wants to be chased by a giant bovine.

As this was Saturday, March 1, skies overcast, mercury hanging at 48°F, the field overflowed.

Cindy Chandler, owner of Foxglove, kept her foxes happy. She had a mating pair under the old schoolhouse, a mile and a half from the main barn. Another male fox lived at the eastern edge of her property and occasionally Comet would travel over from Roughneck Farm.

An accomplished gardener, one with a long knowledge of plants, Foxglove delighted all who hunted there unless they offended Clytemnestra. The clapboard barn, the old clapboard schoolhouse, the clapboard house, all sparkled in good condition, impressive given the hard winter. No paint peeled.

Painted fencecoat black, three-board fences marked off intelligently laid-out pastures and paddocks. However, what always excited comment from newcomers were the two ponds at different levels, a small water wheel between them.

Today, ice rimmed both ponds. The raised walkway between the ponds had some icy spots but the water wheel—quite simple as opposed to the enormous one at Mill Ruins—still flowed, the wheel lazily turning.

Hounds promptly moved off at 10:00 A.M. Shaker included all the young entry in today's draw. They'd been working all season, a couple here, a couple there, then two couple—until now, when all the youngsters could go.

With Clytemnestra at his back, glaring while she chewed expensive hay, Shaker prudently cast in the opposite direction from the brooding beast.

Near the front of First Flight, Phil looked over his shoulder. "That has to be the biggest heifer I have ever seen. Each year she's larger."

"Why does Cindy waste good hay on her?" complained Mercer. "Cows have four stomachs. She doesn't need the pricey stuff," he quipped.

"Oh, yes, she does," said Cindy, riding behind Mercer.

A flush over Mercer's face indicated that once again he had opened his mouth before looking around or thinking. Fortunately, Cindy possessed both charm and a great sense of humor. She wasn't the least offended by his criticism.

"Sorry, Cindy," Mercer apologized instantly. "I didn't realize you were back there."

"If he'd known, he might have babbled even more," Phil tormented Mercer.

"Well, gentlemen, if Clytemnestra eats four-star hay, she behaves herself. If not, she will smash right through a fence. Actually, I believe she could take out the barn if she'd a mind to."

Up front, Sister heard them chattering, as well as others. She loathed a chatty field but hounds had not yet been cast, spirits were high, why squelch them? If the blab continued once hounds were working, well, that's different.

"Lieu in." Shaker put the pack into a thin line of woods below the ponds, using the old Norman term now about one thousand years old.

This woods expanded to the north, providing good hiding places for foxes, bobcats, deer, raccoons, and the occasional weasel.

This morning, red-tailed hawks, red-shouldered hawks, and broad-tailed hawks sat motionless in treetops. All of them hoped hounds would scare up voles, moles, mice, and other little rodents. Perhaps those raptors were the original foodies.

Riding with Sybil today, Tootie trotted at woods' edge as they headed due east. If the pack had turned right, they would be heading south, finally running into Soldier Road. Foxglove Farm boundaries were more natural than man-made, with the exception of Soldier Road. Natural boundaries can be easier to hunt than man-made ones and Shaker was making the most of it.

Hounds worked the edge of the woods; a few, noses down, walked along the pasture by the woods while the bulk of the pack moved through the woods. For Sister, this was a complete cast. She wanted her hounds fanning out. Other Masters and huntsmen did not. Everyone had their own ways and their own reasons. Sister wanted her hounds to do what was called "Make good the ground." She wanted as much ground studied by those superb hound noses as possible.

The ponds—now above the field, to the right—lowered the temperature a bit as they all moved alongside them.

Older Asa, out today for his once-a-week hunt, widened his search heading to the bottom of the ponds' high banks.

Hounds, horses, and people really do become wiser with age and Asa, feeling the slight temperature drop, also could smell more moisture below those banks. He stopped, inhaled deeply, moved a few paces, inhaled again. His tail slowly waved to and fro, then that stern picked up speed.

"Hot. A hot line!" With that, he ran straight up until he was now level with the top pond.

No reason for any hound to check Asa, the pack immediately rushed to him. Shaker didn't even have to say, "Hark."

Within seconds the whole pack opened, the young entry beside themselves with excitement.

On the south side, Betty kept at two o'clock. She wanted to be on somewhat higher ground, which afforded her a wider view. The First Whipper-in, which Betty was, often sees the fox first. If a cast is like the face of a clock, Shaker is in the middle where the two hands meet. Hounds start at twelve o'clock. Betty was to their right at two o'clock. Sybil would ride at ten o'clock. Once a fox tore off, the staff did their best to maintain those positions but ground conditions could make it difficult.

If a hunt is fortunate enough to have a professional whipper-in, that individual is usually given the title of First Whipper-in. A few hunts in North America carried three to four paid whippers-in— wonderful for them and really wonderful for a young person starting out, say, being given the slot of Fourth Whipper-in. There's only one way to learn foxhunting, and that's by doing it.

Sister occasionally dreamed of a paid whipper-in or even two, say, young men or women in their middle twenties, but her two honorary whippers-in—loyal, reliable, shrewd in the ways of quarry—could have been professionals. Sister was proud of Betty and Sybil and knew that putting Tootie out with them would fast-forward the young woman's knowledge.

On a good trail in the woods, Sybil held hard, as did Tootie. A medium-sized red fox shot right in front of them, plunging deep down into a narrow crevice in the land. The two women counted to twenty, then bellowed, "Tallyho!"

The count to twenty is plenty sufficient for a fox.

Hearing the call, Shaker waited. His hounds were turning in that direction. In his mind, to pick them up and throw them into the woods would be to undermine them. Both Shaker and Sister wanted hounds to work on their own, be confident and not dependent on constant human interference.

Asa was no longer in the lead, as he wasn't fast enough. He worked in the middle of the pack. Irritating though it was to fall back to the middle, he knew he did his job. One of the youngsters, Zorro, shot over the line, then pulled up, confused. He wailed.

"Shut up, Zorro," Asa called to the tricolor in his deep voice. *"Come back to the middle."*

Zorro wanted to be first but he returned to the middle, for he had an inkling he'd messed up.

In their prime, Tattoo and Pickens now led the pack with Dreamboat, Diana, and Dasher close behind, the rest of the pack just behind them. They all headed into the woods, where their voices ricocheted off the trees. All slid down into the crevice, then clambered out as the humans circled round, losing time in the process.

Sister knew her fixtures. No need to kick on Matador. Keeping a steady pace, Shaker and hounds in sight, she put the field in a good position. They splashed across the narrow creek, running down the wide path on the other side. Then . . . silence.

Sister pulled up to see the pack gathered at the base of a tree. A fox, a beautiful gray in full winter coat, sat on a wide branch above. This was not the fox Sybil and Tootie had seen. Hounds had been on another fox's line that ended up at the tree.

Shaker blew "Gone to Ground" because there are no special notes for "Climbed a Tree."

Zorro, Zane, and Zandy couldn't believe a fox lounged over their heads. The other hounds, however, had seen this many times.

"You come down, this isn't fair," Zandy bitterly moaned in her high-pitched voice.

"Cheater," Zane added to the disgust of his sister. *"You're a cheater."*

Smiling, the gray called down, *"Well, why don't you get right under me, stand on your hind legs. Maybe you can grab my tail and pull me down."*

"Yeah. Right." Zorro did just that, with his two littermates now on their hind feet.

The fox taunted them a little more, swinging his butt over the tree limb and urinating all over them, laughing loudly.

"Ow, ow, ow. It stings!" Zorro blinked his eyes as the older hounds couldn't believe the youngsters would do what a fox told them to do.

Sitting on his haunches, Asa declared, *"Young and dumb."*

Hounds laughed, horses laughed, and the people laughed, although they had no idea what Asa had said.

Shaker, thumbs-up to the fox, turned his horse Showboat around. "Come along, hounds. Come along. No telling what he'll do next."

Having a girl moment, Tootsie wrinkled her nose at the humiliated Zandy. *"Don't get near me!"*

Poor thing. Zandy dropped her ears, falling back in the pack where Pookah walked beside her without saying a word.

Shaker left the woods and rode up on the hill. The ponds below sparkled as a shaft of light sliced through the clouds; then, like quicksilver, disappeared.

He cast hounds up toward the schoolhouse. Fox scent led to it, a short burst with singing ended at the foundation. A pair lived inside and had no incentive to open the front door.

Shaker sat by the schoolhouse. Sister waited, as did the field. Gray rode up with Phil and Mercer. The Bancrofts rode right behind Sister. Kasmir and Alida rode together behind Gray. As with any hunt, the longer one is out, the more the well-mounted, fit rider and horse move forward. Because of the recent weather, many people had not been able to keep their horses in as good a shape as they wished, but right now, all was well. No one was winded. Bobby Franklin kept an eye on his group, especially since new people usually started in Second Flight. He watched their horses for them. If a horse began to lag or tuck up a bit, Bobby would kindly send them back, with a guide always, at a walk.

Shaker motioned for his whippers-in to come up to him. The pack sat, waiting.

"Betty, go down to the wildflower meadow," he said. "If the pack crosses the road, you'll be with them. Sybil, parallel me on the other side of the fence and Tootie, you take the right. I'm casting west then south once we reach the meadow. Wind's come up a bit. We'll head into it."

He waited as they moved off, giving Betty an extra five minutes. Tootie, first time alone as a whipper-in, actually wasn't nervous. She loved it.

"All right, lieu in." Shaker asked the hounds to draw on the south side of the farm road.

They wiggled under the fence. Five minutes passed, ten, then fifteen. Shaker and Showboat walked on the farm road, ice crystals in the ruts.

A peep, then a bark sent the huntsman into a trot. Showboat took three strides to easily clear the coop, painted black like the fence. Sister and the field followed while Bobby trotted down to a large farm gate.

Hounds worked the line, not enough for a roaring chorus but the scent was warming.

The pack moved into the wildflower meadow, nothing but brown stalks now. Betty crashed through winter's debris, staying tight on their left shoulder while Sybil came out of the woods above her, behind Shaker. As the pack headed straight for the road, so did Sybil.

Betty crossed with them. Sybil—who always rode effortlessly, no fuss—brought up the rear, making certain no hound lagged on the macadam highway. Given that all the young entry hunted today, Sybil correctly flew up there with extra vigilance.

Also over the farm-road coop, Tootie stayed on the right, crossing the road minutes after Sybil. Tootie found herself in the mess below Hangman's Ridge. There was no easy way up or down on either side of the broad flat plateau. Given that she lived at Sister's, she knew where the deer trails were. Finally, on one she headed upward. Already halfway up the steep incline, Betty marveled at the pack. Hangman's Ridge harbors all manner of game and the youngsters, while being exposed to some of the scents, had not yet smelled others. They never took their noses or eyes off the correct line.

As Betty stood in the stirrups, reins in her left hand, right hand entwined in Magellan's mane, she was able to stay over her horse's center of balance.

Sybil picked her way to the left of this, finally reaching the base of the ridge where she, too, picked up a narrow trail to circle the base. Given the distance, she had to move as fast as she could.

Betty finally reached the top of Hangman's Ridge, the wind blowing as always. Minks scattered about as the hounds flew across the flat plain.

Shaker now reached the top, stopped for a moment, saw Betty go down the Roughneck side. He followed. Sound echoed around the ridge but it seemed that hounds moved forward and down.

Sister galloped across the top, the huge centuries-old hangman's tree to her right.

Cursing the hounds, horses, and people all the while, minks ran across the top.

Not one bird sat in the hangman's tree. They didn't like it.

With great effort, Sybil had rounded the base, and now could see the old orchard on the other side of the Roughneck Farm road. To her delight, she also saw Comet. He skimmed the surface of the road as he ran hard, then turned left toward her. He knew who she was and, before he reached her, he zigged right, reached the stone ruins to pop into his den. Sybil remained motionless because she didn't want to cross the line.

Within minutes the pack ran right in front of her, Dreamboat, Giorgio, and young Pickens up front closely followed by the entire pack, Betty immediately behind and Shaker perhaps a football field behind her. Normally Betty would have ridden off the road, parallel to it, but there was no way to do that coming down from the ridge. The minute she hit the farm road, she jumped over the old orchard fence to parallel the pack, then jumped out again and into the stone ruins field, holding up at a bit of distance from the den.

By the time Shaker reached it, hounds dug at the stones, carried on in high excitement.

"Go ahead. Bloody your paws," Comet taunted.

Having been made a fool of once today, Zorro stopped digging at the stones.

Sister and the field came up as Shaker dismounted, blew "Gone to Ground," and praised each hound. He caught his breath as did everyone else.

The distance back to Foxglove Farm was perhaps three miles straight as an arrow and involved climbing, sliding down, rough terrain.

Sister waited for Shaker to mount up. He stood on the stones and stepped onto Showboat who stood still, as a huntsman's horse should. Horses get excited by the chase, too, so staff is always grateful when their mount does what he's supposed to do.

Sister then rode up. "We're near the kennels. Let's put them up and we can drive over to Cindy's to fetch the hound truck and Betty can drive the trailer back."

"Right."

She rode back to the field, telling them to return to Foxglove, she and staff would reach Cindy's place a little later.

Once at Roughneck, Tootie and Betty took care of the horses. Sybil also dismounted, stripped her tack off, sponged her horse, dried him, then borrowed a blanket. She'd come back later with her trailer.

Sister and Shaker walked hounds to the kennels.

"This last month has been so good." Sister beamed.

"Really has," he agreed.

As extra rations and lots of fresh water were poured into the buckets and hound troughs, Sister wiped her eyes. The fox piss scent was overwhelming. "What are we going to do with the smell?"

"Don't pick on me," Zorro cried. *"I didn't know."*

Hearing the puppy cry as he stared directly at her, Sister praised him. "You hunted very well today. And foxes are tricky."

Shaker and Sister praised each hound, calling every name and then when finished with the treats, calling each hound by name again to go to their special runs and petting everyone.

Shaker sniffed his hand. "Let's put these three in the medical run."

"Good idea. Zane, Zandy, Zorro, come along. Special motel tonight." Sister and Shaker walked to one of the doors off the big draw room, opened it, and the three obediently followed.

Once they were given an extra cookie plus fresh straw for bedding in the warm enclosed recovery room, Shaker advised, "We can wash them tomorrow. I'll get the straw out first thing."

Both Shaker and Sister washed their hands in the deep stainless steel sink.

"All right. Tootie can help us." Sister glanced at the wall clock in the special medical room, which even had an operating table. "We'd best get over there. I'll borrow Gray's Land Cruiser. We can all squeeze in there."

"Sister, I'll drive my truck. You know how he is about his Land Cruiser."

She paused. "You're right. The girls and I will bounce over in my truck."

"I'll take Tootie," said Shaker, "then you only have to fit in three."

"Thank you. Good thing we're all slim, isn't it?"

In full swing, the breakfast greeted the staff as they walked into the Foxglove dining room, more eighteenth century than twenty-first.

Alida thanked Sister. "Another wonderful day and Kasmir lent me Mumtaz for Saturdays, Kavita for Tuesdays. And I can use my horse on Thursdays. Such fabulous horses."

Sister looked over the crowd to see Kasmir talking to Gray. "He is a generous soul and a good, good man. We're all lucky to have him in our club." She prayed to herself that perhaps lightning would strike Alida.

The beauty glowed. "Yes. Yes, I can see that. I have never met a kinder man."

"Nor I." Sister took a chance. "You know, Alida, as I have aged I have learned just how sexy kindness and ethics are."

Alida looked into those bright hazel eyes with her own soft brown ones. "Yes. Yes, Master, how very true."

Before more could be said, Mercer charged up. "I have an idea."

"God help me," Sister joked.

Phil hurried over with Cindy, along with Betty and Ben. "Actually, Sister, it's a good one. We've all been discussing it."

"I know you e-mailed your curriculum suggestions to Craw-ford. Right?" Mercer referred to their Custis Hall board duties.

"I did," replied Sister. "Actually, I thought they were creative. At least I hope they are. I suggested we use hunting to teach the girls about the environment. And we don't always need to ride. We can do walking tours."

"Great idea," Phil said supportively.

"Well, here's what we've been thinking," said Mercer. "Next week is our next to last week and Woodford will be here from Kentucky for our Thursday hunt and our Saturday hunt. So why not invite Crawford?" Mercer held his hands together as though suppressing a clap.

"Putting both packs together?" Sister wondered aloud.

Mercer immediately saw the problem. "Well—"

A born mediator, Cindy offered her idea. "Ask him for Thursday to make it a triple meet, even though he's an outlaw pack. We can say he's a farmer pack, which in essence he is if he'd just be halfway decent to the MFHA. They are far more reasonable than he is. Crawford brings his pack; his new huntsman and Sam can whip in if he wants. The fixture is Oakside. Not too far for him."

Sister wasn't entirely convinced. "Well, let me ask Walter. I'm not opposed, but we have to consider how the MFHA will respond to a triple meet with one club being an outlaw pack. My suggestion is just for us and Crawford to go out together the last hunt of the season. This also gives Shaker time to ride with Skiff. Sorry, but it really is politics."

Cindy smiled, realizing Sister wanted to find a middle path, wanted to avoid open conflict with the national organization. "That's why you're the Master. You have to consider everything, but I think doubling up for our last meet is a great idea."

Desperately needing a drink, Sister trod toward the bar once the discussion wrapped up. She heard Phil say to Mercer, "Do you live to make life difficult?"

Mercer replied, "No, but I want to know really what's in my Dixie Do," he said, naming his horse.

"You know he goes back to Dixieland Band. He's a foxhunter, Mercer. It's irrelevant."

"I'm on a DNA kick," Mercer replied defiantly.

Sister thought that Mercer really couldn't let things go. She just hoped he wouldn't blurt out that Ben Sidell had asked them to review pedigrees. "He wouldn't," she thought.

Prudently, she sought out Ben once she had a cup of tea in her hand, and reported what she'd overheard. "Hopefully he'll stick to Dixie Do."

Ben shrugged. "I think he will, but I'll just give him a reminder." With that, the sheriff made straight for Mercer, grabbed his elbow, saying to Phil, "Excuse me one minute, Phil."

"Of course." Phil went looking for Sybil, as he wanted to know what the whipper-in thought of the day.

"Mercer." Ben fixed his gaze on the man. "Best not to discuss DNA or anything."

"I'm not." Mercer's eyes opened wide. "But I'm curious about my horse. That's all."

"Well, keep it at that, will you?"

Sister sidled up to Gray, who inhaled deeply. "Ah, yes, fresh fox."

"Honey, is it that bad? I walked the Z's to the back room. We'll wash them tomorrow."

"I've smelled expensive perfumes that weren't as potent," he teased her. "Hey, you can never predict what will happen."

She put her arm through his. "That's the truth."

CHAPTER 27

"Those little skulls with the glowing eyes have got to go," O.J. whispered as she rode up to the Saddlebred barn with Sister Jane.

"They are creepy," she agreed.

Woodford rode out with The Jefferson Hunt on Thursday at Oakside for the first of two joint meets. The field numbered thirty-five people—good for a cold rainy day.

Vicki Van Mater and Joe Kasputys drove down from Middleburg again to add to the mix. Along with their horses, their two German shepherds, Ben and Gandy Man, rode along. Vicki and Joe would laugh that the dog Ben was smart enough to do police work like the human Ben. While Vicki and Joe were intelligent, neither Ben nor Gandy felt their humans were in the German shepherd league. Much as they loved Vicki and Joe, they felt they needed guidance.

While the rain wasn't pounding, it slid inside collars and down the insides of boots if even the tiniest gap occurred. Cold feet were bad. Cold wet feet were even worse.

The Saddlebred barn emanated fright in the steady rain. The water washed the glowing skulls so the red eyes popped right out at you.

O.J. stiffened in the saddle as she caught sight of the hanging mannequin. "Dear God."

"Startling. I bet those pony clubbers screamed bloody murder when they saw that guy hanging," Joe teased.

Vicki gasped when she saw the hanged man.

Tedi Bancroft chuckled. "It really is awful."

Vicki replied, "I foxhunt so I can legally trespass and enjoy countryside I can only see from horseback. I may revise my opinion."

Joe laughed. "I'll mark the day you revise your opinion." He heard a hound open. "Then again, what's a barn of horrors if hounds open?"

The hound was Cora.

The two Masters shut up and squeezed their horses into a trot.

Hounds sang out but the pace stayed at a trot. Shaker stayed behind them, rain hitting him in the face.

Kasmir, Alida, Freddie, Phil, Mercer, Ronnie, Xavier—the stalwarts—filled First Flight, along with the guests. People in this part of the world organized their work schedules so they could hunt at least one day a week—if lucky, two.

Walter usually kept office hours on Thursdays and Bobby Franklin had an appointment today. He asked Ben Sidell to lead Second Flight, which he happily did.

The field crossed a meadow, took a log jump into another meadow, then threaded through woods, tree bark turning darker. Hounds continued after their fox at the same pace.

When they reached the back of this woods, everyone noticed swirling low mist rolling up from the abutting meadow. The swirl turned into a wall, a dense ground fog. The temperature dropped so rapidly everyone felt it. This wasn't a lower temperature in prox-

imity to water or a dip in the terrain. The mercury headed straight
down, the rain continued, but now a *pip, pip, pip* could be heard
hitting helmets.

Joe tweaked Vicki. "Honey, just remember this was your idea."

As the freezing fog enveloped them, hounds opened wide.

In territory she was learning, Sister stayed on the widest path
she could find. Ahead, she could just make out Shaker, thanks to
the scarlet coat.

Hounds turned toward them, then veered into the woods
again. Staying on the path, Shaker halted a moment to listen.

Twist's voice sounded the closest to Sister, then he, too, moved
away. Sister couldn't see a thing except Rickyroo's ears and neck. If
she stopped, everyone behind her would collide into one another.
She thought moving along the outside of the woods, keeping between the trees and the back fence line might work. If nothing else,
the fence line was a better guide than being in the middle of the
woods in a pogonip.

Did Woodford drag this curse along with them?

No point wondering about that. She trotted along, reached
the corner of the back fence and turned in what she felt was the
direction back to the barn. No way to hunt in this. The problem
now was getting everyone back.

Maria Johnson knew her property but she couldn't see anything either.

Hound voices echoed in the fog, near, then far, then near
again. Sister heard the horn: two beeps to tell hounds and staff
where Shaker was.

She thought she heard galloping hooves, perhaps a whipper-in,
but that faded away.

"Maria," Sister called out loudly.

"Yes," a voice replied, seemingly from the middle of the riders.

"Come up here. Can you?"

"Yes."

As Sister waited, she felt O.J.'s horse now beside her. "Can you believe we're in this freezing pea soup again? I blame it on you."

"And how do I know you didn't bring it to Kentucky?" countered O.J. "Don't blame me if we're in this mess again." Her voice floated toward Sister.

"Can you see me?"

"Not well."

"So you can't see me flip you the bird?"

O.J. laughed. "Sister, I am shocked, deeply shocked."

O.J. felt a horse slide by her, then she saw Maria. O.J. fell back.

Sister minced no words. "How the hell do we get back?"

"We aren't far. I'll ride next to you and when we have to we'll go single file. I'll go up front. All right?" offered the blue-eyed Maria.

Sister kept her sense of humor. "Do I have a choice?"

"Come on." Maria asked her dark bay Thoroughbred, Annie, to walk out.

Ten minutes later they reached another fence corner. Maria turned right, still inside the fence. The freezing rain stung as it turned to sleet, lots of sleet.

People dropped their faces. Gloves became soaked. Those who did as was proper had white string gloves under their girths and pulled them out. They would become soaked, too, but the reins didn't slip.

There was abundant misery for all.

"We're almost there." Maria spoke to Sister.

The next ten minutes seemed like an eon. First one trailer appeared, then disappeared, then another. But everyone did find their trailers.

"Thank you," Sister said to the much younger woman.

"Do you need help? I can go look for hounds," Maria volunteered.

Just then they all heard the horn close by. Giorgio appeared, Sister spied a few tricolor coats next to her. Then Shaker.

She sighed. "How glad I am to see you."

"Damn, this came out of nowhere." Shaker dismounted, walked his horse toward where he thought the trailer was. Wrong trailer. He looked at this one, getting up close, then remembered where the others had parked.

When he finally reached the right trailer, Betty was already there. She held open the door and hounds gratefully hurried inside, snuggling in the straw.

Shaker blew for Sybil and Tootie. "Betty, go on and see to your horse," he said. "I'll wait by the trailer."

Hojo, his mount today, usually rode in the trailer with the horses. Shaker had a divider for the horse so hounds wouldn't get underfoot. The hounds had a second story in the trailer with a rubber-covered walk so everyone could get in and not be crowded. Shaker didn't want to put Hojo inside until his other whippers-in showed up. He prayed they had the hounds Parker and Pickens with them.

As he waited, he threw a blanket over Hojo, over the saddle, too. "Hold on, buddy. Let's hope this doesn't take long. If it does, I promise I'll walk you to their barn, if I can find it."

A hound wiggled between his legs.

Sybil appeared. "That's Pickens. Would you blow again? I think Parker was with me five minutes ago. Lost sight."

Shaker blew three long notes.

As Sybil dismounted, they both waited.

And waited.

Shaker was ready to walk Hojo into the stable, wherever it was, when he heard a little yell.

"Where are you? Where am I?" came Parker's mournful howl.

"Parker. Parker. Come along." Shaker's voice radiated warmth and within seconds, a sleety hound raced up to him, couldn't contain himself, stood on his hind feet to see the huntsman.

"I'm so happy. I was scared!"

"All right, Parker, in we go." Shaker opened the door and the youngster scooted in.

No one wanted to come outside.

"Sybil, go on to your trailer. We've got everyone. I'll see you in the house."

"I think we need a compass," she joked.

Curled up in the straw on the trailer, Ben and Gandy rose to greet their masters, Joe on Ali Kat and Vicki on Boo Bear.

Gandy shook himself. *"You all are crazy."*

"Not me," the TB/Shire mix replied. *"It's her."* The horse indicated the human.

Fortunately Vicki understood nothing of this exchange.

"Joe, hurry up and put me in the trailer," his TB/Hanoverian begged.

The two Middleburg Hunt members hurried as fast as they could. Once the horses were up and wiped down, they looked at the dogs.

"We'll put them in the truck when we leave," Joe said sensibly. "It's warmer here with the horses and the straw than in the truck with the heater turned off."

"Okay," Vicki agreed.

When the humans left to grope their way to the house, Ben lifted his head. *"Hmm."*

Gandy Man inhaled deeply. *"Filthy day but that smells too interesting."* With that, the shepherd left the comfort of the trailer for the driving sleet. Ben followed.

Taking care of their mounts took longer, but after twenty minutes most people had put up their horses and done whatever needed to be done. Then some, holding hands, made their way to the house.

"We could form a chain." Alida smiled.

"If we don't reach the house in the next two minutes, we'd better," Xavier added.

Once inside everyone started talking, hurrying for hot drinks, breathing a sigh of relief.

The Woodford group caught up on the Hinson news, as well as Middleburg Hunt news. Everyone wanted to know about everyone else's season.

Phil made his way through the crowd, looking around. He spoke to people one by one, then came up to Sister and Gray. "Have you all seen Mercer?" he asked.

"No."

"His horse was at the trailer but untied. I put him on the trailer. I figured maybe he slipped the knot. Mercer doesn't always tie the best knot." Phil looked at the door when someone opened it. "It will be a good story when he gets inside." Phil rejoined the circle.

Sister made sure to speak to each Woodford guest, most of whom she knew. Maria, Nate, and Sonia kept a shuttle between the kitchen and the dining room. A good cook, Nate outdid himself.

Sister inhaled. "Did he make shepherd's pie?"

"He knows it's your favorite," Gray replied.

"How did he know that?"

"I told him, and I bet he's saved you a big slice in the kitchen. Otherwise, you won't get any."

True enough, for people stood in line for a slice—plus Sister rarely got to eat much at these gatherings.

A half hour passed with food, drink, chat and feet warming.

Phil returned. "Still no Mercer."

"That is peculiar," Gray said.

"I'm going out to look for him," said Phil. "This isn't like him. Maybe he fell and his horse came back. Who would know?" He walked toward the hall to fetch his jacket.

"I'll come with you." Gray put his plate on a small table and, as he walked away, he said to Sister, "Phil and I are going to look for Mercer."

"I'll come, too." She hurried to them.

Seeing them leave, worry on their faces, Xavier, Ronnie, and Kasmir also followed.

Once outside, the brutal weather hit them again.

"Won't do any good to look for hoofprints," Phil said. "They're all over the place."

"The only thing I can think to do is to backtrack," said Kasmir. "Let's walk down the middle path, then turn toward the fence line. At least I think that's the fence line." He pointed west.

Staying together, they trudged through now stinging sleet. The fog hadn't thinned.

Two dogs howling alerted them to something in the barn.

They reached the edge of the Saddlebred barn but couldn't see the glowing skulls, the sleet was so thick.

"*Blood.*" Ben held his nose up, following the scent inside the barn.

"*Fresh.*" Then Gandy Man shouted, as he heard the humans outside.

The mannequin sprawled on the barn floor. Swinging slightly from the rafter was Mercer, blood dripping down his coat.

"*Terrible trouble.*" The two German shepherds sang a dirge, hoping to hurry along the humans outside.

Following the cry as best they could Sister, Gray, Shaker, Phil, Kasmir, Ronnie, and Xavier stepped into the barn.

"Oh, my God," Phil gasped. "Mercer! Mercer!"

CHAPTER 28

In the old barn, Phil Chetwynd rolled old hay bales under Mercer's body. Being tall, he stepped upon them, holding Mercer's legs and, with great strength, lifted the body so the pressure was off the neck.

Ronnie Haslip, the most nimble, climbed up the rafters. Gray joined Phil. Gray knew Mercer was gone, but Phil, a man possessed, kept pleading, "We have to help him. Help me."

And so the other men did. Ronnie, like most foxhunters, carried a pocketknife. He cut the rope and Mercer dropped down into Gray and Phil's arms, the unexpected weight toppling them off the hay bales.

The two German shepherds, sitting down now, didn't budge.

Kasmir, Shaker, and Xavier, also by the hay bales, did their best to break the fall, trying to prevent Mercer's body from hitting the ground hard.

Xavier left the group to go back to the house and find Ben Sidell. Given the thick fog, he only found his way through the noise coming from the house.

Ben hurried out of the house with Xavier and Sister, groping their way to the Saddlebred barn. Once inside, the sheriff walked over to Mercer, carefully laid on the ground, on his back, bloodshot eyes staring upward.

Ben removed his leather hunting glove, placing his finger on Mercer's neck. He said nothing, for it was obvious that Mercer was dead. He wanted to feel the temperature of the body. His guess was the body had cooled very slightly. Clearly the man's neck was broken. Putting his glove back on so as not to leave more fingerprints, he gingerly tilted Mercer's head to the side where his hair was matted with blood. He'd first been struck by a blunt instrument.

Phil leaned over on the other side of the body. "Let me perform CPR. He's not dead. He can't be dead."

Ben rose, "I'm afraid he is, Phil."

"No!" Phil knelt down to pump on Mercer's chest.

Gray and Shaker had to lift Phil up, protesting.

With kindness but firmness, Ben said, "He's gone. Anything any of us do to him will compromise this crime scene." Turning to Sister, he said, "Will you go inside, tell everyone there has been an accident and no one must leave the house? Oh, Sister, when you get inside stay there until I get there, which will be some time. Don't tell anyone what has happened, only that there has been an accident. I'm going to call the department right now and hope a team makes it out here in this miserable fog before too much time passes. Obviously, the faster we can go over all this, the better."

"He can't be dead." Tears filled Phil's eyes. "He can't really be dead."

"Phil, I'm going to ask you to sit down on one of the hay bales. Xavier, will you sit with him? Oh, Gray, perhaps you'd better go in with Sister. And whose dogs are these?"

Sister, before heading into the slashing weather, answered, "Vicki and Joe's. The Middleburg folks."

"Ah, well, they seem well behaved. They'll have to stay here until folks are free to leave the house."

Fortunately, Ben's team arrived within forty minutes, a good time considering the deplorable conditions. Two law enforcement officers, both women, were sent into the house. Ben knew the women would be very good at calming people and getting statements. The new head of his forensic team went immediately to work and another young man carried a bright flashlight, as the electric power had long ago been cut off in this barn used only for hay storage and odds and ends.

No matter what happens in our life if you're hunt staff, hounds and horses must be attended to. Sister, Shaker, O.J., and Tootie, due to the long delay at Oakside, finally reached Roughneck Farm at 6:00 P.M. The hounds, subdued, ate warm kibble, then quietly returned to their lodges and sleeping quarters. Rickyroo, Hojo, and Iota, Tootie's horse, and O.J.'s mare, told everyone in the stable. Back at Oakside, Sister had asked Kasmir if he would take Phil's horse and Mercer's wonderful Dixie Do, to his farm. With Alida's help, Kasmir loaded them up.

At Tattenhall Station, the Indian gentleman watched as Alida brushed the horses and comforted them.

"My man can do that," Kasmir offered.

"They know something's wrong. Sometimes a bit of attention helps." Alida ran her fingers along Dixie Do's neck.

Kasmir bedded the stalls himself thinking here was a woman not afraid of work and one who was sensitive as well.

Gray called Sam and told him the news. He met his brother as soon as Ben Sidell released him from Oakside. They both drove to Daniella Laprade's. She took the grim news with steely calm, asked where her son's body was, and wanted to know when she could see him. Gray called Ben Sidell, who called back in twenty minutes, saying she could see her son now. Mercer wouldn't be sent to Richmond until tomorrow, assuming the weather improved.

So Gray and Sam drove their aunt to the county morgue. Using only a cane, Daniella stood firm as the large file cabinet, for that's what it looked like, was opened and the body slid out, feet first on the slab.

Both nephews stood on either side of her in case she collapsed.

"He was a good son." She then looked up at Gray. "Who did this?"

"Aunt D, we don't know."

"You'd better find him before I do. And it was a man. Women don't kill like this. Hear me?"

"Yes, ma'am," both brothers said.

Then she turned and walked out, barely using her cane.

Later, Sister, O.J., and Tootie, in the library at Roughneck Farm, discussed the remaining weekend.

O.J. leaned on soft cushions on the sofa. "I understand if you cancel Saturday's hunt, Sister. Perhaps you should."

"Mercer loved hunting. You all drove all the way from Kentucky. I think he'd want the hunt to go on. You know I'm a stickler for things being done properly. I wouldn't do this if I thought it would be slighting him." Sister stood up. "Let me call Walter. Best to discuss this with my Joint Master."

Walter had by now been informed of everything. As Sister sat at the desk, Tootie mulled over the awful happenings while talking to O.J.

"It's a strange coincidence," Tootie said. "The first pogonip and now this one and both—well, awful."

"Two murders." O.J. felt suddenly very tired.

"Three." Sister had hung up the landline. "You didn't know our local vet, Penny Hinson, but three. It can't be a coincidence. It can't be." She then returned to her chair, falling into it, also exhausted. "Walter agrees with me. Mercer would want the joint meet to continue and Saturday is the big day at the Bancrofts'. Always a beautiful fixture."

"Yes, it is," O.J. agreed.

They heard the back door open. The dogs ran to the kitchen, where Gray walked in from the mudroom.

"Gray." Sister rose to greet him. "Let me get you a drink."

He kissed her. "Thank you, honey."

Neither O.J. nor Tootie said anything until Sister handed him his drink and he was comfortably seated in an armchair. She held up an empty glass toward O.J.

"I believe I will." O.J. joined Sister at the bar. "I don't know why but I want an old-fashioned."

"Let's make two." Sister asked Tootie, "You're twenty-one. Anything?"

"No, thanks."

Once they were all seated and Gray had some restorative scotch in him, Sister asked, "How did it go?"

"No tears. No raised voice. She's really a terrifying old woman." He took another deep sip. "But I feel for her. She looked at him and said he was a good son. Then she wanted to know who killed him and told Sam and me to find the killer before she did."

O.J. frowned. "Like a Greek tragedy."

"In a way, yes." Gray set his drink on a coaster. "You know, I keep thinking about that old barn, the House of Horrors barn. Whoever killed Mercer had a kind of sick sense of humor."

O.J. murmured, "I guess."

"And whoever killed him knew the place," Sister added.

Tootie curled her legs under her. "And the killer took advantage of the rotten weather. It doesn't seem like a planned murder."

"No, it doesn't," Sister agreed. "You're right about there being something spontaneous about this. The pogonip provided the chance and he or she was tremendously bold."

"He. Aunt D says women don't kill like that." Gray spoke, having picked up his drink again.

"She's right," O.J. agreed.

The phone rang, Sister got up to answer it. After listening to Greg for a bit, Sister asked, "Eclipse? Eclipse, not Matchem?"

"Yes." On the other end of the line, Greg Schmidt's voice was positive.

"Eclipse." She then recited. "Pot-8-Os, Waxy, Whalebone, Camel, Touchstone, Orlando, the second Eclipse, Alarm, Himyar, then Domino. That line. That Eclipse line?"

"Yes," he repeated.

"I suppose you've heard by now all that's transpired?" said Sister.

Greg replied, "Tedi Bancroft called me. I'm so very sorry."

"Yes, I am, too. Greg, does anyone else know this, know Midshipman's line back?"

"I couldn't rightly say."

"Thank you." Sister hung up the phone, turned to the others and stated definitively, "Benny Glitters."

CHAPTER 29

Daniella appraised Mercer's house as she directed Gray and Sam in the large bedroom. "A place for everything and everything in its place," she said.

"We won't have the body for at least a week, I would think, Aunt D." Gray stood in the large well-lighted closet.

"I want to select his clothes while it's on my mind." She leaned on her cane, the wheelchair in the living room should she tire.

Sam, allowed to go in to work a few hours late this morning, knelt down in the closet as his aunt shuffled through Mercer's shined shoes. "Not a speck of dirt, even on the soles," Sam observed.

"His idol was Cary Grant," Daniella said with uncharacteristic warmth. "Mercer always said if a man can dress half as well as Cary Grant he'll be smashing."

"True," Gray agreed. "Duke Ellington wasn't bad either."

"Those were the days, those were the days," she intoned with a kind of wonderment. "Gray, I don't want him buried in a black suit. The undertaker can wear a black suit, not my boy. He needs color. So"—she flicked her cane right under a navy suit, chalk pinstripes—

"he always looked good in this and we can use an eggshell white shirt and, oh, the tie, the tie will be what makes it—that—and the pocket square."

"A rosebud on the lapel," Sam volunteered.

"I hadn't thought of that." She liked the idea. "Regimental stripes, so many regimental stripes, but I think for this, his last social occasion, we should use a solid-color silk tie. I say a glorious burnt orange or a cerise. Something that just says 'Mercer.'"

"Right." Gray, though not a man for a bright tie, did agree. "And the pocket square can be a darker color or a different color. Mercer always said matchups were boring."

Daniella nodded. "Yes, he did. Now Sam, the rosebud. If we use the cerise tie it could be pink, now that's bold, I think. If we use the burnt orange then I say a creamy white, not stark, and we won't know until we go to the funeral home. We'll have to hold the colors up to his face."

This thought did not appeal to Mercer's cousins, but dressing her son was of paramount importance to the ancient lady. They would do it. Both nodded.

A knock on the front door quieted them.

"I'll get it." Gray strode out of the room, glad for a moment out of the closet.

Opening the door, Phil—strained, drained, but composed—greeted him. "I thought you all would be here. The cars are here. I came to help."

The two men walked to the bedroom.

Phil bent down to hug Daniella. "I am so sorry, so very very sorry. Whatever you want, just ask." Tears rolled down his cheeks.

She kissed him and said, "I am not going to cry. Phil, don't you cry either."

He reached into his jacket, pulled out a linen handkerchief to wipe his eyes. "Yes, ma'am."

"We are going to celebrate him. Perhaps it's easier for me because I know I will be joining him before you all do."

"Auntie D, don't say that." Phil's eyes teared up again.

"It's the plain truth. The boys are helping me assemble his wardrobe. I think we've got it. Sam, why don't you carry his clothing over to my house? In fact, we can all repair there for a drink and to plan the service."

"Yes, but while we are here, I thought perhaps I could be of special service," said Phil. "I know he had quite a few contracts lined up. Usually the bloodline research for the breeding season is over by now so everyone has been billed. But if anything is outstanding, I will call the client."

Gray nodded his assent. "You know most of them anyway."

"Do you know where he kept his important papers? You know, insurance, stuff like that?" Sam asked Daniella.

"He used his computer but he backed up every single thing. I told him all he was doing was making extra work. Just stick to the paperwork and throw out the computer." She paused. "Phil, let Gray call Sheriff Sidell. We want things done properly."

"Sure," Phil assented. "Didn't the sheriff go through his office?"

Daniella nodded. "Yes, but they said they would be back Monday. I guess they're shorthanded." She sighed deeply. "I don't know."

Mercer's small, bright office was as meticulously planned as his closet, where items were divided by season and color. Seeing the office made Phil dab his eyes again. He got hold of himself.

"All the insurance, car title, and tax returns are in that file cabinet. I know it looks like a pie safe but it's really his file cabinet. Phil, you know that," Daniella said.

Having quickly contacted Ben, Gray walked into the office. "Take the billing folder," Gray said to Phil while looking at his aunt. "Surely there's some outstanding monies."

"Mmm," came her compressed reply as the monies would go to her.

Phil opened the double doors, revealing long, thin editing drawers within. "He was certainly imaginative. Did he take in his papers to the accountant for this year's taxes—well, last year's, I mean?"

"Yes, but he made copies of all that, too," said Daniella. "His billings are in the top drawer, marked. Red means unpaid if there's a red tab on the folder. Green, paid." She touched the drawer under that. "He divided his research work up by states. So then he also alphabetized stallions in the drawers. He had cross-references and more cross-references. When a stallion moved, say, to Spendthrift Farm, he kept the former state file, made a new one, plus cited the move in the alphabetized file. His mind was so orderly."

She ran her forefinger lower. "These drawers here are miscellaneous. In his research he'd find a name from the past, like Foxhall Keene, and he'd put that information here. But everything is clearly marked. Owners files, mare files, progeny files, and percent of winners. All broken down and cross-referenced. Phil, take the billings file, but leave everything else. We can all go over that later."

"Quite right," Phil agreed.

"Auntie D, would you like me to take the computer?" asked Sam. "To double-check stuff?"

"No. The Sheriff's Department had a quick look and will return Monday. I told him Mercer backed up everything but Ben Sidell insisted. I suppose they're right." She sighed. "I guess a lot can be hidden in computers, not that he had anything to hide. He was an honest man."

"I'll go over everything the minute I get home and bring it all back by Monday," said Phil. "I'm sure everything is in order but there are always a few laggards when it comes to payments." He frowned for a second.

As Sam helped Daniella on with her coat, Phil opened the front door. Gray quickly walked back into the office. He opened the pie safe, slid open the miscellaneous drawer, snatched the folder on top, sticking it under his jacket.

Once home, Gray smacked the folder on the kitchen table. "Janie! Janie!"

"In the library."

"Come here."

While she walked down the hall he was already recounting what had transpired. "Let's go over this now."

"Yes." Sister needed no prodding.

Gray pulled up a chair next to Sister. They opened the folder. Golly hopped right onto it. *"I love paper,"* she purred.

"Golly, get off," Sister commanded and, of course, the cat paid her no mind. "The things I do to keep peace in this house."

Golly leapt off as Sister had gotten up to give her tiny dried-liver treats. The aroma brought the dogs; out came large GREENIES. The three pets chewed happily.

Sister sat back down, examining each page or newspaper clipping that Gray now handed her.

"A lot of stuff here on the Aga Khan. His breeding theories." She looked over the next paper. "The racing stables of King Edward the Seventh."

"Here you go." Gray slid over a genetic blueprint for Dixie Do, Mercer's hunt horse. "One of the Broad Creek Stables horses Phil called back from the western tracks."

"Right, Dixie had one-fourth Quarter Horse blood. We don't have any Quarter Horse tracks here, as you know. A very nice horse and"—she inhaled sharply—"back to Eclipse. Mercer knew! He knew if the DNA was what it was supposed to be, and you can trace male ancestors back a few centuries, he'd find Matchem. Dixie would go back to Matchem. He figured out that Navigator and Benny Glitters had been switched. Both were handsome bay horses much resembling each other."

"But when did he know?" Gray looked to see if there was a date at the top of the page, tiny print along the top. "He knew Wednesday."

"Let me call Ben."

"Before you do, should we call Meg and Alan?"

"Not until we are 100 percent sure. There's no point in creating uproar at Walnut Hall or worse, danger. A killer can board an airplane as easily as someone else and we don't want to jeopardize anyone at Walnut Hall. We know he was here to kill Penny and Mercer. Let's wait."

She rose, phoned Ben, told him what they had, and her fears for the wonderful people at Walnut Hall. Finally, she sat back down. "We're between the Devil and the deep blue sea."

Gray put his large, strong hand over hers. "Janie, don't go out tomorrow."

"Sweetheart, I have to. It's a big Saturday joint meet. O.J. and Tootie are up there at Horse Country buying out the store with the rest of the Woodford gang. We can't disappoint them. And I suspect we are safer in the hunt field than inside."

"Mercer wasn't."

She thought long and hard. "True, but the pogonip provided opportunity. Tomorrow it's supposed to be clear."

"All we have is circumstantial evidence. With a little luck, maybe we can flush him out in the open. Ben can't make an arrest just yet, but we can help him. It seems impossible and yet . . ." Gray gazed off in the distance for a moment. "And yet it makes sense."

"Let me make a suggestion. Have Sam take Daniella to the home place. Just the outside chance that she might get close to figuring this out and endanger herself—because I know she'll pick the phone right up for a loud accusation."

"Kill Daniella? That's crazy," Gray said.

"Exactly. But he is now a little crazy."

CHAPTER 30

Smoke curled upward, then flattened out from the two chimneys at the Lorillard Farm. Given Saturday off by Crawford so he could help his aunt, Sam fed the wood-burning stove. The fireplace in the living room also roared. The mantelpiece had the flourish of a Grecian scroll. The fire screen, almost as old as the house, had a hunt scene in metalwork across the center. Made at Pattypan Forge along with the fireplace utensils, it bore witness to the artistic urges of those long-dead workers.

Aunt Daniella, wrapped in a rich cashmere shawl, watched him feed more large heavy oak logs to the living room fire, then replace the screen. "You could have ridden today. Mercer would have liked that."

"Mercer would have liked it but Crawford wouldn't. He hunts on Saturdays, too."

She pursed her lips, a thin line of dark lipstick spread on them. "Foolish"—she took a breath—"but entertaining. Mercer never could get him interested in racing. You'd think someone with that big an ego would have jumped right in."

"A big ego but also a big brain. Very few people make money racing. Crawford believes in profit."

"Foxhunting is hardly profitable," she fired back.

"No, but he feels he gets a lot of bang for his buck. His words."

"Common. Such a common expression." She sniffed. She shifted in the comfortable chair placed before the fire. "While I enjoy your company, Sam, I don't see why I must be here. I'm perfectly fine at home."

"Of course you are, Auntie D, but the sheriff thought you might be tempted to go back into Mercer's house before they do."

"He gave us permission to select his funeral attire and Ben allowed Phil to take the current billing file since we have copies and"—she paused—"is there anything else?"

"No." He lied, nor was he about to tell her about Gray taking the miscellaneous file, which he had already replaced. Gray had gone early to Mercer's house, before the hunt. "Auntie D, did Mercer ever talk to you about horses' bloodlines?"

"All the time." She smiled.

"Did it ever interest you?"

She tugged at the corner of the cashmere shawl. "Not so much, although last week he was completely transfixed—transfixed, I tell you—with DNA stuff. Related to bloodlines, but he started off about a horse bone that is seven hundred thousand years old. He was so caught up—truly caught up and excited—I let him rattle on. That was the only way with Mercer. Even as a child. Remember when he decided to become the marbles champion of central Virginia? I told him there was no marbles champion." She waved her hand. "So he trooped down to the county courthouse and wrote out a plan for a marbles tournament, handing it to the county commissioners." She laughed.

"I remember he beat me all the time." Sam stood up, thinking this would be a good day for hunting as opposed to marbles. "But he didn't call your attention to anything peculiar last week?"

"Not in so many words, but he was troubled. Penny Hinson's murder deeply upset him." She sighed. "He was too sensitive. And overly curious about other people's lives." She spoke a bit louder. "Oh, I told Chantal to stay in Atlanta. No need to return. We'll take care of my boy. I think she was offended but she can be claustrophobic. Well, she makes me feel claustrophobic, although I know she means well." She gave Sam a sharp look. "Is there no making peace with her?"

"You can answer that better than I. I'm polite."

"Mmm." She pursed her lips together, one of her signature expressions.

As the two talked, Sam didn't let on that Ben didn't want Aunt Daniella left alone until the department had a bit more clarity, which he hoped might occur today.

Meanwhile, Uncle Yancy had returned to the Lorillards' mudroom. Knowing two people sat in the house, he was circumspect. That quickly evaporated as Aunt Netty popped up through the hole he'd dug in the floorboards, casting away the rag pile.

"How cozy." She beamed.

"Netty, what are you doing here?" Burled up in old saddle pads, he lifted his head.

"I wanted to see your place. You have two dens over here, plus this room. My, aren't you living high? Anyway, I miss you."

He knew that was a major fib. *"What do you want, my beloved?"*

"A little warmth. My den at Pattypan is cold." She was half telling the truth.

"How can it be cold? You've got the den lined with straw and grass, every rag you could find and the old roof and sides still stand. That cuts the wind."

"It's the chill, Yancy. I feel such a chill."

He stated flatly, *"Life gets colder."*

They shut up and listened intently as Sam had walked into the kitchen. He opened the refrigerator door, then closed it.

"Does he ever throw out anything good?"

Yancy whispered, *"Juicy bones, coffee grounds which are too bitter, but he's been eating a lot of soybeans and he throws out the shells. I've gotten fond of them."*

"Enough for two?"

"Netty, you are not living with me. You'll try to throw me out again and I'm not leaving." He paused. *"And I'm not leaving Sam. He's a sweet fellow but sad, so very sad. Every now and then I'll show myself and he stands still as a statue. I make him happy."*

She frowned. *"It doesn't do to care too much about humans."*

"I know, but I like some of them, and look at Inky. She lives in the old orchard and knows the silver-haired Master well. She gets treats all the time."

Aunt Netty considered this. *"That's a Master and a Master takes care of foxes. By and large it's best to be wary of humans, if for no other reason than that they are sublimely stupid. Name another animal that breeds past the food supply or uses up all the water. Remember the new people who ran their well dry, then dammed up the creek? See? No brains."*

"I don't remember that." He stopped, cocked his head. *"The horn. They're at the covered bridge."*

With her fabulous ears she, too, heard the hunting horn. The sound carried this morning. Using the farm roads, After All lay a mile and a half from the Lorillard place.

"They might pick up my line if they head east," Aunt Netty said. *"Doesn't matter, we're safe."*

The "we're" alerted him. *"You can't stay."*

"I need the warmth."

"Then take some rags and be gone. He's got piles of them, the dirty ones and the neatly folded ones."

"Throwing me out when hounds are running? You can't be serious!" She fumed.

"After the hunt then." He listened as Shaker blew for hounds to move off. *"Let's hide on the top shelf. In case Sam opens the mudroom door. He likes to hunt, but today he's got old Auntie D with him."*

"She's two years older than God." Aunt Netty giggled as she leapt from shelf to shelf.

Yancy wanted to say, *"So are you!"* Then realized he was, too. He kept that to himself.

Seventy-one people rode out this Saturday as Sister had sent an e-mail asking members to come to honor Mercer with this joint meet with Woodford hounds. She also requested that The Jefferson Hunt members wear black armbands. Most everyone had to make one, but that was easy enough. Mercer would have been touched.

There were low clouds and decent footing—at least it wasn't icy. A starting temperature of 42°F promised a good day, perhaps even a great one. Sister asked O.J. to ride up with her as always. Other First Flight Woodford people could also ride forward. The Bancrofts, Phil, Ronnie, Gray, Xavier, Kasmir, Alida, Freddie, and Felicity all rode up behind them. Lila Repton was trying First Flight again and After All Farm was a good place for a novice First Flight rider; the jumps were so well set, most creek crossings were solid. Second Flight found Bobby Franklin leading, and Ben Sidell rode with him. If necessary, Ben would move up.

The sheriff had men placed at strategic points in After All, Roughneck Farm, and the Lorillard place, as all abutted one another. He did not put any officers on the other side of Soldier Road, figuring the hunt would stay on the south side.

The clatter of seventy-one sets of hooves reverberated through the red-painted covered bridge. Hounds, sterns held high, couldn't wait to be cast, but all their training ensured they didn't scoot off.

On the right, Betty crossed the creek, as did Sybil on the left, neither one riding through the bridge. The steep crossings didn't faze the whippers-in.

Shaker was on Kilowatt, a Thoroughbred of great power. He had planned to ride to the front fields of After All, then turn inward, avoiding the woods and riding toward Roughneck Farm.

Then he would ultimately turn eastward again after drawing the Roughneck fields, jump back into After All and draw through the woods. Given the promising conditions, he thought this would allow people to see the hound work—at least in the beginning.

And they did, but not as Shaker planned.

Once cast, Diana loped into the middle of the field, streaks of snow still in the deeper folds. She stopped, stern upright. She blew out of her nostrils, then sucked air in. Pickens desperately wanted to be a forward hound, so he immediately ran over to the reliable, driven Diana.

Putting his nose down, he whimpered for a moment, *"Umm."*

Diana sharply told him, *"Open or shut up."*

She continued on, nose down, and he shut up but by now the whole pack spread out around her. Everyone knew she had something, but would it heat up or grow cold?

Aztec jigged a little. He wanted to go and so did Sister.

To Diana's right, Thimble opened, followed by Diana who ran on the line up to where a bouquet of fox scent just burst into her nose. Everyone spoke at once, tore off at first in a line, then bunched up, running a bit like a rugby scrum.

The field witnessed this beautiful sight; it sends chills down a foxhunter's spine and often does the same to someone seeing for the first time hounds work as a team.

The fast pace right off the mark thrilled Sister. Much as she loved hunting, there were times when she was eager to find a line, or disappointed on a poor day. Impatience, a fault with her, had to be curbed. A lovely jump—twenty-four feet long, three fence panels long—sat square in the fence line. Edward Bancroft had built this stone jump thirty-five years ago and it held up. He actually bought the stone because he wanted to practice stone fences. Sister and O.J., grinning and laughing—they couldn't help it—took that fence as a pairs team, as did many of the riders behind them. If two or three people can clear an obstacle together, so much the better. That got everyone high; hearts beat faster. Poor Bobby had to hustle to a gate but many of the Second Flight people managed to catch up, observing the wonderful jumping in pairs and determining then and there they would be doing that next year.

Flying through the second large field, hounds hooked sharply left; they took the hog's-back jump first, followed by Shaker, then Sister, then O.J.—as this jump was maybe twelve feet long. Although three feet by six and using thick railroad ties, it was not a solid jump; one could see through the ties. Not that it was terribly airy, but a horse not encountering a hog's-back before might well put on the brakes. Not one did today because the pace was too good and The Jefferson Hunt horses had flown over this jump many a time. The Woodford horses were Thoroughbreds and that had to count for something.

Those seventy-one people thundered over the field, jumped a coop into the wildflower field between Sister's and the Bancrofts', roared up to the ruins, and stopped. Hounds crawled over the ruins.

Inside his den, Comet remained silent. He'd retreated to the deepest part of his lair. Happy for a rousing start, Shaker dismounted, blew "Gone to Ground," and praised everyone. He took Kilowatt's reins from Kasmir, who had ridden up at Sister's direction to hold Shaker's horse.

Stepping on the wall ruins, Shaker threw his leg over.

"Thanks, Kasmir."

"My pleasure." Kasmir slightly inclined his head, then rode back to Alida Dalzell. He was resplendent in a weazlebelly and top hat, riding his flaming chestnut mare, Lucille Ball. That mare had such a fluid stride the sight of her moving could bring tears to the eyes of any true horseman.

Sister smiled at O.J. As Masters, both knew to be asked to perform any service in the field was a singular honor. The harder, dirtier, or more dangerous the chore, the greater the honor. And while this was an easy chore, it did mean all eyes fell on Kasmir. He was marked by Shaker as a trusted man.

Sometimes, riding back to the trailers after a hard hunt, Sister would muse that this was one of the last sports where the warrior ethic prevailed. The point of foxhunting was not to make the sport easy but to make it superb sport enhanced by elegance. She could hear her mother's words, "Jane, face danger with elegance!"

Not that the blazing run had been particularly dangerous. The footing was pretty good, no steep incline or decline troubled them. Nor had there been any difficult crossings, but people had to put on the afterburners and jump some decent jumps, interesting jumps.

Shaker pointed the stag end of his crop toward Betty, then swept it forward. She moved forward on the right and Sybil shadowed her on the left. They knew he was heading back over the field at the base of Hangman's Ridge, toward the tiger trap into the woods of After All. A hog's-back jump was also placed in this fence line about three football fields farther down, should anyone have difficulty with the tiger trap, which looks like a big coop with logs vertically next to one another. Again, an easy enough jump, but it helps if a horse has seen one before.

Somehow no matter how many gates one puts into a fence line they never seem to be in the right place when hounds are running. Bobby, as Second Flight Master, dealt with this frustration constantly.

Hounds left Comet as they walked along the bottom of Hangman's Ridge.

"Ooo," Pookah exclaimed, "bear tracks."

Feeling especially good today, Dreamboat said, "Pookah, don't fret over a bear. We'll get plenty of fox today. It's a perfect day. Low clouds, the right temperature, moisture in the earth and best of all, no wind. Perfect, perfect, perfect."

As they rode along the foot of the eerie ridge, some trees grew out horizontally from the earth. There were also odd, dark rock formations.

Sister thought it was a perfect day, a day Mercer would have loved. She prayed he could see all this and appreciate the tribute. He was truly loved.

Not one given to expressing deep emotions, she felt them. Irrational as it was, Sister often sensed her son or husband near and she thought other people who had lost someone dearly loved could feel their spirits as well. Somehow she believed Mercer was with them today and if they saw their quarry, she would know it for certain.

Shaker popped over the tiger trap, Kilowatt floating over, followed shortly by Aztec, a smaller horse than Kilowatt, but such a handy fellow. One by one, the field jumped into the woods while Bobby, once through the gate, shepherded the Second Flight toward them by a different trail.

Hounds cleared. Fifteen minutes elapsed, then Dreamboat shifted into third gear, shouted, *"Follow me!"* and once again, all on! The hounds' music swirled around the trees, intensified as they crossed Broad Creek, then moved up along the fast rushing waters only to cross again. Within ten minutes, the pack was at Pattypan, always so difficult.

Athena, the great horned owl, had been lazily dozing inside the forge. Mice were everywhere. It was a bit like taking a nap in the supermarket. She cursed when the hounds lurched through the long high windows. *"Damn you all!"*

No hound bothered to reply because they hurried to Aunt Netty's den—tidy, as always.

"She's not here!" Cora surmised.

"Maybe she'll come back," Pansy said hopefully.

"Oh, we'll give the old girl a run for her money," Ardent promised, for Aunt Netty had teased him many times.

Hounds jumped out the other side of the forge.

Anticipating the direction once Dreamboat headed again into the woods, Sybil loped onto the narrow deer trail to head toward the Lorillard farm. She had to gallop, as this was a longer route, but there was no way through the thick undergrowth, the reason Pattypan was such a good place for a den. There was one way in and pretty much one way out. At least that old farm road ran in both directions.

Sister pushed Aztec onto the road but hounds circled the woods before they shot toward the Lorillard farm. She had a lot of territory to make up. Right behind her, O.J. twisted so many times in the saddle to avoid low-hanging branches, she knew she wouldn't be needing Pilates today. Behind her, Ginny Howard had the same thought, with Walter moving up behind as other people fell back.

Back on the good road between After All and the Lorillard place, hounds could be heard screaming toward the old home place. By the time the entire field reached the white clapboard home, hounds scratched at the back door.

Sam stood outside in front with Aunt Daniella, who used her cane. Hearing the hounds, she wanted to see the show. Sam didn't want to leave her, even though hounds blazed for his mudroom door.

Inside, Uncle Yancy cursed a blue streak. Aunt Netty had led the entire hunt right to his best place! She pretended she hadn't done a thing but she did flatten herself on the top shelf, along with Uncle Yancy.

As the field waited, Shaker dismounted, walked to his hounds. "Good hounds, good hounds. Come along now."

"Two foxes!" Pickens screamed, totally beside himself. *"Two."*

"Open the door," Taz begged. *"Please open the door. Let me at 'em!"*

Tempted as Shaker was because he knew his hounds had to be right, he led them away. If he had opened the door to the Lorillard's mudroom, they would have ripped it up, and it's never a good idea to desecrate a landowner's property.

Waiting, Sister looked back at Ben. Tapping the brim of her hunt cap with her crop, she rode to Phil as Ben came forward.

"Great run," Phil enthused as Gray came alongside him.

"Phil"—Sister leaned forward on Aztec's gleaming neck—"we know that Navigator was actually Benny Glitters. Why don't you tell us about how the horses were switched? That's why Harlan was killed, wasn't it? He knew."

Wedged in, Phil couldn't take off, but he threw his leg over his horse, dropping to one side, and ran like hell toward Aunt Daniella.

Sam stepped in front of her as Sister, also wedged in, tried to stay clear of Phil's horse. Ben, too, but Phil had a head start and they were at this moment encumbered by being mounted. Ben reached inside his coat and took out a .38 from his chest holster, well hidden by his heavy winter frock coat.

A tall man, Phil threw Sam to the ground but the slight man gamely rose to try to fight the bigger, heavier man. Phil reached for Aunt Daniella.

Without flickering an eye, she brought up her ebony cane between his legs with great force.

He bent over and that fast, Sam, using both hands, smashed him with an uppercut that sent teeth flying. Phil hit the ground. Ben dismounted, holding his gun to Phil's temple.

With Kasmir holding Kilowatt, Shaker ran over just as Sam hit Phil again. Shaker put Phil's arm up behind his back, lifted him up and held him tight.

Sam got control of himself.

"You have the right to remain silent . . ." Ben began reading Phil his rights, as Phil would be charged with murder.

It had happened so fast. Not one of those now seventy people said a word. Even the hounds stood still, waiting for a command from the huntsman.

Sam took Aunt Daniella by the elbow, for the exertion had cost her. He supported her while Gray, also dismounted, gently took his aunt's other arm. He handed her her ebony cane, which she had dropped after whacking Phil.

She looked stunned, then looked at all the people wearing black armbands. Her mouth opened. Nothing came out. She put her head on Gray's shoulder and the tears flooded out.

"He would be so proud," she gasped, oblivious of Phil or anything else.

"Yes, he would. And he would be proud of you." Gray kissed her cheek as he and Sam gently walked her to the front door.

Uncle Yancy couldn't help it. All this commotion. He snuck out, creeping around the back of the mudroom to look. Sister saw him and tears came to her eyes. Mercer had indeed sent a sign.

CHAPTER 31

Two weeks later, a lovely service was held for Mercer, who was buried in the Lorillard plot next to his grandfather. Daniella had requested that his horse Dixie Do be at the service, along with the entire pack of The Jefferson Hunt.

Gray held Dixie's reins. Mercer's tack glowed, the run-up stirrups gleamed. The hounds sat silent as stone, with Shaker on foot, in livery, at their head.

The entire hunt club attended, as did many members of Keswick, Farmington, Oak Ridge, Stonewall, Bedford, Deep Run, Casanova, Rockbridge, and Glenmore. Mercer had hunted with so many people over the years.

The glorious day saw a few crocuses peeping up out of the ground. If one stared intently, red could be seen returning to buds, although the trees still looked barren. Spring was stirring.

After the service, everyone retired to the Bancroft residence because the Lorillard place wasn't big enough to hold all these people. The Bancrofts had paid for everything, as well as opening their home.

Uncle Yancy—still stuck with Aunt Netty, and back in the mudroom—was glad the party was held elsewhere.

A large framed photograph of Mercer as a child on his first pony stood next to an identically-sized photograph of Mercer in full formal kit wearing a weazlebelly and top hat on Dixie Do, braided for Opening Hunt.

O.J. had flown back from Kentucky for the service. She talked with guests eager to catch up with her, with Kentucky hunting. Sister, Gray, Betty, and Tootie gathered for a moment by the punch bowl.

"It was an ingenious crime." Betty did give the Chetwynds credit. "And it made their fortune for 121 years."

O.J. joined them. "Alan and Meg did have tests run on Benny's, I mean Navigator's, lineage. Sure enough, he goes back to Matchem. I guess Harlan and who knows, another worker or Old Tom himself, switched the stallions at night. They greatly looked alike. Sometimes the cleverest crimes are the simplest."

Gray shook his head. "Can you imagine the work? Now the Jockey Club has to go through all the pedigrees for the last 121 years to correct them."

"They can do it." Sister smiled. "I have great faith in them. Remember, the founding member of the Jockey Club was Domino's owner, James Keene."

"Lucky Phil confessed," Tootie remarked. "Just spilled it all out."

"Well, honey." Betty put down her punch glass. "He had nothing to lose anymore and I don't think he was in his right mind at the end. The strain of that remarkable dishonesty, the knowledge, the weight of the crime passed to the oldest son from generation to generation, and then the horror of two murders. He told Ben he didn't really want to kill anyone. He couldn't see a way out."

Ben joined them. "I heard my name."

The small group reviewed what they'd just said.

The sheriff sighed, then said, "You know, Phil cried and cried, and said it was like killing his brother. He loved Mercer. And he said they were actually related. His grandfather had a long affair with Mercer's grandmother, Daniella's mother. He said he really felt he'd killed his brother. Obviously, the Chetwynds can afford the best lawyers but he says he wants to be put away." Ben shrugged. "For what, for reputation? For the money? Kill for that? Even if he had to shut down Broad Creek Stables because of the scandal, Phil would never have been poor."

"He couldn't live with the shame," Sister posited quietly. "Old name, old ways, old money."

"It's crazy." Tootie couldn't quite understand it. "So he creates more shame. Crazy."

"That it is." Sister put her arm around Tootie's waist. "People have been doing irrational things for thousands of years. We aren't going to stop now."

O.J. asked Ben, "Okay, the stallions were switched, but why did Old Tom Chetwynd have Harlan Laprade killed when he brought the slate memorial to Walnut Hall?"

"Money," said Sister. "Harlan must have been asking for more and more. Blackmail. Harlan loaded Benny Glitters on a big boxcar full of horses going to Broad Creek. No one would really notice that Navigator, who'd ridden on the train from Virginia, was switched. Harlan was in charge of the shipping. Only Old Tom and Harlan knew."

"And was Harlan a frequenter of houses of ill repute?" Betty couldn't help but ask.

Ben nodded. "Not that his wife didn't know he'd done such things in the past, but no one wanted her to know where his clothes were found. The disappearance was bad enough. Making it look like Harlan died in a whorehouse gave Old Tom a cover. Also, Old

Tom was sleeping with Daniella's mother. He didn't mind getting rid of her husband, who by all accounts was a good horseman but a bad husband. King David did it too, remember?"

"Does Daniella know now?" O.J. asked.

Gray's voice was low. "She probably does but like her own mother, there are some things a lady doesn't want to investigate. All this has been quite enough."

Ben spoke again. "Phil killed Mercer then strung him up. He's a strong man. If the pogonip lifted, he hoped no one would look closely as they'd become accustomed to the hanging dummy. He wanted to go to the breakfast, look for Mercer, then worry about his friend not showing up. Then he could go out and look for him. Bold and clever."

And just then, Sam, next to his aunt, her ebony cane in hand, walked in front of the enormous silver punch bowl.

Ed Bancroft tapped a glass. The room fell silent.

"I thank you all for your tribute to my son," said Daniella. "He was a good son, a good horseman, and a good businessman. I was and will always be proud of him. There are over two hundred years of Laprades and Lorillards buried at the old home place and soon I will rest next to my son." A murmur went up but she held up her hand. "To everything there is a season. I think Mercer went before his time but we do as the Lord commands. So it was his time and I look forward to mine. All good things must come to an end. When I go, don't mourn me. If there is any quality of mine you admire, make it your own. The quality I most admired in my son, apart from his love, was his eagerness for life.

"Thank you again and I especially thank Tedi and Edward Bancroft for giving Mercer his last social engagement." She smiled. "I thank my nephews, Gray and Sam, and I thank Jane Arnold for Mercer's hunt.

"I wish you all a good life and I know Mercer would want me to say, 'Good hunting.'"

Everyone applauded and Daniella was mobbed. Sensing her fatigue, Sam walked her to a chair. Gray left the small group to attend to his aunt, get her another drink, do all the things Mercer used to do.

That night, Sister visited the stables at Roughneck, saying good night to each of her horses, including the two newcomers from Broad Creek. Then she walked across to the kennels, careful not to awaken anyone if possible. She spied Inky looking at her from the edge of the orchard.

She winked at the beautiful vixen who remained motionless. Then Sister walked back up to her house, the pale smoke curling from the chimney.

She thought the Three Fates had cut the threads of two good lives recently as they were spinning out the lives of others. Spinning, spinning, spinning, and she prayed she would live a much longer life to be part of the tapestry.

To the Reader,

You might wonder how The Jefferson Hunt could have such a good season in such nasty weather. I have no idea.

Our season (Oak Ridge Foxhunt Club) from January to March 2014, proved bitter, snowy with odd, wild temperature bounces as in fifty degrees. Yes, fifty degrees. Without gilding the lily, it was the strangest, worst winter I've ever experienced, yet the hunting was terrific. On the days of the huge temperature bounces it was not terrific, granted. The rest of the time, we picked up fox after fox and ran as best we could in snow and sometimes over ice patches. When the snows melted, we ran in mud, returning splattered to the trailers. But when we smiled our teeth were white.

Parking proved more of a problem than hunting.

For those of you who do not foxhunt, most of us who do, do not go out in a deep powdery snow. For one thing, should a fox be out they can't get away from you. Usually they are tight and warm in their dens. If there is a good crust on the snow, I will take hounds out because the fox, being light, can get away. However, one must be careful because if the crust is too thick it will cut hound pads. One has to use judgment, obviously. Also, if the snow is deep it tires horses and hounds quickly.

A light snow, a few inches on the ground is perfect and to hunt while flakes are twirling down is the best. The horses and hounds become so excited, hounds will throw up snow at one another and people ignore the snow sliding down their collars. It's too much fun to complain.

If nothing else, I hope the Sister Jane novels impart the respect we have for our quarry and the care we give to our partners: horses and hounds.

Given that 80 percent plus of the U.S. population lives in cities and suburbs, the connection with nature is fading to the detriment of all living creatures. You and I are medium-sized predators. All mammalian creatures divide into predator and prey. To know where one falls on that scale goes a long way to integration in that scale. In other words, sisters and brothers, we are not the crown of creation. But we sure can be fun.

Up and over,
Rita Mae Brown

During hunt season, mid-September to mid-March, you can follow some of our hunts at http://www.facebook.com/sisterjanearnold

ACKNOWLEDGMENTS

The oldest equine graveyard in the United States is at Walnut Hall. Benny Glitters, however, is a fictional horse.

The owners of Walnut Hall, Meg Jewett and Alan Leavitt, are not fictional, and Lexington, Kentucky, is grateful for this. Their generosity and kindness is legendary. I especially call attention to their support of the library.

And I thank Alan again for the exciting tour he gave me of his stables and its residents.

As for Jane Winegardner, MFH of Woodford Hounds, what can I say about a beloved friend of years and an inspiring Master? Whenever I think of this hard riding lady, I remember the laughter first.

I also thank Robert M. Lyons, MFH, and Justin Sautter, MFH, of Woodford for their hospitality to Oak Ridge members and myself when we visit.

My much abused whipper-in, Dee Phillips, walked me through most of the DNA material, all that stuff about a mother's DNA, etc. Thank God, she is a tolerant soul as well as a terrific whipper-in to myself as well as Deep Run, the grand hunt outside of Richmond. The history of that group alone would make a fabulous novel. Deep Run has experienced everything: war, fast women, beautiful horses, men too handsome for their own good and the good of the ladies, and all of this shining with that Virginia veneer of perfect manners. Ah, yes.

I suspect this could be said of most hunts in the United States and Canada. Dull people don't foxhunt.

Thank you to Kathleen King, Oak Ridge member, and lawyer who digs into my research keeping me this side of trouble. We also hunt bassetts together.

And one last request. Please do not visit Walnut Hall. It is a privae residence and the equine graveyard is also private. Peace should be preserved.

To anyone I might have forgotten, just cuss me out.

Always and Ever,

Rita Mae Brown

About the Author

RITA MAE BROWN is the bestselling author the Sister Jane foxhunting novels—*Let Sleeping Dogs Lie, Fox Tracks, Hounded to Death, The Tell-Tale Horse, The Hounds and the Fury, The Hunt Ball, Full Cry, Hotspur,* and *Outfoxed*—the *New York Times* bestselling Sneaky Pie Brown mysteries, and *Rubyfruit Jungle, In Her Day,* and *Six of One,* among many other novels. An Emmy-nominated screenwriter and a poet, she lives in Afton, Virginia, where she is Master of foxhounds and huntsman of Oak Ridge Hunt Club and one of the directors of Virginia Hunt Week. She founded the first all-women's polo club, Blue Ridge Polo, in 1988. She was also Visiting Faculty at the University of Nebraska in Lincoln.

www.ritamaebrown.com

ABOUT THE TYPE

This book was set in Baskerville, a typeface designed by John Baskerville (1706–75), an amateur printer and typefounder, and cut for him by John Handy in 1750. The type became popular again when the Lanston Monotype Corporation of London revived the classic roman face in 1923. The Mergenthaler Linotype Company in England and the United States cut a version of Baskerville in 1931, making it one of the most widely used typefaces today.